Case Studies in Couple and Family Therapy

THE GUILFORD FAMILY THERAPY SERIES
Michael P. Nichols, Series Editor

Recent Volumes

Case Studies in Couple and Family Therapy

Systemic and Cognitive Perspectives

Edited by
Frank M. Dattilio

Foreword by Marvin R. Goldfried

THE GUILFORD PRESS
New York   London

© 1998 The Guilford Press
A Division of Guilford Publications, Inc.
72 Spring Street, New York, NY 10012
www.guilford.com

Printed in the United States of America

This book is printed on acid-free paper.

Last digit is print number: 9 8 7 6

Library of Congress Cataloging-in-Publication Data

Case studies in couple and family therapy: systemic and cognitive
   perspectives / edited by Frank M. Dattilio; foreword by Marvin R.
   Goldfried.
      p.   cm.
   Includes bibliographical references and index.
   ISBN 1-57230-297-6 (hardcover)—ISBN 1-57230-696-3 (pbk.)
   1. Family psychotherapy—Case studies.   2. Marital
psychotherapy—Case studies.   I. Dattilio, Frank M.   II. Goldfried,
Marvin R.
RC488.5.C368   1998
616.89′156—dc21
                                                     97–40877
                                                        CIP

*To my lovely wife of 20 years, Maryann,
and my three children,
Roseanne, Tara, and Michael, for
allowing me to be part of their lives*

About the Editor

Frank M. Dattilio, PhD, ABPP, is clinical associate in psychiatry at the Center for Cognitive Therapy, University of Pennsylvania School of Medicine. He is also a clinical psychologist in private practice and the clinical director of the Center for Integrative Psychotherapy in Allentown, Pennsylvania. Dr. Dattilio is a clinical member and approved supervisor of the American Association for Marriage and Family Therapy. He is a diplomate of the American Board of Professional Psychology and serves as an adjunct professor of psychology at Lehigh University in Bethlehem, Pennsylvania. Dr. Dattilio has also served as a guest lecturer at Harvard Medical School and a visiting faculty member at several major universities throughout the world.

He has more than 100 professional publications in the areas of anxiety disorders, behavioral problems, and marital and family discord, and has also given numerous presentations worldwide on the cognitive-behavioral treatment of anxiety disorders and cognitive-behavioral marital and family therapy. His works have been translated into more than one dozen languages, and he has served on the editorial board of a number of professional journals. Among his many publications, Dr. Dattilio is coauthor of *Cognitive Therapy with Couples* (with Christine A. Padesky, 1990); he is coeditor of *Comprehensive Casebook of Cognitive Therapy* (with Arthur Freeman, 1992), *Cognitive-Behavioral Strategies in Crisis Intervention* (with Arthur Freeman, 1994), *Cognitive Therapy with Children and Adolescents: A Casebook for Clinical Practice* (with Mark A. Reinecke and Arthur Freeman, 1996), and *Panic Disorder: Multiple Treatment Perspectives* (with Jesus A. Salas, 1998). He has also made audiotapes and filmed three professional videotapes, including the popular series *Five Approaches to Linda* (with Marvin R. Goldfried, Arnold A. Lazarus, William Glasser, and James F. Masterson, 1996).

Contributors

Donald H. Baucom, PhD, is Distinguished Professor of Psychology and director of the Clinical Psychology Program at the University of North Carolina, Chapel Hill. His research has included controlled outcome studies of cognitive-behavioral marital therapy, as well as the development of instruments for assessing couples' standards, attributions, and other cognitions. He has collaborated extensively with Norman B. Epstein on empirical studies of couples' cognitions, as well as on workshops, many book chapters, and the text *Cognitive-Behavioral Marital Therapy* (1990). Dr. Baucom also has won several awards for excellence in undergraduate teaching, and he maintains an active clinical practice.

Insoo Kim Berg, MSSW, is director and cofounder (with Steve de Shaver) of the Brief Family Therapy Center in Milwaukee, Wisconsin. Many of her papers and books have been translated into eight different languages. Her most recent publications include *Family-Based Services: A Solution-Focused Approach* (1994); *Working with the Problem Drinker* (with coauthor S. Miller, 1992); *Interviewing for Solutions* (with coauthor, P. DeJong, 1997); and *Brief Treatment Manual for Substance Abuse* (with coauthor N. Reuss, 1997).

Norman B. Epstein, PhD, is a professor of family studies at the University of Maryland, College Park. He is a fellow of the American Psychological Association and a clinical member of the American Association for Marriage and Family Therapy. A major portion of his teaching, research, scholarly writing, and clinical practice is focused on the assessment and treatment of couple and family problems. His collaboration with Donald H. Baucom has included empirical studies of couple relationships, professional workshops, numerous book chapters, and their book *Cognitive-Behavioral Marital Therapy* (1990).

Joseph B. Eron, PsyD, is founder (1981) and codirector of the Catskill Family Institute (CFI) with offices in New York's Hudson Valley region. In the late 1970s and early 1980s, he wrote several book chapters that contributed to the integration of core concepts and techniques in brief family therapy. In recent years, he has published numerous articles and chapters on CFI's unique narrative solutions approach, and has presented and trained in the United States and Canada. Eron's recent book with coauthor Thomas W.

Lund, *Narrative Solutions in Brief Therapy* (1996), focuses on what works to generate helpful conversations inside and outside the therapy session; it has allowed their approach to reach a broad audience.

Marion S. Forgatch, PhD, is a research scientist at the Oregon Social Learning Center, where she is principal investigator of a 5-year study with Gerald R. Patterson to test an intervention designed to help single mothers prevent and ameliorate their children's conduct problems. Her professional life is divided between basic research and clinical application. She has published numerous journal articles and book chapters in the areas of single parenting, family process, prevention, and therapy process and outcome. Her intervention publications include books, audiotapes, and videotapes that teach principles involved in effective family living.

Paula Hanson-Kahn, MBS, MA, CP, received her legal education in her native Singapore, where she was admitted as advocate and solicitor to the Singapore Supreme Court. After years as a missionary in the Philippines and Taiwan, she moved to the United States (with her husband and daughter) to attend Trinity Evangelical Divinity School, where she obtained a master of arts degree in counseling psychology. She is a licensed professional counselor and has been a senior resident in marriage and family therapy at Cross Keys Counseling Center in Atlanta, Georgia, since 1994, where she works closely with Luciano L'Abate.

Harville Hendrix, PhD, is the president and founder of the Institute for Imago Relationship Therapy in Winter Park, Florida. He is the author of *Getting the Love You Want: A Guide for Couples* (1988) and *Keeping the Love You Find: A Guide for Singles* (1992), and coauthor of *Giving the Love That Heals: A Guide for Parents* (with Helen Hunt, 1997).

Michael F. Hoyt, PhD, is senior staff psychologist and former director of adult psychiatric services at the Kaiser Permanente Medical Center in Hayward, California; and a clinical faculty member of the University of California School of Medicine, San Francisco. He is the author of *Brief Therapy and Managed Care: Readings for Contemporary Practice* (1995); the editor of *Constructive Therapies,* Volumes 1 and 2 (1994 and 1996) and *The Handbook of Constructive Therapies* (1998); and coeditor of *The First Session in Brief Therapy* (with S. H. Budman and S. Friedman, 1992).

Susan Johnson, EdD, is a professor of psychology and psychiatry at the University of Ottawa. She is also director of the Marital and Family Clinic at the Ottawa Civic Hospital, where she supervises a multidisciplinary team within the Department of Psychiatry and conducts a yearly summer externship in emotionally focused therapy. She is an approved clinical supervisor for the American Association for Marriage and Family Therapy and maintains a small private practice. She is actively involved in conference and workshop presentations across North America, most recently at the American Psychological Association conference and the

International Society for Traumatic Stress Studies, where she gave presentations on creating healing relationships for trauma survivors dealing with marital distress. Her most recent publications include *The Heart of the Matter: Perspectives on Emotion in Marital Therapy* (with coeditor L. S. Greenberg, 1994) and *The Practice of Emotionally Focused Marital Therapy: Creating Connection* (1996). She lives in Ottawa with her husband and two children.

James Keim, MSW, LCSW-C, is director of training at the Family Therapy Institute of Washington, D.C., in Rockville, Maryland. He is also founder and director of the Community Health Project, which collaborates with the National Institutes of Health to provide continuing education to public health professionals. He has worked closely with Cloé Madanes and Jay Haley; he is coauthor (with Cloé Madanes and Dinah Smelser) of the book *The Violence of Men* (1996), and has written or contributed to numerous other publications on strategic family therapy.

David V. Keith, MD, is an associate professor of psychiatry, family medicine, and pediatrics, and the director of family therapy, at the State University of New York Health Science Center in Syracuse. He was formerly with the Family Therapy Center in St. Paul, Minnesota and the University of Wisconsin Department of Psychiatry in Madison. Dr. Keith is the author and coauthor (with Carl Whitaker) of numerous journal articles and book chapters in the field of family therapy. Dr. Keith is one of the leading figures of experiential family therapy and for years was a close colleague and cotherapist with Carl Whitaker.

Luciano L'Abate, PhD, ABPP, was educated in his native Italy until moving to the United States as an exchange student. He received his doctorate in clinical psychology from Duke University. He has retired from Georgia State University as professor emeritus, and has been consultant at Cross Keys Counseling Center in Atlanta, Georgia, for the past 18 years, and director of multicultural services at Cross Keys for the last 3 years. He is a diplomate of the American Board of Professional Psychology and an approved supervisor of the American Association for Marriage and Family Therapy. In 1994, he received the "Family Psychologist of the Year" award from Division 43 (Family Psychology) of the American Psychological Association. He is widely published, and his many works have been translated into several languages.

Thomas W. Lund, PsyD, has been a child and family psychologist for 23 years. For the past 11 years, he has been codirector of the Catskill Family Institute (CFI), providing direct services to individuals, couples, and families. During this time, he worked at developing CFI's narrative solutions approach and has published numerous articles on its principles and practices. Over the past 7 years, he has trained psychotherapists in the United States and Canada in the CFI approach, and recently coauthored a book with Joseph B. Eron entitled *Narrative Solutions in Brief Therapy* (1996). Dr. Lund also teaches clergy, caseworkers in children's services, family specialists in family-based treatment programs, and other nontherapists the principles of the narrative solutions approach as they apply to the task of having helpful conversations.

Wade Luquet, ACSW, is on the faculty of the Institute for Imago Relationship Therapy and has worked closely with Harville Hendrix. He is the author of *Short-Term Couples Therapy: The Imago Model in Action* (1996) and coeditor of *Healing in the Relational Paradigm: The Imago Relationship Therapy Casebook* (1998). Luquet maintains a private practice with his wife, Marianne, in North Wales, Pennsylvania.

Terry MacCormack, PhD (candidate), currently teaches with the Department of Health Studies at the University of New England in Armidale, Australia. A former doctoral student in clinical psychology at the University of Ottawa, he completed his internship in the Family Therapy Program at the University of Calgary School of Medicine. His work with Karl Tomm is part of a larger qualitative study comparing the experiences of couples and therapists working from either a narrative or an emotion-focused approach. His interests also include working with individuals, couples, and families coping with life-threatening illness, and what this is like both for clients and for those who counsel them.

Salvador Minuchin, MD, has been at the forefront of family therapy since the early 1960s. He first developed his structural model while working at the Wiltwyck School for Boys, and in 1965 he was invited to become the director of the Philadelphia Child Guidance Clinic. In 1981 Minuchin moved to New York and founded Family Studies, Inc., where he pursued his dedication to teaching family therapists from all over the world and his commitment to social justice by working with the foster care system. His 1974 book *Families and Family Therapy* is the most popular volume ever written in family therapy; his 1993 book with coauthor Michael P. Nichols, *Family Healing,* features moving descriptions of his clinical artistry. His latest book, *Mastering Family Therapy* (with W. Y. Lee and G. M. Simon, 1996), is a complex study of the supervision and learning process. Dr. Minuchin retired in 1996 and now lives with his wife, Patricia, in Boston.

Michael P. Nichols, PhD, has been practicing and teaching family therapy since 1973. In addition to his psychoanalytic training, Dr. Nichols studied with Murray Bowen and Salvador Minuchin. Among his many books are *Family Therapy: Concepts and Methods,* fourth edition (with coauthor Richard C. Schwartz, 1998), which has been one of the most widely read textbooks in family therapy; *The Self in the System; No Place to Hide; The Lost Art of Listening*; and *Family Healing* (with Salvador Minuchin, 1993). After 17 years at Albany Medical College, Dr. Nichols recently resettled in Virginia and now teaches psychology and family therapy at the College of William and Mary.

William C. Nichols, EdD, ABPP, is a fellow of the American Psychological Association, the American Psychological Society, and the American Association for Marriage and Family Therapy (AAMFT). He is also a diplomate of the American Board of Professional Psychology. Currently an adjunct professor of child and family development and a member of the graduate faculty at the University of Georgia, he is also a consultant with The Nichols Group. A former president of both the AAMFT and the National Council of Family Relations and president-elect of the International Family Therapy Association, he is currently editor of the journal *Contemporary Family Therapy* and the International Family Therapy Association's *International Connection*. Dr. Nichols is also the author of numerous articles and book chapters, as well as two books—*Marital Therapy: An Integrative Approach* (1988) and *Treating People in Families: An Integrative Approach* (1996).

Gerald R. Patterson, PhD, is a research psychologist at the Oregon Social Learning Center (OSLC), Eugene, Oregon, and one of the foremost behavioral family therapists in the world. He received his doctorate from the University of Minnesota; prior to the establishment of OSLC, he was a research scientist at the Oregon Research Institute and served in various professional capacities at the University of Oregon for 13 years. He founded OSLC in 1977 to focus upon the family interaction process as it relates to aggressive children, marital conflict, and parent training therapy with antisocial youths. Dr. Patterson has authored and coauthored numerous professional articles and book chapters; he is also the sole author of the book *Families: Applications of Social Learning to Life* (1971). Dr. Patterson is a past president of Association for the Advancement of Behavior Therapy. He is the recipient of the Distinguished Professional Contribution Award from the Division of Clinical Child Psychology of the American Psychological Association (APA); the Distinguished Scientist Award from the Division of Clinical Psychology of the APA; the Distinguished Scientist Award for the Applications of Psychology from the APA, and the award for Distinguished Scientific Contributions to Developmental Psychology from the Society for Research in Child Development.

Cheryl Rampage, PhD, is a clinical psychologist and senior therapist at the Family Institute at Northwestern University, Evanston, Illinois, where she provides psychotherapy to individuals and couples; supervises family therapy trainees; and teaches courses on family therapy, ethics, and gender issues. She has previously served as the director of graduate education at the Family Institute, and also spent 11 years on the faculty of the University of Houston–Clear Lake. Dr. Rampage is a graduate of Marquette University, and received her doctorate from Loyola University of Chicago. She is the coauthor (with T. J. Goodrich, B. Ellman, and K. Halstead) of *Feminist*

Family Therapy: A Casebook (1988), as well as numerous articles and book chapters on gender and family therapy. She is a frequent presenter at national conferences.

Laura Giat Roberto, PsyD, (now Laura Roberto Forman), is professor of psychiatry and behavioral sciences at Eastern Virginia Medical School. She has also served on the psychology faculties of the Eastern Virginia Family Therapy Institute, Old Dominion University, and the College of William and Mary. She is the founder of the Center for Eating Disorders in Norfolk, Virginia. She is a graduate of the University of Connecticut, received her doctorate from the University of Illinois, and served her internship, residency, and postdoctoral fellowships in family research at the University of Wisconsin School of Medicine. She is the author of *Transgenerational Family Therapies* (1992). Dr. Roberto is a member of several journal editorial boards, and is an approved supervisor and a site visitor for postgraduate training programs for the American Association for Marriage and Family Therapy. She was book review editor for the *Journal of Feminist Family Therapy* from 1993 through 1996. She maintains an active practice of marital, family, and individual psychotherapy, and has written extensively on women in families.

Fred M. Sander, MD, is associate clinical professor of psychiatry at the Mount Sinai School of Medicine in New York. He received his psychiatric training at the Albert Einstein College of Medicine in New York, and he is a graduate of the New York Psychoanalytic Institute. In addition to his 1979 book *Individual and Family Therapy: Toward an Integration,* he has written extensively on the integration of psychoanalytic theory and family therapy, and has taught on this topic for several years. In "off hours," Dr. Sander leads audience discussions after theater productions in New York.

Richard C. Schwartz, PhD, received his doctorate in marriage and family therapy from Purdue University; he then worked for the Institute for Juvenile Research in the Department of Psychiatry, University of Illinois at Chicago, for 16 years. In 1996, he moved to the Family Institute of Northwestern University. In addition, to writing numerous articles on a variety of topics related to psychotherapy, he is author of the book *Internal Family Systems Therapy* (1994) and coauthor of the books *Mosaic Mind: Empowering the Tormented Selves of Child Abuse Survivors* (with R. Goulding, 1995); *Family Therapy: Concepts and Methods,* fourth edition (with Michael P. Nichols, in press); and *Metaframeworks: Transcending the Models of Family Therapy* (with D. Breunlin and B. MacKune-Karrer, 1992). He is also coeditor of the *Handbook of Family Therapy Training and Supervision* (with H. A. Liddle and D. Breunlin, 1988). He is on the editorial board of five professional journals, including the *Journal of Marital and Family Therapy,* and is a fellow of the American Association for Marriage and Family Therapy.

Karl Tomm, MD, is a professor of psychiatry and director of the Family Therapy Program at the University of Calgary Faculty of Medicine. He has published and presented widely, and over the years has introduced a number of influential ideas and approaches to the family therapy field. He is currently developing and refining his ideas about psychiatric assessment with his "pathologizing interpersonal patterns" (PIPs) and "healing interpersonal patterns" (HIPs) approach. Chapter 13 is his first published work on his use of the Internalized Other Interview.

David N. Ulrich, PhD, ABPP, received his doctorate in clinical psychology from Harvard University in 1956. He is a diplomate of the American Board of Professional Psychology, and is also a charter member of the American Family Therapy Academy. Between 1956 and 1982, he served as a staff member of Judge Baker Guidance Center, Boston, and the Child Guidance Center of Southwestern Connecticut, in Stamford. Dr. Ulrich currently maintains a staff position with the Northeast Center for Trauma Recovery, Greenwich, Connecticut, and also maintains a private practice in Stamford, Connecticut. He has authored and coauthored numerous publications on contextual family therapy, one of which is a chapter with I. Boszormenyi-Nagy and J. Grunebaum in the *Handbook of Family Therapy,* Volume 2, edited by A. Gurman and B. Kniskern (1991).

Acknowledgments

I owe much to my early mentors, Joseph Wolpe and Aaron T. Beck, who have taught me most of what I know about cognitive-behavioral therapy. I am also indebted to Thomas A. Seay, who taught me a great deal about psychotherapy integration as well as couple and family therapy during my early graduate school training. Additional thanks goes to Wallace E. Crider for his supervision of my early work with couples and families. Along the way in the development of my work, personal conversations with noted figures such as Harry Aponte, Norman B. Epstein, James Framo, Cloé Madanes, Donald Meichenbaum, John C. Norcross, Arnold A. Lazarus, and Peggy Papp have also helped me tremendously in understanding the potential role of cognitive-behavioral techniques in couple and family therapy. I also thank the many couples and families who have served as the pioneering samples for my early work in the refinement of the cognitive-behavioral approach.

Compiling a major casebook such as this is not possible without the aid of many talented contributors. The chapters in this book have been written by some of the finest couple and family therapists in the world. In addition, a tremendous debt of gratitude is owed to the series editor, Michael P. Nichols, who has provided tireless effort and superb editorial suggestions that helped to shape this text into what is (in my opinion) one of the finest collection of case studies in the couple and family therapy literature. Staff members at The Guilford Press who deserve acknowledgment are Jodi Creditor and Anna Nelson for their outstanding work as the production editors, and Seymour Weingarten, the editor-in-chief, who has been extremely supportive and patient with my ideas. It is because of Seymour's open-mindedness and flexibility that this project has become a reality.

I also profusely thank my personal secretary, Carol "Fingers" Jaskolka, for her long hours of typing and her excellent computer skills. Her expertise in coordinating all of the details with this book is appreciated more than she will ever know. Her patience in enduring the stressful periods during this project was remarkable and has also earned her the guarantee of a lifetime supply of Prozac.

Finally, I owe the greatest acknowledgment to my children, Roseanne, Tara, and Michael, as well as my wife, Maryann, who endured my many absences during the preparation of this text. They have also taught me the true meaning and beauty of being a father and husband.

Foreword

From its very inception a century ago, the field of psychotherapy has resembled a dysfunctional family—with covert and overt antagonism among those representing different orientations, and few if any attempts made to comprehend or value the points of view held by others. It has operated on a win–lose basis, and the real losers have unfortunately been our clients. However, there is nothing like an attack from the outside—taking the form of third-party payments, biological psychiatry, and pressures for accountability—to facilitate cooperation within the system. This attack may very well have helped facilitate the interest in integration among therapists of different orientations and modalities. Other forces that have caused the long-term latent interest in psychotherapy integration to evolve into a more visible movement have been the proliferation of different schools of therapy; the realization that no one approach is capable of dealing with everything that therapists encounter clinically; and the formation in 1983 of the Society for the Exploration of Psychotherapy Integration (SEPI), an interdisciplinary organization dedicated to the development of clinically meaningful and empirically informed interventions that are not necessarily constrained by theoretical schools.

Although most of the attention of the psychotherapy movement has been paid to the integration of different schools of thought associated with individual therapy, a small but energetic group of clinicians has been interested in applying integrative thinking to family and couple therapy. Contributions by Alan Gurman, Jay Lebow, and William Pinsof have dealt with the integration of different theoretical approaches, and work by Larry Feldman, Ellen Wachtel, and Paul Wachtel has focused on the conjoint use of different modalities, such as individual along with couple/family interventions. The present casebook, edited by Frank M. Dattilio, is a very clear illustration of how an integrative stance can be used when couple/family work is approached from within a cognitive-behavioral orientation.

In commenting on the developmental status of behavior therapy in the early 1980s, Philip Kendall observed that as a result of years of industry and hard work, the behavioral approach—including cognitive-behavior therapy—had finally achieved its own personal identity. With this sense of security, he went on to add, it was now ready to become more intimate with other orientations. Even the very fact that Kendall, a behavior therapist, used this Eriksonian metaphor in his formulation attested to the readiness of behavior therapy for psychotherapy integration.

Kendall's characterization of the developmental status of behavior therapy is very much in accord with my own personal experience. Indeed, behavior therapy and I grew up together. Although originally trained within a psychodynamic orientation, I arrived at the State University of New York at Stony Brook in the mid-1960s, shortly after the birth of behavior therapy. I was both a participant in and an observer of its development over the years, with my clinical writings focusing on behavioral assessment and case formulation; the incorporation of cognitive factors into behavioral interventions; the conception of cognitive-behavior therapy as training in coping skills; and the incorporation into cognitive-behavior therapy of contributions from other orientations. The openness of cognitive-behavior therapy to what therapists from other schools of thought might have to say can be seen in Gerald C. Davison's and my book, *Clinical Behavior Therapy,* originally published in the mid-1970s. In retrospect, it was probably the incorporation of cognition into behavior therapy that provided a bridge to other orientations, and many behavior therapists who championed the cause of cognitive-behavior therapy (e.g., myself, Gerald C. Davison, Arnold A. Lazarus, Michael J. Mahoney, and Donald Meichenbaum) have since moved on to develop an interest in psychotherapy integration.

In their earlier conception of how cognition might be integrated into behavior therapy, behavior therapists found the contributions of Albert Ellis and Aaron T. Beck to be particularly significant. As more clinical attempts were made to make use of cognitive variables, it became evident that clients were not always able to articulate the "self-statements" that were at the root of their problematic emotional reactions and behavior. More often, it was "as if" they were saying certain things to themselves. The recognition that the meaning clients attributed to events was often implicit soon led to the incorporation of concepts developed in cognitive science, such as the "schema" construct. Of particular significance for psychotherapy integration is the fact that cognitive-behavior therapists began attending to those very same clinical phenomena that had long been of interest to their psychodynamic colleagues (e.g., clients' distorted perceptions of others). The fact that psychodynamic therapists were independently drawing on the cognitive sciences—similarly using the notion of "schema"—even further facilitated a link between the two orientations. In light of this, it is not at all surprising that many of the contributions to this volume make use of the schema concept.

The possibility that clients' views of themselves and others might mediate their clinical problem and constitute a focus for change has provided a common ground among psychodynamic, behavioral, cognitive, and experiential therapists. Although the means by which such change can be brought about are believed to vary—with behavioral approaches emphasizing action, psychodynamic and cognitive orientations stressing thinking, and experiential interventions focusing on emotion—it is nonetheless possible to induce a common set of change principles. Thus, in the context of a positive therapeutic alliance consisting of a good interpersonal bond, with therapists and clients agreeing on the goals of therapy and how they may be approached, therapists attempt to increase clients' awareness of themselves and others in regard to factors that may be creating difficulties in their lives. By becoming better aware of what they are thinking and not thinking, doing and not doing, and feeling and not feeling, clients are in a better position to take risks that can change their maladaptive patterns of thinking, behaving, and feeling. This risk taking, which we can refer to as the "corrective experience," is at the very heart of the change process.

The corrective experience begins with clients having certain expectations about themselves and the impact that they are likely to have on their world and on others. These expectations are typically schema-driven, based on early ways they may have learned for dealing with others. By now, however, these methods of coping are maladaptive. For example, clients with a history of parental abuse may approach current interactions with their significant others with this expectation: "If I tell my partner what I really feel or want, something bad will happen." This expectation, be it explicit or implicit, typically occurs with accompanying affect, such as fear, guilt, or anger. Within the context of a good therapeutic alliance, and once the clients have become more fully aware of the anachronistic nature of this perception of intimate relationships in their current life situation, they are in a better position to take the risk and recognize the invalidity of this "if–then" expectation.

In the case of clients who have experienced parental abuse, the risk may involve expressing their feelings or needs in a close interpersonal interaction, even though at some level the clients may still perceive this as being somewhat dangerous—hence the "risk." Telling their partners that they would prefer not to spend the weekend doing something they don't want to do, or expressing displeasure or disappointment about something without any major negative consequence occurring, provides the clients with a corrective experience containing cognitive, affective, and behavioral evidence that goes counter to their maladaptive schema. In the context of individual psychodynamic therapy, the corrective experience typically involves interaction with the therapist. In cognitive-behavior therapy carried out individually, this is more likely to occur between sessions, as in a homework assignment to assert oneself to a spouse. As so vividly illustrated in many of the cases described in this book, couple or family therapy allows the corrective experience to take place within the session itself and with the very individuals with whom clients' interactions, attitudes, and feelings have been problematic. Regardless of where this cognitive–affective–behavioral risk takes place, or how it is brought about, the corrective experience is at the core of therapeutic change.

In this collection of cases, Dattilio and his contributors have demonstrated in a direct clinical way how change occurs and how psychotherapy integration may be implemented. When therapists actually *show* rather than *say* what they do, it is far easier to draw out the points of similarity among the different schools of thought and to see how one approach can complement another. In editing this volume of cases, in providing commentary for each, and in obtaining the authors' responses to this commentary, Dattilio has taken an important step in this process of psychotherapy integration.

MARVIN R. GOLDFRIED, PHD
State University of New York at Stony Brook

Preface

In-te-grate (iń ti grāt): To bring together or incorporate into a unified, harmonious, or interrelated whole.

This book is the result of almost 10 years of contemplation, reflection, and debate on integrating various approaches to couple and family therapy. The contents contain most of the major theories along with a number of innovative and nontraditional approaches to working with couples and families, including the cognitive-behavioral modality.

As a young doctoral student in the early 1980s, I received my formal training in behavior therapy at Temple University from Joseph Wolpe, who is now regarded as the father of behavior therapy. It was through him that I was introduced to the application of behavioral principles in the treatment of individual and marital problems. At that time, very little was known about the true efficacy of behavior therapy with couples and families.

During my training, I was always struck by how little emphasis the behavioral strategies received in my courses in family therapy, particularly in light of how effective some of the strategies proved to be. Much of the general thinking in the field at that time was that behaviorists were naive about couple and family dynamics, and that their techniques were only effective when a family presented with an acting-out child or adolescent. In my opinion, much of the fine work done by such individuals as Gerald Patterson (1971), Richard Stuart (1969), and Robert Liberman (1970) in the late 1960s and early 1970s got little attention from many in the field of marriage and family therapy, even as an ancillary mode of treatment.

As the 1980s came to a close, I began to read more about psychotherapy integration. I read works by such individuals as Arnold A. Lazarus, Marvin R. Goldfried, and John C. Norcross, who promoted a distinct model of psychotherapy integration (e.g., Norcross & Goldfried, 1992). I also become keenly interested in writings by James Coyne and Howard Liddle, who spoke specifically about a technical eclecticism in the field of couple and family therapy (e.g., Coyne & Liddle, 1992).

I had always agreed with the notion that cognitive-behavioral therapy fell somewhat short of being a comprehensive mode of treatment for couples and families. As I began to read works by Donald H. Baucom

(1981) and Norman B. Epstein (1982), I began to see how effective cognitive-behavioral techniques could be when used within a systems framework or in combination with other modalities. By the mid-1980s, I also had the honor of working with Aaron T. Beck at the University of Pennsylvania School of Medicine on the development of his theories of cognitive therapy and the application to distressed couples. This effort subsequently spawned his popular book *Love Is Never Enough* (Beck, 1988), as well as my coauthored text *Cognitive Therapy with Couples* (Dattilio & Padesky, 1990).

By the 1990s I, like many psychotherapists, was feeling overwhelmed by the bewildering array of therapeutic approaches that had become available to couple and family therapists. This therapeutic morass was both a cause and consequence of the often-repeated research finding that no one modality was ideal or superior in addressing the broad range of couple and family dysfunctions. A summer lecture tour to southern Italy came at about the right time during this period. At one point, I had the good fortune to be invited on an outing to a Sicilian farm that had several hundred acres of vineyards. An Italian farmer was explaining to me in his native tongue how he combined the use of hybrid vines or *meritage* blends to produce an extraordinarily robust wine. It struck me that his thoughtful hybrids were analogous to the integration of psychotherapy models and to the blending of techniques to achieve a common goal—unique and robust results.

As I continued my European travels, this notion of blending various therapies sparked more thought on the idea of using cognitive-behavioral techniques as an integrative component with other models of couple and family therapy. This idea of integration was particularly intriguing, since Aaron Beck had always taught me how cognitive therapy was one of the most "integratable" of therapeutic modalities. Beck drew from various schools of thought in developing cognitive therapy, which rendered it compatible with many other psychotherapies.

In the past decade, cognitive-behavioral therapy with couples and families has gained tremendous popularity worldwide (Dattilio, 1990, 1992; Dattilio & Padesky, 1995, 1996). Many fine researchers and clinicians have been making an indelible impact throughout the world on practitioners of couple and family therapy. This comes primarily as a result of its adaptability to other modalities as well as to other cultures.

The early 1990s witnessed the beginning of a strong movement toward psychotherapy integration, which has led practitioners to explore various schools of thought that were once viewed as incompatible.

The primary focus of this book is theoretical integration. Previously, structural therapy and strategic therapy, the primary influences in the early development of couple and family therapy, have been combined in an attempt to maximize the effective components of both theories (Coyne & Liddle, 1992; Haley, 1976; Stanton, 1981). This theoretical melding has also been the case with concepts and techniques of the psychodynamic orientation (Norcross & Prochaska, 1988; Pitta, 1997), as well as those of other schools of thought (Kirschner & Kirschner, 1993; Lazarus, 1992; Christensen, Jacobson, & Babcock, 1995). Such hybrid forms of intervention appear to be on the increase, as practitioners become more aware of their potential effectiveness with individuals as well as with couples and families. In fact, the modal orientation of family therapists is now eclecticism/integration (Prochaska & Norcross, 1994). Within systemic therapy alone, there has been a decided breakdown of schoolism and a movement toward integration. In a survey of 900 family therapists, nearly one-third described their theoretical orientation as eclectic (Rait, 1988).

One of the beauties of integrating theories is that the essential framework of the primary theory need not be abandoned in order to integrate other techniques or strategies. These techniques may be augmented in various fashions and forms, depending on the vitality of the basic therapy model. Cognitive-behavioral therapy has received increasing support in the professional literature as a highly "integratable" theory in work with couples and families (Beck, 1988; Dattilio & Padesky, 1990; Dattilio, 1989, 1990, 1994, 1997; Lombana & Frazier, 1994). In fact, two recent articles addressed the question of whether or not *all* therapies are cognitive (Alford & Norcross, 1991; Persons, 1995), particularly since cognitive components appear to be part of the fabric of most modalities. Clinicians may selectively choose various cognitive-behavioral techniques to incorporate into their primary approach as the need arises. (This integration is particularly important in short-term treatment, due to the effective results achieved with cognitive-behavioral techniques.) Interestingly, this phenomenon was often mentioned during the process of choosing contributors for this book. After I explained to authors my idea for the work, many of them spontaneously said, "Oh, I use cognitive-behavioral strategies in my work all the time."

In addition to the concept of integration, this book also provides detailed case analysis from more than 16 different perspectives of couple and family therapy, with elaborate commentary by both the authors and the editor.

Laurence Sterne, the 18th-century novelist, said that writing is just a different name for conversation—a conversation that takes place between the author and the reader. The present book transcends this definition by providing a conversation among the authors, the editor, and (in a tacit sense) the reader. In this text, the symbol "†" denotes my comments as the editor, and these are highlighted in italics. The author or authors of each chapter were also invited to submit a follow-up commentary after receiving a copy of my editorial comments.[1] The primary intention was to create a dialogue that would help readers draw their own conclusions regarding the integration of cognitive-behavioral strategies with other therapies as presented in this book.

FRANK M. DATTILIO
September 1997

NOTE

1. The author or authors of each chapter were provided with a copy of *Cognitive Therapy with Couples* (Dattilio & Padesky, 1990), which contains the basic philosophy and theory of cognitive-behavioral therapy with couples and families. They were also provided with a uniform list of questions to answer when composing their "authors' reply to the editor's comments," along with a guideline for disguising case material to ensure confidentiality.

REFERENCES

Alford, B. A., & Norcross, J. C. (1991). Cognitive therapy as integrative therapy. *Journal of Psychotherapy Integration, 1*(3), 175–190.

Beck, A. T. (1988). *Love is never enough.* New York: Harper & Row.

Coyne, J. C., & Liddle, H. A. (1992). The future systems therapy: Shedding myths and facing opportunities *Psychotherapy, 29*(1), 44–50.

Christensen, A., Jacobson, N. S., & Babcock, J. C. (1995). Integrative behavioral couple therapy. In N. S. Jacobson & A. S. Gurman (Eds.), *Clinical handbook of couples therapy* (pp. 31–64). New York: Guilford Press.

Dattilio, F. M. (1989). A guide to cognitive marital therapy. In P. A. Keller & S. R. Heyman (Eds.), *Innovations in clinical practice: A source book* (Vol. 8, pp. 27–42). Sarasota, FL: Professional Resource Exchange.

Dattilio, F. M. (1994). Families in crisis. In F. M. Dattilio & A. Freeman (Eds.), *Cognitive-behavioral strategies in crisis intervention* (pp. 278–301). New York: Guilford Press.

Dattilio, F. M. (1997). Family therapy. In R. Leahy (Ed.), *Practicing cognitive therapy: A guide to interventions* (pp. 409–450). Northvale, NJ: Jason Aronson.

Dattilio, F. M., & Padesky, C. A. (1990). *Cognitive therapy with couples.* Sarasota, FL: Professional Resource Exchange.

Haley, J. (1976). *Problem-solving therapy: New strategies for effective family therapy.* San Francisco: Jossey-Bass.

Kirschner, S., & Kirschner, D. A. (1993). Couples and families. In G. Stricker & J. R. Gold (Eds.), *Comprehensive handbook of psychotherapy integration* (pp. 401–412). New York: Plenum Press.

Lazarus, A. A. (1992). When is couples therapy necessary and sufficient? *Psychological Reports, 70,* 787–790.

Liberman, R. P. (1970). Behavioral approaches to couples and family therapy. *American Journal of Orthopsychiatry, 40,* 106–118.

Lombana, J. H., & Frazier, F. B. (1994). Cognitive–systems therapy: A case excerpt. *Journal of Mental Health Counseling, 16*(4), 434–444.

Norcross, J. C., & Goldfried, M. R. (Eds.). (1992). *Handbook of psychotherapy integration.* New York: Basic Books.

Norcross, J. C., & Newman, C. F. (1992). Psychotherapy integrations: Setting the context. In J. C. Norcross & M. R. Goldfried (Eds.), *Handbook of psychotherapy integration* (pp. 3–45). New York: Basic Books.

Norcross, J. C., & Prochaska, J. O. (1988). A study of eclectic (and integrative) views revisited. *Professional Psychology: Research and Practice, 19,* 170–174.

Patterson, G. R. (1971). *Families: Applications of social learning to life*. Champaign, IL: Research Press.

Persons, J. (1995). Are all psychotherapies cognitive? *Journal of Cognitive Psychotherapy, 9*(3), 185–194.

Pitta, P. (1997). Marital therapy: A systemic psychodynamic integrated approach: A case study. *Psychotherapy Bulletin, 32*(1), 45–48.

Prochaska, J. O., & Norcross, J. C. (1994). *Systems of psychotherapy: A transtheoretical analysis* (3rd ed.). Pacific Grove, CA: Brooks/Cole.

Rait, D. (1988). Survey results. *The Family Networker, 12*, 52–56.

Stanton, M. (1981). An integrated structural/strategic approach to family therapy. *Journal of Marital and Family Therapy, 7*, 427–439.

Stuart, R. B. (1969). Operant–interpersonal treatment of marital discord. *Journal of Consulting and Clinical Psychology, 33*, 675—682.

Contents

*Marriages and families
are not as they are made,
but as they turn out.*

—Italian proverb

Chapter 1

An Introduction to Cognitive-Behavioral Therapy with Couples and Families

FRANK M. DATTILIO
NORMAN B. EPSTEIN
DONALD H. BAUCOM

Cognitive-behavioral therapy has now gained recognition among mental health theorists, researchers, and practitioners as a mainstream approach to psychotherapy. Even though the various forms of cognitive-behavioral therapy are in their infancy as compared to some other schools, they have generated more empirical research and resulted in more outcome studies than any other psychotherapeutic modality (Beck, 1991a).

Albert Ellis was among the first to publish descriptions of the application of cognitive-behavioral therapy to problems in intimate relationships. Ellis applied his A-B-C theory[1] of rational–emotive therapy (RET) to distressed couples (Ellis, 1977; Ellis & Harper, 1961), in an attempt to modify their thoughts and subsequently their emotions and behaviors. Ellis contended that marital dysfunction occurs when partners hold unrealistic beliefs about their relationship and make extreme negative evaluations once dissatisfied. He further proposed that disturbed feelings in a relationship are not caused merely by partners' actions or other adverse events, but by their particular views of each other's actions and other life stressors (Ellis, Sichel, Yeager, DiMattia, & DiGiuseppe, 1989). Ellis introduced the notion of "irrational beliefs" and defined them as highly exaggerated, inappropriately rigid, and illogical contentions that produce disappointment and frustration. In an individual, these negative cognitions and emotions then lead to negative behavior toward another person, causing a vicious cycle of disturbance. Ellis (1995) has recently renamed his approach rational–emotive behavior therapy (REBT) in order to acknowledge more fully the role of behavioral responses in individuals' interpersonal problems. This suggests that he places equal emphasis on the role of such responses in couple and family relationships.

Unfortunately, the RET model of relationship dysfunction may have been perceived as simplistic when it first appeared in the literature, and consequently there was little discussion of it in the literature until much later. Moreover, at the time that Ellis first introduced his model, the systems theory approaches to marriage and family therapy had already gained substantial popularity; thus, they overshadowed the RET approach. Furthermore, because the RET model tended to emphasize linear, intrapsychic causation, it had limited appeal among family therapists, who focused on circular interaction processes with family members.

At about the same time, during the 1960s, modern behaviorists were utilizing principles of learning theory to assess and treat adults and children who displayed behavioral problems. Behavior therapists' work with children led them to observe parent–child interaction patterns and to train parents in principles of behavior modification to alter their children's negative actions (Berkowitz & Graziano, 1972; Patterson & Hops, 1972). Similarly, Richard Stuart (1969) described the use of operant learning strategies to produce more satisfying interactions in distressed couples. Observations of parents and their children with behavioral problems also led behavior therapists to begin to address issues in the parents' own relationships, as they began to realize how marital discord contributes to inconsistent parenting (Gordon & Davidson, 1981). The movement toward applying principles of operant conditioning and social learning developed into a more comprehensive theory of marital and family discord and therapy (e.g., Liberman, 1970; Patterson, 1971). Initially, behavioral treatment approaches placed emphasis on the components of operant conditioning, social exchange theory, and contingency contracting with couples and parent–child relationships (Gordon & Davidson, 1981; Stuart, 1969); they later included an increased focus on communication and problem-solving skills (Falloon, 1991; Jacobson, 1981; Jacobson & Margolin, 1979).

Even though nonbehavioral marital and family therapists long ago recognized the importance of intervention with cognitive factors, such as family members' interpretations of one another's behavior (Dicks, 1953; Satir, 1964; Haley & Hoffman, 1968), only in the late 1970s did clinical researchers begin to add cognitive components to behavioral treatment in controlled outcome studies. Initially, aspects of cognition were introduced as auxiliary components of treatment within the behavioral approach (Margolin, Christensen, & Weiss, 1975). A study by Margolin and Weiss

(1978) compared behavioral marital therapy with a treatment in which behavioral marital therapy was supplemented with cognitive restructuring techniques. The results suggested that the cognitive restructuring significantly enhanced the effectiveness of traditional behavioral 'marital therapy on several outcome measures. During the 1980s, cognitive factors became more of a focus in the couple research and therapy literature (e.g., Baucom, 1987; Baucom, Epstein, Sayers, & Sher, 1989; Beck, 1988; Dattilio, 1989; Doherty, 1981a, 1981b; Eidelson & Epstein, 1982; Epstein, 1982; Epstein & Eidelson, 1981; Fincham, Beach, & Nelson, 1987; Fincham & O'Leary, 1983; Jacobson, 1984; Jacobson, McDonald, Follette, & Berley, 1985; Margolin, 1983; Schindler & Vollmer, 1984; Weiss, 1980, 1984). This movement underscored the need for couple treatment procedures to include a focus on the partners' cognitions regarding each other's actions, and led to the application of established cognitive interventions in conjoint couple therapy (Baucom & Epstein, 1990; Dattilio & Padesky, 1990; Epstein, 1992; Epstein & Baucom, 1989).

Similarly, cognitive-behavioral family therapy evolved from behavioral approaches to research and intervention with families. Whereas early work by Patterson and his associates (e.g., Patterson, 1971, 1982; Patterson, McNeal, Hawkins, & Phelps, 1967) emphasized contingency contracting and operant learning procedures, the theoretical, research, and clinical literature broadened to include family members' cognitions about one another. Once again, Albert Ellis was one of the first to introduce a cognitive approach to family therapy, in an article that discussed the significant difference between RET and systems-oriented therapy (Ellis, 1982). At about the same time, a chapter by Richard Bedrosian (1983) addressed the notion of cognition in family dynamics. Subsequently, the 1980s and 1990s saw a rapid growth in the literature on cognitive-behavioral approaches to therapy with families (Alexander, 1988; Dattilio, 1993, 1994, 1996a, 1997; Epstein & Schlesinger, 1995; Epstein, Schlesinger, & Dryden, 1988; Falloon, Boyd, & McGill, 1984; Huber & Baruth, 1989; Robin & Foster, 1989; Schwebel & Fine, 1994; Teichman, 1981, 1992).

BEHAVIORAL FACTORS IN COUPLE AND FAMILY PROBLEMS

A basic tenet of the cognitive-behavioral model of couple and family dysfunction is that relationship distress and conflict are directly influenced by an interaction of cognitive, behavioral, and affective factors (Epstein et al., 1988). Considerable evidence suggests that exchanges of negative behavior among family members are associated with relationship distress, and that members' use of aversive control is associated with a variety of dysfunctional outcomes for children, such as school, work, and interpersonal problems (Biglan, Lewin, & Hops, 1990). Consequently, traditional behavioral family therapy methods of assessment and modification of behavioral interactions remain important components of the cognitive-behavioral approach. In particular, the cognitive-behavioral family therapist pays attention to family members' (1) frequencies and patterns of antagonistic/discordant behavior exchanges, (2) expressive and listening skills for communicating thoughts and feelings, and (3) problem-solving skills (Baucom & Epstein, 1990; Epstein et al., 1988; Robin & Foster, 1989). Concerning exchanges of aversive behavior, evidence that distressed couples and families engage in circular, escalating antagonistic/discordant interaction patterns (e.g., Patterson, 1982; Revenstorf, Hahlweg, Schindler, & Vogel, 1984) is consistent with a systems theory conceptualization of reciprocal influences among family members. Similar to other family therapists who focus on the "process" of family interactions, cognitive-behavioral therapists carefully observe sequences of behavior and interaction among family members during conjoint sessions, noting how each person's behavior is a response to others' actions and serves as a stimulus that elicits further responses from other members. Concerning communication skills, cognitive-behavioral therapists assume that effective communication is the mutual responsibility of the speaker, who intends to express his or her thoughts and feelings, and the listener, whose role is to understand what is being expressed (Guerney, 1977). In addition, it is assumed that in order to resolve the problems of daily living (ranging from relatively trivial matters to major issues), family members require skills for defining problems clearly, identifying mutually acceptable and appropriate re-solutions or problem-solving strategies, and implementing these solutions effectively. These assumptions of cognitive-behavioral therapy are supported by empirical findings that couples and families referred for relationship distress exhibit more dysfunctional communication and less constructive problem-solving behavior than do satisfied couples and families (Baucom & Epstein, 1990; Robin & Foster, 1989; Weiss & Heyman, 1990).

COGNITIVE FACTORS IN COUPLE AND FAMILY PROBLEMS

Cognitive factors involved in couple and family distress have been conceptualized in varying ways by cognitive-behavioral theorists and therapists. The central principle, however, is that family members' appraisals and interpretations of one another's behavior influence the nature and extent of their emotional and behavioral responses to one another.

Beck's Cognitive Model

Beck's cognitive model (Beck, 1991b; Beck, Rush, Shaw, & Emery, 1979) has been expanded to focus on cognitive variables that shape an individual's reactions to life events, in order to provide a better understanding of cognitive mediation in interpersonal relationships. Those who have applied Beck's model to couple and family interaction (Beck, 1988; Bedrosian, 1983; Bedrosian & Bozicas, 1994; Dattilio, 1989, 1990, 1997; Dattilio & Padesky, 1990; Epstein, 1982, 1986) have described the assessment and modification of "automatic thoughts" and "cognitive distortions" that are involved in faulty information processing, as well as of unrealistic, extreme, or inappropriate "schemas."

Automatic Thoughts

"Automatic thoughts" are defined as stream-of-consciousness ideas, beliefs, or images that individuals have from moment to moment, often elicited by specific situations (e.g., "My wife is late again—she doesn't care about my feelings," or "My parents are setting a curfew for me because they like hassling me"). The word "automatic" indicates the spontaneous quality of these cognitions, and cognitive therapists (e.g., Beck et al., 1979) have noted how individuals commonly accept them as plausible rather than questioning their validity. A perfect example of this is portrayed by an incident that occurred with a newly married couple. During working hours, a gentleman had received a call from a distant relative who had arrived in town unexpectedly. She asked if he and his wife were available for lunch. The gentleman attempted to call his wife at home, but since it was short notice, she was not available for lunch. However, he made plans to meet the relative for lunch by himself. Ironically, the gentleman's wife had been out shopping and saw him leaving a restaurant with his relative, who happened to be an attractive young female. Upon seeing her husband with another woman, the wife immediately flew into a rage. She began catastrophizing that her husband was having an affair, and she became emotionally distraught. After she confronted her husband, he informed her of the situation and arranged for an opportunity to introduce his wife to his relative later that same day. This is a clear example of a woman engaging in the distortion of "jumping to conclusions," which led to the automatic erroneous belief that her husband was being unfaithful.

Cognitive Distortions in Automatic Thoughts

The same cognitive distortions contributing to depression that were identified in early writings on cognitive therapy (Beck et al., 1979) are likely to contribute to distorted automatic thoughts and thus to be sources of relationship discord. Below is a list of eight common cognitive distortions (many others could be described), with examples of how they may occur in couple or family interaction:

1. *Arbitrary inference.* A conclusion is drawn from an event, in the absence of supporting substantiating evidence. For example, a man whose

wife arrives home 30 minutes late from work concludes, "She must be having an affair," or parents whose son or daughter was 15 minutes late for curfew conclude that the child is engaging in inappropriate activities with friends.

2. *Selective abstraction.* Information is perceived out of context; certain details are noticed or highlighted, while other important information is ignored. For example, an individual may focus on the negative behavior of other family members, but fail to notice their positive actions. In distressed families, it's common to hear the members whose positive acts go unnoticed complaining, "You never notice the good things that I do!"

3. *Overgeneralization.* An isolated incident or two is allowed to serve as a representation of similar situations, whether or not they are truly related. For example, after her husband fails to complete one household chore, a woman concludes, "He is totally unreliable."

4. *Magnification and minimization.* A case or circumstance is perceived as having greater or lesser significance than is appropriate. For example, an angry husband becomes enraged upon discovering that his wife has overspent the weekly budget for groceries, and magnifies this event by concluding, "We're doomed financially." In contrast, he may engage in minimization when his wife spends less than the budgeted amount the next time she does the grocery shopping, as he concludes, "That hardly saved us any money."

5. *Personalization.* This is a form of arbitrary inference, in which external events are attributed to oneself when insufficient evidence exists to render a conclusion. For example, a woman finds her husband remaking the bed after she previously spent time making it herself and concludes, "He is dissatisfied with the way I did it."

6. *Dichotomous thinking.* Experiences are classified as either all or nothing—as complete successes or total failures. This is otherwise known as "all-or-nothing" or "polarized thinking." For example, a mother who states to her son who is cleaning his room, "There is still dust on your bureau," elicits this reaction from her son: "She's never satisfied with anything I do."

7. *Labeling and mislabeling.* Behaviors such as mistakes made in the past are generalized as traits to define oneself or another family member. For example, subsequent to making repeated errors in balancing the checkbook, a partner states, "I'm really stupid," as opposed to recognizing the errors as situational behavior (perhaps influenced by fatigue). Similarly, a parent who observes a child dragging along in the morning as he or she gets ready for school concludes, "This kid is really lazy."

8. *Mind reading.* This is another special case of arbitrary inference, in which an individual believes that he or she is able to know what another family member is thinking or will do in the near or distant future, without the aid of direct verbal communication between the parties. Members of distressed couples and families often make negative predictions about each

other. For example, a woman says to herself, "I know what Tom is going to say when he hears that I'll be working late tomorrow." Although such predictions may be accurate, based on past experiences with the other person, mind reading involves going beyond the available data and risking erroneous conclusions.

Schemas

Research on human cognition (Fiske & Taylor, 1991) supports the premise that moment-to-moment automatic thoughts and the cognitive distortions on which they are based tend to be shaped by the individual's "schemas," which are underlying core beliefs that the person has developed about characteristics of the world and how it functions. Schemas are relatively stable cognitive structures that may become inflexible and unconditional in character. Many schemas about relationships and the nature of family members' interactions are learned early in life from primary sources, such as family of origin, cultural mores, the mass media, and early dating experiences (Dattilio, 1993, 1994). These schemas or dysfunctional beliefs about relationships are often not articulated clearly in an individual's mind, but exist as vague concepts of what "should be" (Beck, 1988). For example, some men believe that holding a door open for a woman is a way of being polite or showing courtesy—something that has been taught in many American households. A woman who was brought up in a different environment, however, may interpret this gesture as not respecting her independence, particularly if it is overdone.

These kinds of schemas are the basis for coding, categorizing, and evaluating experiences during the course of one's life. Central to Beck's cognitive theory of depression is the concept of the "negative triad"—pessimistic schemas about the self, world, and future. Schemas that have been previously developed influence how an individual subsequently processes information in new situations. A basic tenet of cognitive-behavioral family therapy is that each individual family member maintains schemas about every member of the family unit (including himself or herself), in addition to schemata about family interaction in general. These schemas are sometimes conscious and overtly expressed, but more often individuals aren't fully aware of the basic beliefs that guide their responses to family interactions.

When a couple forms a relationship, each partner brings some schemas from his or her family of origin and other life experiences (e.g., schemas about the characteristics that each individual assumes are typical of an intimate relationship). Although these schemas influence each partner's perceptions and inferences about events in the current relationship, events in the current relationship can also modify preexisting schemas (Epstein & Baucom, 1993). For example, even though an individual who grew up with abusive parents may have developed a schema involving danger in family interaction, and years later this schema may lead the individual to make arbitrary inferences about malevolent intent by his or her adult partner, current experiences with a safe and supportive partner may alter the negative schema. However, preexisting schemas may be difficult to modify, particularly if they are associated with strong feelings.

In addition to the schemas that partners or mates bring to their relationship, each member of a couple develops schemas specific to the current partner and relationship. Consistent with empirical findings concerning schemas as templates according to which individuals process new information, Beck (1988) describes how each partner develops a "frame" or stable schema concerning the other's characteristics, and how subsequent perceptions and interpretations of the other's behavior tend to be shaped by the frame. For example, when a woman's observations of her partner produce a schema in which he is viewed as "selfish," the woman is likely to notice future partner behaviors that seem consistent with the schema, to ignore actions that are inconsistent with the schema, and to attribute other negative partner behavior to the trait of "selfishness."

Members of a couple are also likely to develop schemas about themselves as a couple (e.g., "We share a lot of interests," "We're from two different worlds," "Our goal is to raise children with high moral standards"). The couple dyad is modified with the birth of any offspring and the development of a triad or larger family unit. Here the development of "triangles" becomes important, because they contribute profoundly to the development of family members' cognitions (Procter, 1985; Guerin, Fogarty, Fay, & Kautto, 1996). For example, consistent with systems theory, when family members form coalitions against other members, each individual develops schemas concerning the conflict and power dynamics involved in such coalitions. Moreover, cognitive-behavioral therapists are particularly interested in helping individuals link such schemas to experiences in their families of origin (Dattilio, 1997). As a result of years of integrated interaction among family members, the individuals develop jointly held beliefs, which constitute the "family schema" (Dattilio, 1994). To the extent that the family schema involves cognitive distortions, it may result in dysfunctional interaction (e.g., when all members of a family view a particular child as irresponsible and therefore behave in ways that constrain the child's development of autonomy). Figure 1.1 depicts the evolution of a family schema from the schemas the partners bring from their families of origin, and the blending of their life experiences and beliefs.

Baucom and Epstein's Typology of Cognitions

Baucom and Epstein (1990; Baucom et al., 1989) have presented a typology of cognitions that have been implicated in relationship conflict and distress: (1) "selective attention," in which each member of a relationship tends to notice some aspects of the events occurring in their interactions but not

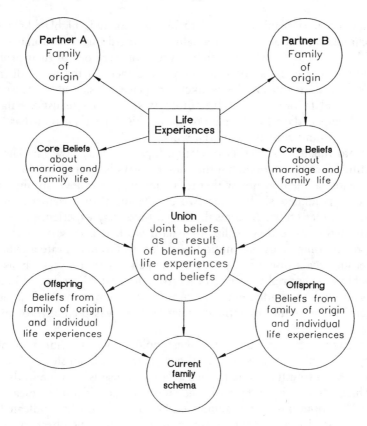

FIGURE 1.1. The development of a family schema.

others; (2) "attributions," or inferences that individuals make about causes of events in their relationship; (3) "expectancies," or predictions about the probabilities of particular events' occurring in the future; (4) "assumptions," which involve beliefs about the characteristics of relationships and how relationships work; and (5) "standards," or family members' beliefs about the ways relationships in general, or their own relationships in particular, "should" be. These typologies are based largely on the schemas and automatic thoughts discussed on the preceding pages.

Cognitive-behavioral theorists propose that these five types of cognitions have the potential to erode satisfaction in family relationships and to elicit dysfunctional family interactions. In particular, assumptions and standards can be problematic if they are unrealistic or distorted; in such cases, they are based on misinformation or faulty thinking and usually rooted in circumstantial evidence. For example, the assumption "Women like to control men's lives" carries negative connotations and involves the cognitive distortion of overgeneralization. If an individual applies such an assumption in a blanket manner to all women, it is highly likely to be inaccurate. An example of an unrealistic standard might be a man's belief that "I must help my wife and children resolve every one of their problems in life in order to be a good husband and father." If the man adheres to this standard steadfastly, he is likely to place considerable pressure on himself, and failure is inevitable. In contrast, a more realistic, balanced, conditional standard for the man might be this: "It's important that I offer assistance to my wife and children when I can."

Unfortunately, sometimes relationships are like flowers: They are beautiful when they bloom, but they don't always last very long. Individuals often enter a relationship with the assumption that love springs up or develops spontaneously between two people and thrives that way forever without further effort. As a result, the partners may experience a decrease in satisfaction once they realize that hard work is necessary to maintain their relationship. This assumption may also lead to inaccurate attributions concerning the cause of any strains in their relationship, such as "We probably were not right for each other from the start." Epstein and Eidelson (1981) found that adherence to unrealistic assumptions and standards concerning the nature of intimate relationships was predictive of marital distress.

Attributions that family members hold about determinants of the happy and unhappy events that occur in their relationships have been demonstrated to influence both their relationship satisfaction and the ways in which they behave toward one another. Considerable research on couples' attributions (see Bradbury & Fincham, 1990) has indicated that members of distressed couples are more likely than members of nondis-tressed couples to attribute their partners' negative behavior to global, stable traits, negative intent, selfish motivation, and a lack of love. In addition, members of distressed couples are less likely to attribute positive partner behaviors to global, stable causes. The unfortunate implications of these findings are that distressed partners tend to view each other's negative behavior as due to relatively unchangeable negative factors, and that they tend to discount each other's positive behavior as transitory and atypical. Similarly, there is empirical evidence (Morton, Twentyman, & Azar, 1988) that parents who tend to use coercive and abusive corporal punishment are more likely than nonabusive parents to attribute their children's negative behavior to stable, global negative traits (e.g., "He just loves to frustrate me"). Thus, the common refrain of distressed partners, as well as many children, that "You just focus on the negatives and don't give me any credit for the good things I do" may accurately describe the occurrence of biased attributions (which may lead to selective attention to behaviors consistent with the attributed negative traits).

Concerning expectancies, Doherty (1981b) proposed that family members who believe that there is a low probability that they will engage in effective problem-solving behavior together tend to behave as if they are helpless, rather than making active attempts to resolve family conflicts. Another possible negative outcome of negative expectancies in family relationships is the "self-fulfilling prophecy," in which an individual predicts that other family members will behave negatively, responds negatively toward the others, and thereby elicits the predicted behavior from them.

More extensive reviews of empirical findings concerning the roles of these five types of cognitions in marital distress can be found in Baucom and Epstein (1990), Epstein and Baucom (1993), and Fincham, Bradbury, and Scott (1990). Although Baucom and Epstein's (1990) typology of cognitions differs somewhat from Beck et al.'s (1979) model of automatic thoughts, cognitive distortions, and underlying schemas, the two conceptualizations are compatible. Both include stable types of cognitions about relationships and involve the same type of distortions that are often based on poor reality testing. The two theories also include the moment-to-moment influences and other fledgling cognitions that are present in more stable belief systems. One of the main differences between the two theories, however, is that Beck places less emphasis on the behavioral aspect of change than does Baucom and Epstein's model. Since Beck is more rooted in the notion that cognitions place the heaviest influence on emotion and behavior, his emphasis is on specific schemas and distorted beliefs.

ASSESSMENT OF COUPLES AND FAMILIES

Because of the high rate of divorce and the heavy emphasis in the mass media on troubled relationships, most of the existing literature on cognitive-behavioral assessment of intimate relationships has focused on couples; relatively little has been published regarding the assessment of families. Although cognitive-behavioral family assessment is similar to that with couples, less emphasis is placed on the use of structured inventories and questionnaires, particularly because some family members may be too young to complete such forms or simply may find this to be a monotonous process. Nevertheless, inventories may be useful with older family members who can appreciate the benefit of identifying cognitions and behavioral interaction patterns on paper. This is particularly so with more nonverbal family members. This section describes representative methods for assessing couples' and families' relationship cognitions and behavioral interactions.

Assessment of Relationship Cognitions

Self-Report Questionnaires

Eidelson and Epstein's (1982) Relationship Belief Inventory was developed to tap unrealistic beliefs about close relationships. It includes subscales assessing the assumptions that partners cannot change a relationship, that disagreement is always destructive, and that heterosexual relationship problems are due to innate differences between men and women, as well as standards that partners should be able to mind-read each other's thoughts and emotions and that one should be a perfect sexual partner.

Baucom, Epstein, Rankin, and Burnett's (1996) Inventory of Specific Relationship Standards (ISRS) assesses an individual's personal standards concerning major relationship themes, including the nature of boundaries between partners (autonomy vs. sharing), distribution of control (equal vs. skewed) and partners' levels of instrumental and expressive investment in their relationship, as the individual applies the standards to his or her own relationship.

The Family Beliefs Inventory (Vincent-Roehling & Robin, 1986) assesses 10 potentially unrealistic beliefs that parents and adolescents maintain about their relationships, and that are likely to contribute to parent–adolescent conflict. Respondents read vignettes describing areas of conflict (e.g., choice of friends, spending time away from home) and then indicate their degree of agreement or disagreement with each of several beliefs.

Several attribution scales have been developed for use in clinical research, and these can be applied in clinical practice as well. Pretzer, Epstein, and Fleming's (1991) Marital Attitude Survey (MAS) includes subscales assessing attributions for relationship problems to one's own behavior, one's own personality, the partner's behavior, the partner's personality, the partner's lack of love, and the partner's malicious intent. Fincham and Bradbury's (1992) Relationship Attribution Measure asks the respondent to rate his or her agreement with statements reflecting attributions about 10 hypothetical negative partner behaviors (e.g., "Your husband/wife criticizes something you say"). Baucom, Epstein, Daiuto, et al. (1996) developed the Relationship Attribution Questionnaire, with which the respondent rates causal and responsibility attributions for real problems in his or her relationship, as well as the degrees to which the problems are attributed to boundary, control, and investment factors similar to those assessed in relationship standards by the ISRS.

Concerning the assessment of expectancies, Pretzer et al.'s (1991) MAS also includes subscales assessing partners' generalized expectancies for overcoming relationship problems, including the perceived ability of the partners to change their relationship and the expectancy that they actually will improve the relationship. At present there are no measures of partners' expectancies concerning more specific positive and negative events that may occur in their relationships.

There are no parallel forms of these attribution and expectancy measures designed to assess cognitions in parent–child relationships. However, in clinical practice one could adapt the couple-oriented items for family assessment.

Numerous other self-report questionnaires have been developed to assess aspects of parent–child relationships and general family functioning, and excellent reviews of these measures can be found in the texts by Grotevant and Carlson (1989), Touliatos, Perlmutter, and Straus (1990), and Jacob and Tennenbaum (1988). Some instruments, such as the Family Environment Scale (Moos & Moos, 1986), the McMaster Family Assessment Device (Epstein, Baldwin, & Bishop, 1983), and the Family Adaptability and Cohesion Evaluation Scales III (Olson, Portner, & Lavee, 1985), assess family members' global perceptions of such family characteristics as cohesion, problem solving, communication quality, role clarity, emotional expression, and values. Other scales, such as the Family Inventory of Life Events and Changes (McCubbin, Patterson, & Wilson, 1985), and the Family Crisis-Oriented Personal Evaluation Scales (McCubbin, Larsen, & Olson, 1985), provide more specialized assessment of family functioning (e.g., members' perceptions of particular stressors and family coping strategies). Because the family of origin is also an important factor in the cognitive-behavioral approach, the Family-of-Origin Scale (Hovestadt, Anderson, Piercy, Cochran, & Fine, 1985) is an excellent tool to measure the self-perceived levels of health in one's family of origin. In general, these scales do not provide data about specific cognitive, behavioral, and affective variables central to a cognitive-behavioral assessment, but they do tap a variety of important components of family functioning likely to be of interest to all family therapists. A few instruments tap family members' attitudes about parenting roles and thus are more directly relevant to cognitive assessment.

Interview Assessment of Cognitions

Clinical interviews with members of a couple or family, together or individually, provide the opportunity to elicit idiosyncratic cognitions and to track inferential processes that cannot be assessed by standardized questionnaires. Using Socratic questioning methods, which are the hallmark of cognitive therapy (Beck, 1995; Beck et al., 1979), the clinician inquires about the chains of thoughts that mediate between events in the relationship and each individual's emotional and behavioral responses. Beck et al. (1979) developed the "downward arrow" technique to identify the underlying schemas (e.g., assumptions and standards) beneath an individual's automatic thoughts. This is done by identifying the initial thought—for example, "I need to scream because Harry doesn't always listen to me"—and then asking the individual, "If he doesn't listen to you, then what does that mean?" and following up each of the individual's subsequent responses with another question that probes for his or her "underlying" cognitions.

As Figure 1.2 demonstrates, screaming at Harry was this woman's way of avoiding her perceived vulnerability and expressing the pervasive frustration that she experienced in relationships with others. The use of the downward arrow exercise served to uncover an underlying schema (assumption) of vulnerability and helplessness, along with her fear of not being

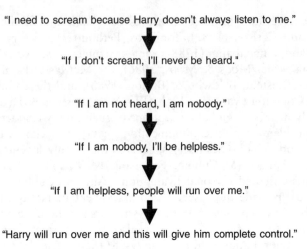

"I need to scream because Harry doesn't always listen to me."

"If I don't scream, I'll never be heard."

"If I am not heard, I am nobody."

"If I am nobody, I'll be helpless."

"If I am helpless, people will run over me."

"Harry will run over me and this will give him complete control."

FIGURE 1.2. Example of the "downward arrow" technique.

responded to. This technique allows the individual, his or her partner or family, and the therapist to become aware of the chain of thoughts and to see how it can lead to erroneous conclusions and reinforce long-standing assumptions. This technique is demonstrated very clearly on video by Dattilio (1996b).

In another example, a husband initially felt angry when his wife complained about being too busy to work on the family finances. When the therapist asked what thoughts occurred as the husband heard his wife's complaint, he reported thinking, "She's always too busy for things that don't interest her." When the therapist next asked what it meant to the husband if that was in fact true of his wife, the husband responded, "It means she's selfish and doesn't care about how things affect me" (negative attributions). Another "What if" question by the therapist elicited this response from the husband: "She doesn't really love me, and I can't count on her when I really need her" (another negative attribution, followed by a negative expectancy). The therapist now had a sense of why the husband had such a strong emotional response to his wife. He interpreted her behavior as reflecting a lack of investment in their relationship and a threat to the bond between them. (The therapist might also have determined that the husband's repeated inferences that his wife had low investment in their relationship constituted a theme underlying his annoyance with her.)

At this point, the therapist still needed to collaborate with both partners to gather information for testing the validity of the husband's attributions and expectancies. The goals of the treatment plan would depend on how much his inferences reflected real negative motives on his wife's part as opposed to cognitive distortions on his part. The therapist also probably noted the extreme wording of the husband's phrase, "She's *always* too busy," and thus could ask other questions to assess possible selective attention on his part.

The example above illustrates how a clinician attempts to gather information about family members' cognitions *as they occur* during family interactions, rather than relying on the clients' retrospective accounts (of what they might have been thinking about each other). The therapist can look for behavioral cues of individuals' emotional responses as the family members interact during sessions, and can interrupt them selectively in order to inquire about the emotions and any associated cognitions. Family members can also be given forms for recording distressing events between sessions, with instructions to write details about the situation, their cognitions, their emotions, and their behavioral responses (see Baucom & Epstein, 1990, for details).

Assessment of Couple and Family Behavioral Interactions

Given the consistent evidence that exchanges of negative behavior among family members are associated with relationship distress, traditional behavioral marital and family therapy methods of assessment and modification of behavioral interactions remain important components of a cognitive-behavioral approach.

Therefore, when a clinician is assessing a couple's or family's exchanges of positive and negative behavior, it is important to gather information about the situation specificity of any negative interactions. The basic question to be answered is the degree to which the negative interactions have generalized over time and settings. For example, when asked systematically for details, members of many couples and families report that there have been times in the past when they have behaved more positively, or they report instances in which they have behaved more positively with other people. The clinician can conduct a "functional analysis," collecting information about antecedent events/conditions and consequences that are associated with more positive and less negative behaviors. Evidence that negative behaviors are less likely to occur under particular circumstances suggests that family members possess constructive skills that are elicited by certain conditions but not by others. The fact that each member of a couple or family uses good communication skills when talking with the therapist often provides this sort of data. The therapist can point to such contrasting behavior when providing a rationale to the partners or family members for exploring changes in their relationships that could create conditions more likely to elicit the types of positive behaviors they direct toward therapists and other people.

Thus, the assessment of a couple's or family's behavioral interactions includes collecting information about the frequencies and reciprocal patterns of positive and negative behaviors that the individuals exchange;

about situational variations in those behaviors; and about any nonbehavioral factors (cognitions and emotions) that influence the behavioral variations. Behavioral assessment typically includes both self-report questionnaires administered to the family members and some form of behavioral observation conducted by the therapist.

Self-Report Questionnaires

Many self-report questionnaires have been developed by providing data on behavioral interactions between members of couples and between parents and children; they vary in the degree to which their items describe specific behaviors versus a respondent's global assessment of interaction quality. However, given various sources of potential bias in self-reports of one's own and others' behavior (e.g., inaccurate memories, social desirability), and a long history of only modest correlations between self-reports and behavioral observations, a clinician must use considerable caution in interpreting responses to these instruments. For these reasons, and because of space limitations in this chapter, we do not discuss such instruments in detail here. Nevertheless, cognitive-behavioral therapists consider it very important to assess how family members *perceive* one another's behavior, and self-report measures can be a useful source of information about cognitive appraisals. (For more detailed information on self-report questionnaires, see Fischer & Corcoran, 1987.)

Behavioral Observation

Because of the limitations of self-report assessments, it is important for the clinician to observe samples of a family's interactions directly. A common misconception about behavior therapy is that it is a "technology of techniques." Actually, one of behavior therapy's essential ingredients is careful and detailed observation of behavior and its consequences. Opportunities for behavioral observation exist from the first moment that a couple or family enters the therapist's office, and experienced couple/family therapists become adept at noticing the process of verbal and nonverbal behaviors that occur between partners or among family members as they talk to the therapist and to one another. Although the topics (content) of family discussions are important (and are foci of cognitive assessment and intervention), the goal of systematic behavioral observation is to identify specific acts by each individual, and the sequences of acts among family members, that are constructive and pleasing or destructive and aversive. The observation of family interactions can vary according to (1) the amount of structure the clinician imposes on the interaction and (2) the amount of structure in the clinician's observational criteria or coding system.

Even though a couple's or family's behavior in the therapist's office is likely to differ to some degree from typical interactions at home, many couples and families reveal significant patterns when given an opportunity to talk about issues in their relationships with minimal intervention by the therapist. We have found that as members of couples and families become more comfortable with the office setting and with our presence, they tend to focus their attention on and respond more spontaneously to one another. If the therapist "fades into the background" for a while, he or she can observe the behavioral interactions. The goal of imposing little structure on the interaction is to sample a couple's or family's communication in as naturalistic a way as possible in the office setting.

In contrast to relatively unstructured interactions, the clinician can provide a couple or family with specific topics for discussions and even with a goal, such as trying to understand one another's thoughts and feelings or to resolve a particular relationship problem. For example, each member of a couple can be asked to complete an inventory, such as Spanier's (1976) Dyadic Adjustment Scale, with which they rate the degree to which there is conflict in their relationship in each of several areas (e.g., demonstration of affection, household tasks, amount of time spent together). The clinician then selects a topic on which both partners have reported at least moderate disagreement, and asks the couple to spend 10 minutes trying to resolve the conflict. Similarly, parents and adolescents can be given the Issues Checklist (Robin & Foster, 1989); the clinician then picks a topic that they have identified as a source of conflict, and asks them either to discuss their feelings about the issue or to try to find a solution to the issue.

Often it is only when a couple or family has been instructed to engage in a problem-solving discussion that the clinician is able to identify a specific difficulty with this specialized form of communication. This is similar to the "enactment" that Minuchin and other family therapists use in family therapy (Minuchin, 1974). A difference, however, is that a cognitive-behavioral therapist may be more directive in this process than a structural family therapist. For example, some clients fail to define a problem in specific behavioral terms, which handicaps them when they attempt to generate a feasible solution. Others fail to evaluate advantages and disadvantages of a proposed solution, and subsequently become discouraged when they try to carry out the solution and encounter unanticipated obstacles or drawbacks. By observing the clients' discussion in the therapy session, the clinician can identify the specific problematic behaviors and can plan interventions to improve their problem-solving skills.

The clinician's own observational criteria for assessing a couple's or family's interactions can vary in detail and structure as well. On the one hand, the clinician can begin the observation with no predetermined categories of behavior to focus on, and can look for repetitive patterns that appear to play roles in the couple's or family's presenting complaints. Using the basic principle of functional analysis, the clinician observes antecedent events and consequences that may be controlling the occurrence of each member's negative behavior. For example, a husband may have complained that his wife rarely reveals or talks about her feelings, but the clinician may observe that whenever the wife does express her feelings, the husband turns away. Similarly, circular causal processes in couple or family interaction can be observed, as when a clinician identifies how one individual's tendency to pursue tends to prompt the other's withdrawal, and vice versa.

Alternatively, observation of a couple's or family's interactions can be guided in varying degrees by behavioral coding systems developed by clinical researchers. An advantage of standardized coding systems is that they help focus the clinician's attention on behaviors that have been demonstrated in empirical studies to be problematic, and that might otherwise be overlooked in an unstructured assessment. For a more detailed description of coding systems, see Baucom and Epstein (1990).

COGNITIVE-BEHAVIORAL TREATMENT OF COUPLE AND FAMILY PROBLEMS

As noted earlier, a cognitive-behavioral model of couple and family dysfunction takes into account complex interactions among family members' cognitions, emotional responses, and behaviors toward one another. Consequently, even when a therapist is focusing on an intervention that may be primarily behavioral or cognitive, he or she assumes that the intervention is likely to affect all three realms of family interaction. For the sake of clarity, we present major forms of cognitive and behavioral intervention separately in the sections below. It's important to note that cognitive-behavioral therapists commonly focus on clients' emotions, but that most intervention procedures involve modifying behaviors (e.g., skills for expressing and listening to each other's emotions) and cognitions (e.g., unrealistic standards that elicit frustration and anger toward other family members). Techniques for accessing family members' unrecognized or unstated emotions, such as those used in emotionally focused couple therapy (Johnson & Greenberg, 1995; see Chapter 19, this volume), are valuable adjuncts to the cognitive and behavioral approaches described below.

Behavioral Interventions

Because of space limitations, we provide only an overview of the major forms of behavioral intervention in cognitive-behavioral couple and family therapy. More detailed descriptions of therapeutic procedures can be found in the texts by Baucom and Epstein (1990), Dattilio and Padesky (1990), Bornstein and Bornstein (1986), Falloon et al. (1984), Jacobson and Margolin (1979), Robin and Foster (1989), Sanders and Dadds (1993), and

Stuart (1980). The degree to which any of these interventions is used with a particular couple or family varies considerably, depending on the clinician's assessment of the clients' needs. The major forms of behavioral intervention are communication training, problem-solving training, and behavior change agreements designed to increase exchanges of positive behaviors and decrease negative exchanges among family members. In addition, in families characterized by coercive exchanges between parents and children, training in parenting skills is likely to be appropriate.

Communication Training

The goals of communication training are to increase family members' skills in expressing their thoughts and emotions clearly, listening to others' messages effectively, and sending constructive rather than aversive messages. Central to achieving these goals is training the members in expressive and listening skills. Guerney's (1977) educational approach is widely used by couple and family therapists for teaching clients to take turns acting as expresser and as empathic listener, according to specific behavioral guidelines. For example, in the expresser role, one's job is to state views as subjective perceptions rather than as facts; to include any positive feelings about the listener when expressing criticisms; to use brief, specific descriptions of thoughts and feelings; and to convey empathy for the other person's feelings as well. In turn, the listener is to try to empathize with the expresser's thoughts and emotions (even though this need not indicate agreement with the expresser's ideas) and to convey that empathy to the expresser. The listener is to avoid distracting the expresser by asking questions or giving opinions that shift the topic; to avoid judging the expresser's ideas and emotions; and to convey understanding of the expresser's experience by reflecting back (summarizing and restating) the key thoughts and emotions expressed. Detailed guidelines for the expresser and empathic listener, as well as procedures for teaching these skills, can be found in Baucom and Epstein (1990) and Guerney (1977). The therapist typically presents instructions about the specific behaviors involved in each type of skill, both orally and in written handouts that the family members can take home. The therapist can also model expressive and listening skills or show the clients videotaped samples, such as the tape that accompanies Markman, Stanley, and Blumberg's (1994) book *Fighting for Your Marriage*. The clients then practice the communication skills repeatedly, with the therapist coaching them in following the guidelines. Typically, a therapist asks the clients to begin their practice of the skills with relatively benign topics, so that any strong emotions associated with highly conflictual topics do not produce "sentiment override" and interfere with the learning process. Once the family members are able to enact expressive and listening skills effectively, they proceed to more difficult topics.

In addition to reducing misunderstandings among family members, use of expressive and listening skills reduces the emotional intensity of conflictual discussions, and increases each person's perception that the others are willing to respect his or her ideas and emotions. Even when family members are expressing negative feelings about one another's actions, the polite and structured interactions created by the procedures often reduce destructive messages.

Problem-Solving Training

Problem-solving skills constitute a special class of communication that the members of a couple or family can use to identify a specific problem in their relationship that requires a solution, to generate a potential solution that is feasible and attractive to all parties, and to implement the chosen solution. Problem solving is cognitive and oriented toward resolving issues, in contrast to the skills described above, which focus on emotional and empathic listening.

As they do in teaching expressive and listening skills, cognitive-behavioral therapists use verbal and written instructions, modeling, and behavioral rehearsal with coaching to help family members develop effective problem-solving communication. The major steps involved in problem solving include (1) achieving a clear, specific definition of the problem, in terms of behaviors that are or are not occurring (and that family members agree is a problem in their relationships); (2) generating one or more specific behavioral solutions to the problem (using a creative "brainstorming" period if necessary), without evaluating one's own or other family members' ideas; (3) evaluating each alternative solution that has been proposed, identifying advantages and disadvantages to it, and selecting a solution that appears to be feasible and attractive to all of the involved parties; and (4) agreeing on a trial period for implementing the solution and evaluating its effectiveness. Details on conducting problem-solving training can be found in texts such as Baucom and Epstein (1990) and Robin and Foster (1989).

Behavior Change Agreements

Even though formal behavioral contracts have become less central to behavioral couple therapy than they were previously (e.g., Jacobson & Margolin, 1979), the general strategy of devising "homework" assignments that clients agree to carry out between sessions is key to the learning-based model underlying cognitive-behavioral therapy, and behavior change agreements are still used extensively with parent–child relationships. Therefore, it is common to end each therapy session with an agreement specifying what behaviors each family member will enact during the period between sessions. A written record of the agreement (with a copy for the therapist and a copy that the family takes home for daily reference) is very helpful when the therapist checks on the success of the homework at the next session.

If a therapist attempts to set up an agreement among family members that they will decrease particular negative behaviors, it is important to define the behaviors clearly, and to devise a more positive behavior that each individual can substitute for the negative one. The therapist can also ask each person to list some positive behaviors that he or she would enjoy receiving from the others. Behavioral couple therapists sometimes ask each partner to engage in "love days" (Weiss, Hops, & Patterson, 1973) or "caring days" (Stuart, 1980), in which he or she enacts some positive behaviors from the other person's "desired" list.

Webster-Stratton and Herbert (1994) provide detailed guidelines for setting up written contracts between parents and children. They note that some parents may at first find the idea of written, business-like contracts an odd way to resolve emotion-laden issues with their children; however, they emphasize that it is exactly the detached, objective aspect of behavioral contracts that can counteract long-standing patterns of anger, criticism, yelling, and hitting, which are common in coercive families. The therapist coaches the family members in a process of discussion and negotiation that may be quite new and reinforcing to them. With families where parents have given their children little opportunity to share some degree of power and decision making in daily life, a therapist may need to discuss with the parents how they can encourage self-esteem and mature behavior in the children by including them in the construction of contracts.

Another type of behavior change agreement is focused on increasing a couple's or family's positive shared activities. Distressed couples and families commonly complain of a lack of intimacy and of little positive time together. Whether the current lack of shared time and activities is a result of members' negative feelings toward one another or of competing demands on their time (jobs, school activities, friends), the therapist discusses with them the role that continued behavioral disengagement would have in maintaining their lack of intimacy. Often family members who have shared few activities for some time become concerned that if they finally do spend time together, they will discover that they have little in common. Consequently, the therapist can engage them in a problem-solving session in which a variety of activities that they might share are considered. A written list of joint activities (e.g., Baucom & Epstein, 1990) can help clients identify activities that appeal to all members. Homework involves an agreement to engage in one or more of the joint activities for a specified amount of time, on a particular day or days. For families with a history of conflict, a contingency plan for how to handle any tension or conflict during the shared times is an important component of the behavioral agreement.

Training in Parenting Skills

Parents who have relied on verbal and physical forms of coercion to attempt to control their children's behavior often lack knowledge of alternative methods for parenting. A therapist can educate and coach parents in alternative methods, such as using positive reinforcement to increase desired child behaviors, paying differential attention (reinforcing positive behavior and ignoring misbehavior), shaping a child's successive approximations to a desired behavior, setting clear guidelines and limits for children's behavior, modeling desired behavior for a child, allowing a child to learn from the "natural consequences" of his or her behavior (e.g., rough play with a toy results in breakage), and using time outs for misbehavior (Webster-Stratton & Herbert, 1994). Webster-Stratton and Herbert's (1994) text is an excellent manual for parent training, as well as a source of references to books and videotapes produced as learning guides for parents.

Cognitive Interventions

Cognitive restructuring techniques, which have been applied to the management of depression, anxiety, and other disorders, are equally applicable for changing dysfunctional interactional patterns in couples and families. Cognitive interventions are designed to increase family members' skills at monitoring and testing the validity and appropriateness of their own cognitions. The issue of appropriateness is often relevant when one individual holds a standard so stringent that the family members will probably not be able to relate in a manner that the individual will find satisfactory. At times an intervention with cognitions may be the primary focus of part or all of a therapy session, as when members of a couple are exploring differences in their relationship standards. At other times, the therapist may shift temporarily to cognitive exploration and intervention from a primary focus on behavior when it appears that the family members' interactions are being affected by their cognitive responses. For example, some family members have difficulty in the practice of expressive and listening skills because they become upset by one another's behavior in that situation. Thus, a wife may become angry and unable to provide empathic listening when she hears her husband describing critical feelings about an aspect of their relationship. At that point, the skills training may be futile unless the therapist points out the difficulty and explores the wife's cognitions (e.g., her expectancy that her husband won't be willing to hear her side of the issue).

In work with family members who have anger control problems, cognitive and behavioral interventions are commonly combined. For example, behavior change agreements can be used to structure a couple's interactions, including the use of "time-out" periods where either partner can request that the two of them spend some time apart in order to calm down and prevent destructive expressions of anger (e.g., verbal or physical abuse). Similarly, parents can be coached to take a "time out" to cool down when angry at their children, in order to avoid abusive behavior. Training in expressive, listening, and problem-solving skills can be used to give family members constructive alternatives for managing their conflicts. Cognitive interventions that can be integrated with these behavioral strategies include teaching family members how to use self-instruction to reduce anger and to focus on constructive behaviors (see Deffenbacher, 1996); coaching them in challenging their negative attributions about one another's motives; and helping them identify standards for their relationship that are less stringent (and thus less anger-eliciting), but still acceptable and satisfying to them. Such techniques are described in more detail in Chapters 2 and 3 of this volume.

Training Clients to Identify Automatic Thoughts

Increasing family members' abilities to monitor their own automatic thoughts is a prerequisite for modifying distorted or inappropriate cognitions. Again, "automatic thoughts" are defined as thoughts that occur spontaneously about certain life circumstances, including family interactions. They are often stereotyped and biased; they may be either negative or positive, but in most conflictual situations they are negative. An early goal of cognitive intervention is to help family members develop the skill of identifying automatic thoughts (including visual images) that spontaneously flash through their minds. These are the cognitions that can trigger charged emotional responses and negative behaviors toward other family members.

Because many of these automatic thoughts arise from underlying schemas (e.g., assumptions, standards) that have developed over time, their restructuring is likely to require repeated identification and challenging over time. In lay terms, such identification allows individuals to "think about what they are telling themselves" about the situation or circumstance, and to learn new or alternative ways of processing what they are thinking.

In order to improve the skill of identifying automatic thoughts, individuals are typically instructed to keep a pad or notebook handy and to jot down a brief description of the circumstances surrounding a conflictual period in their relationships. Included in this notation should be a description of the situation, the automatic thoughts that came to mind, and the resulting emotional responses. The Dysfunctional Thought Record, a version of the Daily Record of Dysfunctional Thoughts (Beck et al., 1979), may be used for this purpose (see Figure 1.3). Below are some examples of automatic thoughts, adapted from clients' notebooks:

Directions: When you notice your mood getting worse, ask yourself, "What's going through my mind right now?" and as soon as possible jot down the thought or mental image in the "automatic thoughts" column.

Date/ Time	Situation	Automatic Thoughts	Emotion(s)	Distortion	Alternative Thoughts	Outcome
	DESCRIBE: 1. Actual event leading to unpleasant emotion, or 2. Stream of thoughts, daydreams, or recollections leading to an unpleasant emotion, or 3. Distressing physical sensations.	1. Write automatic thought(s) that preceded emotion(s). 2. Rate belief in automatic thought(s) 0%–100%.	DESCRIBE: 1. Specify sad, anxious /angry, etc. 2. Rate degree of emotion 0% –100%.	1. All-or-nothing thinking 2. Overgeneralization 3. Mental filter 4. Disqualifying the positive 5. Jumping to conclusions 6. Magnification or minimization 7. Emotional reasoning 8. "Should" statements 9. Labeling and mislabeling 10. Personalization	1. Write rational response to automatic thought(s). 2. Rate belief in alternative response 0%–100%.	1. Re-rate belief in automatic thought(s) 0%–100%. 2. Specify and rate subsequent emotions 0% – 100%.

Questions to help formulate the Alternative Thoughts: (1) What is the evidence that the automatic thought is true? Not true? (2) Is there an alternative explanation? (3) What's the *worst* that could happen? Could I live through it? What's the *best* that could happen? What's the *most realistic* outcome? (4) What should I do about it? (5) What's the effect of my believing the automatic thought? What could be the effect of changing my thinking? (6) If _____ (person's name) was in this situation and had this thought, what would I tell him or her?

FIGURE 1.3. The Dysfunctional Thought Record. Adapted by Aaron T. Beck. Adapted by F. M. Dattilio from the Daily Record of Dysfunctional Thoughts, developed by Aaron T. Beck and the Center for Cognitive Therapy, University of Pennsylvania School of Medicine. Adapted by permission of the Center for Cognitive Therapy.

Relevant situation/event	Automatic thought	Emotional response
1. "John came home and started to recut the chicken parts that I had previously cut for dinner without saying a word to me."	"The way I cut them wasn't good enough for John. He's hypercritical!" "I can't do anything that satisfies him."	Anger Dejection
2. "Johnny failed to take the dog out for a walk again last night."	"He expects us to do his chore for him." "He's lazy and doesn't care."	Resentment Anger and rejection

Through this type of record keeping, the therapist is able to demonstrate to the members of a couple or family how automatic thoughts are linked to emotional responses, and how this contributes to each member's negative frame concerning the other(s). Once individuals have learned to identify automatic thoughts accurately, more emphasis is placed on linking thoughts to emotional and behavioral responses. This can help counteract a common tendency for family members to disown any responsibility for being able to influence how they feel. For example, one husband stated that he failed to see the point of trying to work out his marital problems because he felt so depressed about his relationship with his wife. Once his automatic thoughts associated with the depressed feelings were identified (e.g., an expectancy that any attempt he might make to express his sources of dissatisfaction would be ignored by his wife), the therapist was able to describe communication and problem-solving skills that the spouses could try using, on an experimental basis, to determine whether they could find common ground and resolve their conflicts. The therapist was also able to discuss with the husband how his negative expectancy tended to produce a self-fulfilling prophecy when he held in his feelings and then watched his wife do things her own way.

Strategies for Challenging Dysfunctional Cognitions

Because an individual's cognitions about an intimate relationship generally seem plausible to him or her, in a cognitive-behavioral approach it is assumed that the probability of altering such views depends on each client's playing a major role in gathering data that are more supportive of a modified perception, attribution, or expectancy. Such cognitions are often a projection of the client's own conflicts and need to be addressed directly in the therapy sessions. Consequently, the therapist's role is to use Socratic questioning and related procedures to guide the client toward broadening his or her cognitions and possibly dealing with some of his or her own issues. For example, when it appears that one member of a couple is attending selectively to particular aspects of the other's behavior (e.g., noticing instances when the partner forgets to complete tasks, but overlooking instances when the partner follows through on stated plans), the therapist may ask the first individual to focus on recalling any exceptions to his or her view of the other as "always forgetting." This contrast may actually fortify the point that the therapist is attempting to make. Another strategy is to ask the person who is attending selectively to keep a daily written log of instances when the other person fails to follow through with tasks and instances when the other completes tasks. The goal of these interventions is for the client to draw his or her own conclusion that the narrow view of the other partner is inaccurate. This also facilitates an inroad for the therapist to begin to investigate further some aspects of the client's own conflicts that may be projected onto the situation.

It is important to note here that biased perceptions such as the example above can be associated with other issues in the relationships among family members that require intervention as well, and that coaching a client in observing information that disconfirms a narrow view may not be sufficient to produce a cognitive shift. In the example above, if a "forgetful" spouse has broken his or her partner's trust in the past (perhaps through a sexual affair), the partner may attribute any of the unfaithful individual's current memory lapses to a lack of commitment to their relationship, and may also hold a generalized expectancy that the partner is likely to be unreliable in the future. The mistrustful partner may not express these cognitions directly during therapy sessions and may only exhibit reluctance to pay attention to instances in which the partner follows through on tasks. In such a case, the therapist needs to pursue sources of the client's "resistance" to shifting the narrow perception, through exploration of related cognitions and past events in the couple's relationship.

The amount of restructuring that is required with each couple or family varies, but it is recommended that the restructuring process occur with each person in the presence of the mate or other family members. When members witness the testing and restructuring of one another's cognitions, they are better able to provide support to one another later in the treatment process. Family members are also valuable sources of information that may disconfirm negative cognitions. For example, a parent may attribute a child's failure to complete a household chore to "laziness," but may shift his or her negative attribution when the child reports that he or she interrupted the chore to work on a new school assignment that was due the next day. Hence the therapist works directly in the family unit, having each member test the validity of his or her attributions, expectancies, and perceptions about others' actions. In this way, the therapist helps family members test the validity of their thought processes and weigh the evidence supporting them, in an attempt to yield more balanced interaction. Epstein et al. (1988) emphasize the notion of counteracting the feedback loops that serve to reinforce dysfunctional thinking by working conjointly with individual family members to track ongoing interactions and identify sources of feedback that strengthen a member's negative cognitions. This is done by coaching family members in providing information to one another that may confirm or contradict their cognitions. Individual members are also instructed in identifying and processing their *own* automatic thoughts in the same fashion that clients in individual cognitive therapy are, as illustrated in Figure 1.4.

Concerning potentially biased attributions and expectancies, Socratic questioning can again be used to coach the clients in considering other possible determinants of their family members' behaviors, or other possible outcomes than the ones they anticipate. Expectancies can also be challenged by encouraging a client to devise "behavioral experiments" in which he or she behaves in a particular way and observes whether the other family members respond in the predicted manner. Detailed examples of these

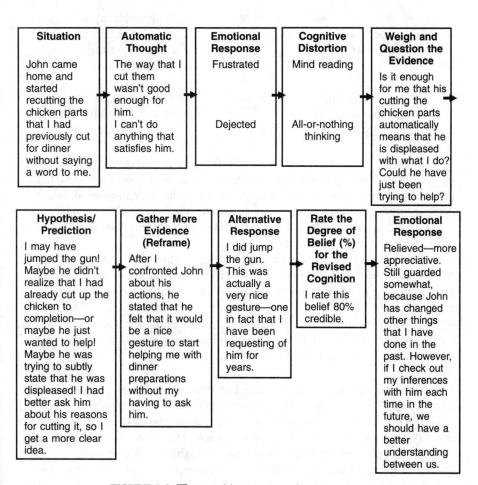

FIGURE 1.4. The cognitive restructuring sequence.

cognitive restructuring techniques can be found in Baucom and Epstein (1990), Dattilio and Padesky (1990), and Beck (1995), as well as in Chapters 2 and 3 of this text.

An Example of the Cognitive Restructuring Process

In an example of this approach to cognitive restructuring, a preadolescent girl developed the belief that her parents no longer trusted her, as a result of an incident in which she disobeyed them. The parents responded by saying, "We just can't trust you," and grounding her for a week. Her automatic thoughts and associated emotional responses to the situation, as well as the cognitive distortions involved in the thoughts, were as follows:

Automatic thought	Emotion	Cognitive distortion
1. "Now that I went out against their orders, they will never trust me."	Worried	An expectancy involving an arbitrary inference and all-or-nothing thinking
2. "They will treat me like a criminal. I'll never have any freedom."	Depressed	An expectancy involving an arbitrary inference and overgeneralization

In this example, the first automatic thought was accompanied by an emotion of worry because the young girl had an expectancy that her parents' behavior was permanent, with no room for redemption. She then drew another arbitrary inference from what she observed, and made a global negative prediction—"I'll never have any freedom," with the term "never" carrying the connotation "forever."

The therapist's next step was to ask the daughter to test her thoughts by weighing the existing evidence and considering alternative explanations. She could do this by asking herself the following questions:

1. What evidence exists to substantiate this thought?
2. Might there be an alternative explanation for my parents' behavior? What other possible outcomes could occur?

After weighing the evidence that existed and seeing that it was actually insufficient to support any strong conclusion about the ways her parents would think about her and treat her in the future, the daughter was more open to considering alternative expectancies. This reduced her negative view of her relationship with her parents until she had the opportunity to gather additional data. She collected additional data by observing her parents' behavior for a longer period of time and by asking them, in a nonthreatening manner, about their attitudes and intentions toward her. The therapist also encouraged the parents and daughter to discuss this issue in session, and coached them in the use of good communication skills.

When clients challenge their automatic thoughts with alternative explanations, the therapist should ask them to rate the credibility of the alternative cognitions. This is important, because these new cognitions may not become assimilated into the clients' thinking unless they are at least moderately believable. For example, after talking with her parents in a therapy session and hearing that they were upset with her but willing to give her opportunities to demonstrate more responsible behavior, the daughter in the example above came up with this alternative cognition: "Now that I went out against their orders, they have less trust in me, but they are open to having me show them that I can be trusted again. I will be able to have more freedom in the future if I follow their directions now." When the daughter rated her degree of belief in the alternative cognition 50% on a scale of 0–100%, the therapist asked her what limited her belief in it. She replied that in the past her parents had been slow to forgive her for breaking their rules. The therapist noted the importance of having credible alternative cognitions in order for the daughter to feel motivated to cooperate with her parents. He then initiated a discussion with the family about a behavioral contract that would specify the behavior the parents expected from their daughter, as well as the privileges the parents agreed to give her if she exhibited the desired behavior. After the family had successfully worked out a behavioral contract, the daughter re-rated her belief in her alternative cognition as 80%. Thus, the therapist's use of contracting with the family provided crucial information that modified the daughter's cognitions.

Therapists should keep in mind that in cognitive restructuring, it's essential to help individuals learn to rely on solid evidence to support the correction of distorted or inappropriate cognitions. The collection of substantial evidence allows individuals to weigh contrasting information against both their current thoughts and their long-standing schemas. Weighing the evidence is a skill that needs to be developed. Each family member must act in a manner similar to a prosecuting attorney or a forensic pathologist, who needs to weigh each piece of evidence carefully prior to rendering a decision or gathering more data. Taking the time initially to review each piece of information enables the individual to consider its validity carefully. Once this process has been practiced, it will occur more spontaneously. It is especially helpful in the beginning for clients to write this reasoning process down, so that they can objectively consider what is actually known about their views of family interactions.

In addition to logical analysis of existing information, clients can be coached in testing their cognitions (e.g., negative expectancies of how other family members will behave in the future) by creating "behavioral experiments." In the example above, the therapist initiated such a behavioral test by engaging the family members in negotiation and having them draw up a behavioral contract. This provided evidence for the daughter that her negative expectancy about her parents' potential for forgiveness was inaccurate.

Couples and family members thus learn to counteract distorted thinking by gathering information and focusing on alternative cognitions on a daily basis. Reframing involves a client's taking all of the data gathered, weighing the evidence, and developing alternative explanations and constructing a new view of a partner or family member. As illustrated in Figure 1.4, the modified cognitions replaces the negative frame once held by the client. The therapist can have couples or family members practice these alternative responses and explanations as homework assignments until they are fully assimilated into their thought processes.

Modification of long-standing assumptions and standards commonly requires the therapist to coach individuals repeatedly in examining the advantages and disadvantages of living according to distorted beliefs or perceptions.

CONCLUSION

A cognitive-behavioral approach to couple or family therapy integrates a consideration of intrapsychic processes (individual's cognitions—though these are often influenced by other family members' schemas—and emotional responses) with one of interpersonal processes (behavioral interaction patterns). It is an educational and skill-building approach that emphasizes collaboration between the therapist and family members in identifying and modifying factors that contribute to conflict and distress in daily family interactions. Although cognitive-behavioral couple and family therapists conduct careful assessments to identify any severe psychopathology in individual family members that may require individual treatment, they also recognize the strong influences of family interaction processes on the functioning of each family member. Just as early family-of-origin and current family experiences shape individuals' schemas about intimate relationships, family processes can be used in the therapeutic setting to modify dysfunctional cognitions and behavioral responses. The clinical case examples in this book illustrate the great potential of couple and family therapy for addressing a wide range of intrapersonal and relationship problems.

NOTE

1. Ellis's A-B-C Theory of Personality is central to REBT. A is the existence of a fact, an event, or the behavior or attitude of an individual. C is the emotional and behavioral consequence or reaction of the individual; the reactions can be either

appropriate or inappropriate. B is the belief about A which is said to largely cause C, the emotional reaction.

REFERENCES

Alexander, P. C. (1988). The therapeutic implications of family cognitions and constructs. *Journal of Cognitive Psychotherapy, 2,* 219–236.

Baucom, D. H. (1987). Attributions in distressed relations: How can we explain them? In S. Duck & D. Perlman (Eds.), *Heterosexual relations, marriage and divorce* (pp. 177–206). London: Sage.

Baucom, D. H., & Epstein, N. (1990). *Cognitive-behavioral marital therapy.* New York: Brunner/Mazel.

Baucom, D. H., Epstein, N., Daiuto, A. D., Carels, R. A., Rankin, L. A., & Burnett, C. K. (1996). Cognitions in marriage: The relationship between standards and attributions. *Journal of Family Psychology, 10,* 209–222.

Baucom, D. H., Epstein, N., Rankin, L. A., & Burnett, C. K. (1996). Assessing relationship standards: The Inventory of Specific Relationship Standards. *Journal of Family Psychology, 10,* 72–88.

Baucom, D. H., Epstein, N., Sayers, S., & Sher, T. G. (1989). The role of cognitions in marital relationships: Definitional, methodological, and conceptual issues. *Journal of Consulting and Clinical Psychology, 57,* 31–38.

Beck, A. T. (1988). *Love is never enough.* New York: Harper & Row.

Beck, A. T. (1991a). Cognitive therapy: A 30 year retrospective. *American Psychologist, 46,* 368–375.

Beck, A. T. (1991b). Cognitive therapy as the integrative therapy. *Journal of Psychotherapy Integration, 1,* 191–198.

Beck, A. T., Rush, A. J., Shaw, B. F., & Emery, G. (1979). *Cognitive therapy of depression.* New York: Guilford Press.

Beck, J. S. (1995). *Cognitive therapy: Basics and beyond.* New York: Guilford Press.

Bedrosian, R. C. (1983). Cognitive therapy in the family system. In A. Freeman (Ed.), *Cognitive therapy with couples and groups* (pp. 95–106). New York: Plenum Press.

Bedrosian, R. C., & Bozicas, G. D. (1994). *Treating family of origin problems: A cognitive approach.* New York: Guilford Press.

Berkowitz, B. P., & Graziano, A. M. (1972). Training parents as behaviour therapists: A review. *Behaviour Research and Therapy, 10,* 297–317.

Biglan, A., Lewin, L., & Hops, H. (1990). A contextual approach to the problem of aversive practices in families. In G. R. Patterson (Ed.), *Depression and aggression in family interaction* (pp. 103–129). Hillsdale, NJ: Erlbaum.

Bornstein, P. H., & Bornstein, M. T. (1986). *Marital therapy: A behavioral-communications approach.* New York: Pergamon Press.

Bradbury, T. N., & Fincham, F. D. (1990). Attributions in marriage: Review and critique. *Psychological Bulletin, 107,* 3–33.

Dattilio, F. M. (1989). A guide to cognitive marital therapy. In P. A. Keller & S. R. Heyman (Eds.), *Innovations in clinical practice: A source book* (Vol. 8, pp. 27–42). Sarasota, FL: Professional Resource Exchange.

Dattilio, F. M. (1990). Cognitive marital therapy: A case study. *Journal of Family Psychotherapy, 1,* 15–31.

Dattilio, F. M. (1993). Cognitive techniques with couples and families. *The Family Journal, 1*(1), 51–56.

Dattilio, F. M. (1994). Families in crisis. In F. M. Dattilio & A. Freeman (Eds.), *Cognitive-behavioral strategies in crisis intervention* (pp. 278–301). New York: Guilford Press.

Dattilio, F. M. (1996a). A cognitive-behavioral approach to family therapy with Ruth. In G. Corey (Ed.), *Case approaches to counseling and psychotherapy* (4th ed., pp. 282–298). Pacific Grove, CA: Brooks/Cole.

Dattilio, F. M. (1996b). *Cognitive therapy with couples: The initial phase of treatment* [Videotape]. Sarasota, FL: Professional Resource Exchange.

Dattilio, F. M. (1997). Family therapy. In R. L. Leahy (Ed.), *Practicing cognitive therapy: A guide to interventions* (pp. 409–450). Northvale, NJ: Jason Aronson.

Dattilio, F. M., & Padesky, C. A. (1990). *Cognitive therapy with couples*. Sarasota, FL: Professional Resource Exchange.

Deffenbacher, J. L. (1996). Cognitive-behavioral approaches to anger reduction. In K. S. Dobson & K. D. Craig (Eds.), *Advances in cognitive-behavioral therapy* (pp. 31–62). Thousand Oaks, CA: Sage.

Dicks, H. (1953). Experiences with marital tension seen in the psychological clinic in "Clinical studies in marriage and the family: A symposium on methods." *British Journal of Medical Psychology, 26,* 181–196.

Doherty, W. J. (1981a). Cognitive processes in intimate conflict: I. Extending attribution theory. *American Journal of Family Therapy, 9*(1), 3–13.

Doherty, W. J. (1981b). Cognitive processes in intimate conflict: II. Efficacy and learned helplessness. *American Journal of Family Therapy, 9*(2), 35–44.

Eidelson, R. J., & Epstein, N. (1982). Cognition and relationship maladjustment: Development of a measure of dysfunctional relationship beliefs. *Journal of Consulting and Clinical Psychology, 50,* 715–720.

Ellis, A. (1977). The nature of disturbed marital interactions. In A. Ellis & R. Grieger (Eds.), *Handbook of rational–emotive therapy* (pp. 170–176). New York: Springer.

Ellis, A. (1982). Rational–emotive family therapy. In A. M. Horne & M. M. Ohlsen (Eds.), *Family counseling and therapy* (pp. 302–328). Itasca, IL: Peacock.

Ellis, A. (1995). Rational–emotive behavior therapy. In R. J. Corsini & D. Wedding (Eds.), *Current psychotherapies* (5th ed., pp. 162–196). Itasca, IL: F. E. Peacock.

Ellis, A., & Harper, R. A. (1961). *A guide to rational living*. Englewood Cliffs, NJ: Prentice-Hall.

Ellis, A., Sichel, J. L., Yeager, R. J., DiMattia, D. J., & DiGiuseppe, R. (1989). *Rational–emotive couples therapy*. New York: Pergamon Press.

Epstein, N. (1982). Cognitive therapy with couples. *American Journal of Family Therapy, 10*(1), 5–16.

Epstein, N. (1986). Cognitive marital therapy: Multilevel assessment and intervention. *Journal of Rational–Emotive Therapy, 4,* 68–81.

Epstein, N. (1992). Marital therapy. In A. Freeman & F. M. Dattilio (Eds.), *Comprehensive casebook of cognitive therapy* (pp. 267–275). New York: Plenum Press.

Epstein, N., & Baucom, D. H. (1989). Cognitive-behavioral marital therapy. In A. Freeman, K. M. Simon, L. E. Beutler, & H. Arkowitz (Eds.), *Comprehensive handbook of cognitive therapy* (pp. 491–513). New York: Plenum Press.

Epstein, N., & Baucom, D. H. (1993). Cognitive factors in marital disturbance. In K. S. Dobson & P. C. Kendall (Eds.), *Psychopathology and cognition* (pp. 351–385). San Diego: Academic Press.

Epstein, N., & Eidelson, R. J. (1981). Unrealistic beliefs of clinical couples: Their relationship to expectations, goals and satisfaction. *American Journal of Family Therapy, 9*(4), 13–22.

Epstein, N., & Schlesinger, S. E. (1996). Treatment of family problems. In M. A. Reinecke, F. M. Dattilio, & A. Freeman (Eds.), *Cognitive therapy with children and adolescents: A casebook for clinical practice* (pp. 299–326). New York: Guilford Press.

Epstein, N., Schlesinger, S. E., & Dryden, W. (1988). Concepts and methods of cognitive-behavioral family treatment. In N. Epstein, S. E. Schlesinger, & W. Dryden (Eds.), *Cognitive-behavioral therapy with families* (pp. 5–48). New York: Brunner/Mazel.

Epstein, N. B., Baldwin, L. M., & Bishop, D. (1983). The McMaster Family Assessment Device. *Journal of Marital and Family Therapy, 9*(2), 171–180.

Falloon, I. R. H. (1991). Behavioral family therapy. In A. S. Gurman & D. P. Kniskern (Eds.), *Handbook of family therapy* (Vol. 2, pp. 65–95). New York: Brunner/Mazel.

Falloon, I. R. H., Boyd, J. L., & McGill, C. W. (1984). *Family care of schizophrenia.* New York: Guilford Press.

Fincham, F. D., Beach, S. R. H., & Nelson, G. (1987). Attribution processes in distressed and nondistressed couples: 3. Causal and responsibility attributions for spouse behavior. *Cognitive Therapy and Research, 11,* 71–86.

Fincham, F. D., & Bradbury, T. N. (1992). Assessing attributions in marriage: The Relationship Attribution Measure. *Journal of Personality and Social Psychology, 62,* 457–468.

Fincham, F. D., Bradbury, T. N., & Scott, C. K. (1990). Cognition in marriage. In F. D. Fincham & T. N. Bradbury (Eds.), *The psychology of marriage: Basic issues and applications* (pp. 118–149). New York: Guilford Press.

Fincham, F. D., & O'Leary, K. D. (1983). Casual inferences for spouse behavior in maritally distressed and nondistressed couples. *Journal of Social and Clinical Psychology, 1,* 42–57.

Fischer, J., & Corcoran, K. (1987). *Measures for clinical practice: A sourcebook. Vol. 1. Couples, families and children.* New York: Free Press.

Fiske, S. T., & Taylor, S. E. (1991). *Social cognition* (2nd ed.). New York: McGraw-Hill.

Gordon, S. B., & Davidson, N. (1981). Behavioral parenting training. In A. S. Gurman & D. P. Kniskern (Eds.), *Handbook of family therapy* (pp. 517–577). New York: Brunner/Mazel.

Grotevant, H. D., & Carlson, C. I. (1989). *Family assessment: A guide to methods and measures.* New York: Guilford Press.

Guerin, P. J., Fogarty, T. F., Fay, L. F., & Kautto, J. G. (1996). *Working with relationship triangles: The one-two-three of psychotherapy.* New York: Guilford Press.

Guerney, B. G., Jr. (1977). *Relationship enhancement.* San Francisco: Jossey-Bass.

Haley, J., & Hoffman, L. (Eds.). (1968). *Techniques of family therapy.* New York: Basic Books.

Hovestadt, A. J., Anderson, W. T., Piercy, F. A., Cochran, S. W., & Fine, M. (1985). Family-of-Origin Scale. *Journal of Marital and Family Therapy, 11*(3), 287–297.

Huber, C. H., & Baruth, L. G. (1989). *Rational–emotive family therapy: A systems perspective.* New York: Springer.

Jacob, T., & Tennenbaum, D. L. (1988). *Family assessment: Rationale, methods, and future directions.* New York: Plenum Press.

Jacobson, N. S. (1981). Behavioral marital therapy. In A. S. Gurman & D. P. Kniskern (Eds.), *Handbook of family therapy* (Vol. 1, pp. 556–591). New York: Brunner/Mazel.

Jacobson, N. S. (1984). The modification of cognitive processes in behavioral marital therapy: Integrating cognitive and behavioral intervention strategies. In K. Hahlweg & N. S. Jacobson (Eds.), *Marital interaction: Analysis and modification* (pp. 285–308). New York: Guilford Press.

Jacobson, N. S., & Margolin, G. (1979). *Marital therapy: Strategies based on social learning and behavior exchange principles.* New York: Brunner/Mazel.

Jacobson, N. S., McDonald, D. W., Follette, W. C., & Berley, R. A. (1985). Attributional processes in distressed and nondistressed married couples. *Cognitive Therapy and Research, 9,* 35–50.

Johnson, S. M., & Greenberg, L. S. (1995). The emotionally focused approach to problems in adult attachment. In N. S. Jacobson & A. S. Gurman (Eds.), *Clinical handbook of couple therapy* (pp. 121–141). New York: Guilford Press.

Liberman, R. P. (1970). Behavioral approaches to couple and family therapy. *American Journal of Orthopsychiatry, 40,* 106–118.

Margolin, G. (1983). Behavioral marital therapy: Is there a place for passion, play, and other non-negotiable dimensions? *The Behavior Therapist, 6,* 65–68.

Margolin, G., Christensen, A., & Weiss, R. L. (1975). Contracts, cognition and change: A behavioral approach to marriage therapy. *Counseling Psychologist, 5,* 15–25.

Margolin, G., & Weiss, R. L. (1978). Comparative evaluation of therapeutic components associated with behavioral marital treatments. *Journal of Consulting and Clinical Psychology, 46,* 1476–1486.

Markman, H. J., Stanley, S., & Blumberg, S. L. (1994). *Fighting for your marriage.* San Francisco: Jossey-Bass.

McCubbin, H. I., Larsen, A., & Olsen, D. H. (1985). F-COPES: Family Crisis Oriented Personal Evaluation Scales. In D. H. Olsen, H. I. McCubbin, H. Barnes, A. Larsen, M. Muxen, & M. Wilson (Eds.), *Family inventories* (rev. ed., pp. 215–218). St. Paul: Family Social Science, University of Minnesota.

McCubbin, H. I., Patterson, J. M., & Wilson, L. R. (1985). FILE: Family Inventory of Life Events and Changes. In D. H. Olson, H. I. McCubbin, H. Barnes, A. Larsen, M. Muxen, & M. Wilson (Eds.), *Family inventories* (rev. ed., pp. 272–275). St. Paul: Family Social Science, University of Minnesota.

Minuchin, S. (1974). *Families and family therapy.* Cambridge, MA: Harvard University Press.

Moos, R. H., & Moos, B. S. (1986). *Family Environment Scale manual* (2nd ed.). Palo Alto, CA: Consulting Psychologists Press.

Morton, T. L., Twentyman, C. T., & Azar, S. T. (1988). Cognitive-behavioral assessment and treatment of child abuse. In N. Epstein, S. E. Schlesinger, &

W. Dryden (Eds.), *Cognitive-behavioral therapy with families* (pp. 87–117). New York: Brunner/Mazel.

Olson, D. H., Portner, J., & Lavee, Y. (1985). *FACES-III manual*. St. Paul: Family Social Science, University of Minnesota.

Patterson, G. R. (1971). *Families: Applications of social learning to family life*. Champaign, IL: Research Press.

Patterson, G. R. (1982). *Coercive family processes*. Eugene, OR: Castalia.

Patterson, G. R., & Hops, H. (1972). Coercion, a game for two: Intervention techniques for marital conflict. In R. E. Urich & P. Mounjoy (Eds.), *The experimental analysis of social behavior* (pp. 424–440). New York: Appleton-Century-Crofts.

Patterson, G. R., McNeal, S., Hawkins, N., & Phelps, R. (1967). Reprogramming the social environment. *Journal of Child Psychology and Psychiatry, 8,* 181–195.

Pretzer, J. L., Epstein, N., & Fleming, B. (1991). The Marital Attitude Survey: A measure of dysfunctional attributions and expectancies. *Journal of Cognitive Psychotherapy, 5,* 131–148.

Procter, H. (1985). A construct approach to family therapy and systems intervention. In E. Button (Ed.), *Personal construct theory and mental health* (pp. 327–350). Cambridge, MA: Brookline Books.

Revenstorf, D., Hahlweg, K., Schindler, L., & Vogel, B. (1984). Interaction analysis of marital conflict. In K. Hahlweg & N. S. Jacobson (Eds.), *Marital interaction: Analysis and modification* (pp. 159–181). New York: Guilford Press.

Robin, A. L., & Foster, S. L. (1989). *Negotiating parent–adolescent conflict: A behavioral–family systems approach*. New York: Guilford Press.

Satir, V. (1964). *Conjoint family therapy*. Palo Alto, CA: Science & Behavioral Books.

Sanders, M. R., & Dadds, M. R. (1993). *Behavioral family intervention*. Needham Heights, MA: Allyn & Bacon.

Schindler, L., & Vollmer, M. (1984). Cognitive perspectives in behavioral marital therapy: Some proposals for bridging theory, research and practice. In K. Hahlweg & N. S. Jacobson (Eds.), *Marital interaction: Analysis and modification* (pp. 309–324). New York: Guilford Press.

Schwebel, A. I., & Fine, M. A. (1994). *Understanding and helping families: A cognitive-behavioral approach*. Hillsdale, NJ: Erlbaum.

Spanier, G. B. (1976). Measuring dyadic adjustment: New scales for assessing the quality of marriage and similar dyads. *Journal of Marriage and the Family, 38,* 15–28.

Stuart, R. B. (1969). Operant–interpersonal treatment for marital discord. *Journal of Consulting and Clinical Psychology, 33,* 675–682.

Stuart, R. B. (1980). *Helping couples change: A social learning approach to marital therapy*. New York: Guilford Press.

Teichman, Y. (1981). Family therapy with adolescents. *Journal of Adolescence, 4,* 87–92.

Teichman, Y. (1992). Family treatment with an acting-out adolescent. In A. Freeman & F. M. Dattilio (Eds.), *Comprehensive casebook of cognitive therapy* (pp. 331–346). New York: Plenum Press.

Touliatos, J., Perlmutter, B. F., & Straus, M. A. (Eds.). (1990). *Handbook of family measurement techniques*. Newbury Park, CA: Sage.

Vincent-Roehling, P. V., & Robin, A. L. (1986). Development and validation of the Family Beliefs Inventory: A measure of unrealistic beliefs among parents and adolescents. *Journal of Consulting and Clinical Psychology, 54,* 693–697.

Webster-Stratton, C., & Herbert, M. (1994). *Troubled families—problem children.* Chichester, England: Wiley.

Weiss, R. L. (1980). Strategic behavioral marital therapy: Toward a model for assessment and intervention. In J. P. Vincent (Ed.), *Advances in family intervention, assessment, and theory* (Vol. 1, pp. 229–271). Greenwich, CT: JAI Press.

Weiss, R. L. (1984). Cognitive and strategic interventions in behavioral marital therapy. In K. Hahlweg & N. S. Jacobson (Eds.), *Marital interaction: Analysis and modification* (pp. 309–324). New York: Guilford Press.

Weiss, R. L., & Heyman, R. E. (1990). Observation of marital interaction. In F. D. Fincham & T. N. Bradbury (Eds.), *The psychology of marriage* (pp. 87–117). New York: Guilford Press.

Weiss, R. L., Hops, H., & Patterson, G. R. (1973). A framework for conceptualizing marital conflict, a technology for altering it, some data for evaluating it. In L. A. Hamerlynck, L. C. Handy, & E. J. Mash, (Eds.), *Behavior change: Methodology, concepts, and practice* (pp. 309–342). Champaign, IL: Research Press.

Chapter 2

Cognitive-Behavioral Couple Therapy

NORMAN B. EPSTEIN
DONALD H. BAUCOM

As noted in Chapter 1, the rapid growth of cognitive-behavioral therapies, including their applications to couples and families, has been based on practical as well as empirical grounds. Research has documented how couples' behavioral interaction patterns, cognitions, and emotional responses have important impacts on the quality of their intimate relationships (Epstein & Baucom, 1993; Fincham, Bradbury, & Scott, 1990; Gottman, 1993a; Weiss & Heyman, 1990). In addition to its strong empirical base, cognitive-behavioral couple therapy (CBCT) has the appeal of a relatively short-term, structured approach that is consistent with managed care demands for specific treatment plans and assessment of defined therapeutic goal attainment.

In this chapter, we only briefly describe the central concepts and methods of CBCT (Baucom & Epstein, 1990; Baucom, Epstein, & Rankin, 1995; Dattilio & Padesky, 1990; Epstein & Baucom, 1989). The reader is referred to Chapter 1 for a more detailed discussion, with references to relevant empirical findings. The main focus of the present chapter is a detailed case example that illustrates the application of a cognitive-behavioral approach with a distressed couple.

PRINCIPLES AND METHODS OF
COGNITIVE-BEHAVIORAL COUPLE THERAPY

CBCT has its roots in behavioral approaches to relationship problems, cognitive psychology, and cognitive therapy. Early formulations of behavioral marital therapy (Liberman, 1970; Stuart, 1969; Weiss, Hops, & Patterson, 1973) focused on the association between marital satisfaction and the exchange of pleasing versus aversive behavior between partners. Research studies confirmed the premise of social exchange theory (Thibaut & Kelley, 1959) that distressed partners exchange more displeasing and less pleasing behavior than members of nondistressed relationships (see Baucom & Epstein, 1990). In Gottman's (1993b) longitudinal research, spouses' behavioral responses to each other during discussions of relationship problems were predictive of their relationship stability, such that more stable couples exhibited higher ratios of positive to negative behavior than did unstable couples (those in which the spouses seriously considered divorce or actually divorced). Furthermore, research has supported the observation of clinical writers (e.g., Stuart, 1980) that behavioral exchanges between partners tend to be reciprocal, in that a negative communication from one spouse increases the probability that the other spouse will respond negatively (see Baucom & Epstein, 1990). The reciprocity of positive behavior tends to be equal or greater in nondistressed than in distressed couples. However, Stuart (1980) noted that members of a relationship need not achieve total equality in the ratios of positives and negatives they exchange in order to be happy; the key is finding a balance of exchange over time that each person finds acceptable. Based on the social exchange model of relationships, assessment instruments such as the Spouse Observation Checklist and the Areas-of-Change Questionnaire (Weiss et al., 1973) were developed to identify frequencies with which partners exchange specific types of pleasing and displeasing behavior, and specific behaviors that spouses want each other to increase or decrease. Behavioral marital therapists also developed interventions for shifting distressed couples toward more satisfying ratios of pleasing to displeasing behavior. These interventions included behavioral contracts (commonly, written agreements for both partners to behave in ways that their mates identified as pleasing), and procedures for training couples in more constructive communication and problem-solving skills (Jacobson & Margolin, 1979; O'Leary & Turkewitz, 1978; Stuart, 1980; Weiss et al., 1973). More recently, research indicating that patterns of withdrawal and defensiveness are associated with marital distress and dissolution (Christensen, 1988; Gottman, 1993a, 1993b) has led behavioral couple therapists to pay more attention to these avoidant responses.

Reviews of empirical studies on the outcome of behavioral couple therapy (e.g., Baucom, Epstein, Rankin, & Burnett, 1996a; Jacobson et al., 1984) have indicated that it is more effective than no treatment or nonspecific treatments in reducing marital distress, and that its components (communication training, problem-solving training, behavioral contracts) tend to be equally effective. Nevertheless, because a sizable minority of treated couples did not score in the nondistressed range on outcome measures (Jacobson et al., 1984), it is clear that at least some factors contributing to relationship distress have not been addressed sufficiently by traditional behavioral marital therapy. Efforts to identify these factors and to incorporate them into the assessment and treatment of couples' problems have focused primarily on partners' cognitions, and more recently on emotions. Initial outcome studies have demonstrated the efficacy of CBCT in modifying couples' negative relationship cognitions (Baucom & Epstein, 1990; Baucom et al., 1996a). Our cognitive-behavioral approach is designed to address the interrelations among partners' behaviors, cognitions, and affects, as they influence the quality of couples' marriages and other intimate relationships. The following case study illustrates how a cognitive-behavioral therapist takes behavioral patterns, cognitions, and affect into account in the assessment and treatment of a distressed couple.

CASE EXAMPLE

Although no brief case description can capture all of the complexities of two individuals and the ways in which their interactions produce joys and frustrations in daily living, we have attempted to convey the essential elements of a cognitive-behavioral assessment and treatment of one such couple. Our case example illustrates how the therapist conceptualizes couple problems, what types of current and historical data he or she considers important in the assessment process, and representative interventions. Concerning assessment, some of the representative aspects of CBCT illustrated in the case include observation of the partners' communication patterns in the clinician's office; an interview about the history of their relationship (including the development of the current problems); systematic questioning to reveal each partner's relationship cognitions (selective attention, expectancies, attributions, assumptions, and standards), both in retrospect and as they occur during therapy sessions; and monitoring of the partners' mood states and their associations with negative cognitions and behaviors. Representative CBCT interventions illustrated include coaching the partners in more constructive expressive, listening, and problem-solving communications; challenging their biased cognitions about each other by exploring contradictory evidence (including "behavioral experiments" that provide new evidence to disconfirm such cognitions as negative expectancies); and fostering mutual empathy between the partners by focusing them on each other's positive intentions and vulnerable feelings.

Wayne (age 37) and Sharon (age 32) were referred for couple therapy by Wayne's individual therapist, who had worked with him on issues of depression for the past several months. Wayne's individual cognitive therapy, in combination with antidepressant medication, was proving successful in alleviating a major depressive episode, apparently triggered by chronic work stress. Wayne reported that his therapist had also diagnosed him as dysthymic. As Wayne began to respond positively to his individual treatment, it became clear to him and his therapist that an unresolved source of distress in his life was his 5-year marriage to Sharon. He described chronic bickering, significant arguments about finances, and a lack of sexual interest on Sharon's part. Wayne's therapist scheduled a joint session with the couple to discuss their relationship problems, but during that meeting it became clear that both spouses felt uncomfortable focusing on marital issues in the conjoint setting, given Wayne's long-standing therapeutic relationship with the therapist. When the therapist suggested a referral for CBCT, both Wayne and Sharon expressed their desire to follow through with the recommendation.

Assessment of Presenting Problems and Relationship History

During the first session, the couple therapist asked Wayne and Sharon to describe the concerns that brought them to therapy and to provide a brief history of their relationship, from the time they met up to the present. The therapist noted that the relationship history would help him to know them better and to place their current difficulties in perspective.

Wayne began by describing how they were referred by his individual therapist because of chronic arguments and Sharon's lack of sexual desire. Sharon concurred with Wayne's summary of their tendency to be irritable with each other, their apparently different "personalities," and their sexual problem. Sharon stressed that she was unhappy about their infrequent sex, but she said that her desire had decreased because of the chronic tension between her and Wayne. Sharon elaborated on sources of conflict in the relationship, including a history of Wayne's coming home tense and irritable from his job (as an administrator in a government agency), his tendency to leave most of the rearing of their 2-year-old daughter to her, and his jealousy whenever she was around other men. Wayne responded to this description by defending himself, stating that his job often was so stressful that he could not hide his bad moods when he arrived at home after work, and that he loved their daughter but often felt too tired to cope with her energy. He also said that he felt his attractive wife might be unaware that her friendliness could be misinterpreted by other men as interest in them. He described how he had been distressed when he learned, after they had begun dating and had initiated their sexual relationship, that Sharon had been sexually active since her teens and had had more sexual partners than he'd had. Now, when his wife dressed in what he considered sexy clothing, and especially when he noticed other men paying attention to her, he felt a combination of anxiety and anger. As is common in jealous responses,

Wayne's anxiety was associated with his perception that other men posed a threat to his relationship with his wife. He felt angry at Sharon for what he considered intentionally dressing in a provocative manner, and at the men who he believed were staring at Sharon even when they knew she was not single (i.e., he took it as a personal affront). Sharon insisted that she had no interest in other men and bitterly resented Wayne's judgmental comments.

Wayne and Sharon agreed that the most difficult times in their marriage had been associated with Wayne's job stress and depression; their conflicts about priorities for spending money; and their conflicts over child rearing. In addition, they argued about when Sharon might go back to work at least part-time. Wayne noted that Sharon had left her job as a department supervisor in another government agency toward the end of her pregnancy with Sarah, and that she had not returned to work since. He was not opposed to Sharon's staying at home with their child, but said that the trend toward government downsizing might threaten his job, and that the loss of Sharon's income had made their finances tighter and put pressure on him as the sole wage earner. He was upset that Sharon had no clear plan about returning to work. Sharon said that she still felt a need to be at home with Sarah, and that she did not know when she would feel ready to put her in child care. Sharon expressed annoyance about Wayne's "judgmental and critical" manner. According to her, he often made critical remarks about her staying at home, especially because he thought their house should look cleaner since she spent so much time there. She also said that she felt blamed by Wayne for her decrease in sexual interest, particularly when he suggested that she consult her gynecologist about "her problem." Wayne replied that he did not understand how Sharon could have such little interest in sex now, when over the years she had been active sexually. When the therapist asked whether Wayne assumed that Sharon now had virtually no interest in sex, Wayne replied that he sometimes wondered whether her wearing sexy clothes indicated that she might be interested in attracting other men, and that he was concerned that her low level of interest might be restricted to himself. Sharon expressed anger that Wayne mistrusted her, and she repeated that she had no interest in other men. She argued that in her view her clothing was not provocative, merely stylish, and that Wayne's insecurity was the real issue. She stressed that he seemed to expect sexual interest from her in the absence of his relating to her with respect and emotional intimacy.

One of the goals of CBCT is to shift the partners' tendencies to hold each other responsible for their relationship problems toward more circular causal attributions, in which the two individuals are aware of how each person is both reacting to and eliciting responses from the other. At this point, the therapist already had some hints that Sharon and Wayne had developed some circular patterns that contributed to their chronic conflict, but that each person tended to view the other as primarily responsible for their relationship problems. Upon observing how the partners talked to each other in the session, the therapist also formed an initial impression that their communication was characterized by mutual criticism and defensiveness, rather than by constructive expression and listening. At this point, the therapist wanted to get more information and develop a clearer conceptualization before providing any feedback to the couple about these observations.

The therapist then gathered more information about the couple's relationship history by asking the partners to describe how they met, what attracted them to each other, and what events during their years together they saw as influencing their relationship in a positive or negative way. Wayne described how he had been married once previously, and that his first wife had been unsympathetic about his depression and left him after 3 years of marriage. When he and Sharon met at a party, he had been divorced for 6 months and had not dated much. He was very attracted to her physically (particularly her pretty face and slim figure) and by her friendly, warm manner. He said that she seemed "sweet and sheltered, rather than worldly." The therapist asked Wayne whether the friendly manner that had attracted him to Sharon was similar to her friendliness toward other men that he found threatening now, and Wayne replied that it was. The therapist responded that this was a point they should return to later, because it appeared that a quality that Wayne had initially liked in Sharon had become a source of conflict.

Wayne continued his description of the couple's history, saying that he asked Sharon to go out to dinner, and that this led to their dating on a regular basis. The two of them spent a great deal of time together and enjoyed each other's company (Sharon agreed with this description). The therapist asked whether Sharon had been sympathetic when Wayne was depressed, and Wayne said that she had been supportive. However, Wayne noted that his new relationship with Sharon had lifted his spirits so much that she probably did not see him very depressed until after they were married. Wayne also said that the couple's sexual relationship seemed to be very good initially, with both of them satisfied and free of any sexual dysfunctions (e.g., low desire, arousal problems).

Sharon noted that she had met Wayne at a time when she was frustrated by a series of relationships with men who did not treat her well. In particular, she described them as domineering, verbally abusive, and much more interested in sex than in emotional intimacy. She added that she enjoyed sex with these men, but became increasingly frustrated at their unwillingness to share feelings and move toward a committed relationship. She had maintained a very active social life since high school and had enjoyed frequenting parties and bars. However, as she reached her late 20s, she decided that she wanted to meet someone on whom she could rely and with whom she could have a family. When she met Wayne at the party, she was attracted by his good looks, intelligence, sense of humor, and firm sense of direction in life. She was impressed with the way he had established himself in his career, and she appreciated how he treated her in a respectful manner. She could tell that he had somewhat more conservative attitudes than she did about politics, sex, and other things, but she did not expect these to affect their relationship in a significant way. When the therapist asked whether Wayne had seemed less focused on sex and more interested in emotional intimacy than other men she had dated, Sharon said that it had seemed so initially but was less true of him in recent times. The therapist suggested that they have a more in-depth discussion of the change that she perceived in Wayne later.

Sharon then described that because she knew that Wayne was "family-oriented" and eager to have children, she was surprised and upset that he was not available to share the child-rearing tasks after Sarah was born. Similarly, she felt a lack of support from Wayne concerning her strong desire to stay home with Sarah, at least until she had started school. Sharon described her own parents as both having been actively involved with her and her two siblings. When the therapist inquired about factors that might be associated with her decreased sexual desire, Sharon reported that she had consulted her gynecologist, and the evaluation suggested that it was primarily influenced by marital distress rather than by hormonal or other factors following Sarah's birth. Sharon reported only mild, situational depression that seemed to fluctuate with ups and downs in the couple's relationship.

Although the partners' open-ended descriptions of the relationship problems provided some information about their cognitions, the therapist asked a number of questions to elicit more details. For example, he probed for attributions by asking each of them, "When you think about the problems between the two of you, what do you tend to think the cause or causes of the problems are?" Expectancies concerning their ability to effect change in their problems were assessed by asking each partner questions such as "When you think about ways to try to improve your relationship, how do you anticipate your partner will respond to your efforts, and how well do you think your approach will work?" More information about the spouses' relationship standards was elicited through questions such as "If things could be just the way you'd really like them to be between the two of you, how would you relate to each other? For example, how would you demonstrate caring for each other? When you disagree about an important issue, how would the two of you handle it?" The therapist also gave the couple copies of the Inventory of Specific Relationship Standards (ISRS; Baucom, Epstein, Rankin, & Burnett, 1996b) to complete at home, noting that discussing their responses during subsequent therapy sessions would be valuable in identifying standards that were met in satisfying ways in their marriage and any that were not.†

†*This is an excellent way of eliciting cognitive schemas that each partner maintains about a relationship. This is a crux of the cognitive-behavioral model—to uncover each spouse's view of how the relationship should be and what standards the spouses hold for themselves and each other.*

The partners' responses to the interview questions revealed a variety of cognitions associated with their distress. For example, Wayne stated that when he thought about the contrast between Sharon's history of sexual activity, which he labeled as "fairly promiscuous," and her current lack of desire, he inferred that she was "turning herself off intentionally, out of spite." Sharon revealed a somewhat similar attribution about Wayne's depression, stating, "He just lets things bother him too much. When I see him come home and mope around the house and ignore Sarah, I just want to shake him and make him get his priorities straight."

It also became clear that the partners had different standards concerning certain aspects of their relationship. Wayne had more traditional beliefs than Sharon about gender roles in responsibility for household chores and child care. He also had more traditional standards about the relative amounts of prior sexual experience that men and women should have. On the other hand, apparently based on their experiences in their families of origin, Sharon wanted more nonsexual affection than Wayne did, and Wayne described how it had been highly unusual for his parents to hug or kiss him (he was an only child) as he was growing up. He added that he felt fairly comfortable being affectionate with Sarah, but felt awkward expressing physical affection with adults or older children.

Sharon revealed a personal standard that members of a couple should have few boundaries between them, which for her translated into an expectation that Wayne would spend most of his free time with her and Sarah. Consequently, she often became angry when Wayne arrived home from work and sat by himself watching news and sports on television. Wayne described his standard concerning boundaries, stating that he believed it is important for each person to have some time alone, either to unwind from life's stresses or just to have the freedom to explore his or her thoughts.

In CBCT, it is important to conduct some systematic assessment of cognitions in order to identify targets for treatment. However, assessment is ongoing throughout the course of therapy, and the clinician is continually attentive to each partner's expressions of selective attention, attributions, expectancies, assumptions, and standards. For example, during one of the early treatment sessions, Wayne reported his anger about an incident that had occurred the previous night. He said that after Sarah was asleep, he had begun hinting to Sharon that he was interested in sex; when he walked up behind her and began to caress her, however, she pulled away and told him that she was not in the mood. Wayne complained, "She wants me to be affectionate with her, but when I do anything physical, she keeps me at arm's length. That doesn't make me feel very affectionate." The therapist then initiated the following exchange:

THERAPIST: Wayne, do you remember what went through your mind when you caressed Sharon and she pulled away?

WAYNE: I was thinking, "Here we go again. She has no interest in me, as a person or sexually, and she doesn't care what it's like for me to have so little sex in our marriage."

THERAPIST: So, then, what's your impression of how Sharon *does* view you?

WAYNE: I think she mainly sees me as someone to bring home a paycheck and to do chores around the house, and sometimes as somebody to socialize with.

THERAPIST: Can you tell me what you meant when you said that she has no interest in you as a person?

WAYNE: I meant that she sees me as someone who fulfills certain roles, like the family breadwinner, but she's not interested in what I think or feel. She doesn't seem to want to be close to me.

THERAPIST: A bit earlier, you mentioned that Sharon wants you to be affectionate with her. Can you give me an example of how she conveys that to you?

WAYNE: Mostly she just tells me.

THERAPIST: What's your impression of what she would like from you?

WAYNE: I'm not sure. It's probably what we discussed earlier, about me not giving hugs and kisses.

THERAPIST: Sharon, is Wayne right about that?

SHARON: That's definitely part of it. The incident he described, when he came up behind me and started touching me, wasn't affection—it was foreplay. It really irritated me.

THERAPIST: What was it about Wayne's touching that led you to consider it foreplay rather than affection, and what irritated you about that? I'm asking because I want to be sure I understand the distinction you're making, and I get the sense that you and Wayne haven't clarified that difference between you.

SHARON: Well, what made it foreplay was that he started touching my breasts, and he was talking about really wanting to touch me. What was irritating was that he does that kind of thing from time to time, even though I've told him that when he comes on like that after not being close with me emotionally, it feels like he's just using me.†

†*This is a common dilemma in relationships. In fact, it appears to involve a basic difference in the manner in which men and women tend to perceive sex and intimacy. The two sexes often operate on the basis of different philosophies of what constitutes affection as opposed to foreplay. This is a very important issue to address in relationships, and the therapist here did this nicely in a clear manner during the therapeutic process. In the cognitive-behavioral model, it is important to explore each partner's assumptions about which behaviors reflect emotional intimacy and affection, and which reflect sexual arousal and intent. Because there are many verbal and non-verbal behaviors that can be either affectionate or sexual (or both simultaneously), there is great potential for misunderstandings between partners. Even if Wayne felt a combination of affection and lust for Sharon, if she attributed his behavior exclusively to lust, then she could feel that he did not care about her or understand her need for emotional intimacy. In turn, Wayne's inexperience with emotional intimacy in his family of origin and subsequent relationships probably led him to equate sexual behavior with affection more than Sharon did, and he interpreted her rejection of his sexual advances as a lack of love. It was important for the therapist to help the partners understand each other's assumptions and attributions, as well as the emotions that these elicited.*

THERAPIST: What other ways could Wayne behave toward you that would make you feel more like he was being close emotionally?

SHARON: He could spend more time just sitting and talking with me rather than going off and doing things by himself, and he could hug me or kiss me like he was glad to be with me.

WAYNE: You know that doesn't come naturally for me. Anyway, why can't you understand that when I want to touch you sexually, that is also because I love you, and it's my feelings for you that make me want to be sexual with you? I see other good-looking women, but I don't have the strong attraction to them that I have to you, because they aren't special to me.

THERAPIST: There are a number of important things that I've been hearing, and I'd like us to take a closer look at each of them. First, during incidents like the one you just described, each of you draws conclusions about what the other's actions mean about his or her feelings about you, and your conclusions tend to be pretty negative. One thing you *both* expressed is your impression that the other person doesn't value you as a person the way that you want him or her to. Did I get the right impression about that?

Both partners agreed that the therapist's description of their inferences was accurate. Please note that the therapist not only was checking the validity of his assessment, but also was modeling the use of language about the subjectivity of cognitions (e.g., the term "impression") and modeling the process of asking for feedback about the accuracy of one's perceptions. Often, a cognitive-behavioral therapist will not only model constructive behavior, but also draw the couple's attention to the example that he or she is providing and discuss the advantages of the modeled behavior. In this instance, the therapist did not want to shift the focus of his feedback, and therefore did not discuss the modeled behaviors. Instead, he continued his observations about what the partners seemed to desire from each other. He began by providing a "reframe" or reattribution intended to draw the couple's attention to the possibility that there might be alternative (and more positive) explanations for each other's behaviors than the negative attributions that they were making.

THERAPIST: I'm not sure that you two have been aware of it, but you may want something very similar from each other—signs that the other person really values you and likes to spend time with you. You've both described how bad it feels when you get the impression that the other person doesn't think of you in those positive ways. Unfortunately, you've described a pattern in which each of you tends to back off when your partner behaves in what you perceive to be an uncaring way, and then the other person sees that backing off, interprets it as uncaring, and backs off as well. For example, Sharon, when you experience Wayne's sexual overtures as uncaring, you feel bad about it and back off. Wayne, you tend to interpret Sharon's backing off as meaning that she has no personal interest in you, and you get upset and withdraw. Sharon, it appears that you then tend to view Wayne's distancing as further evidence that he's only interested in sex, which contributes to your distress and continues this negative cycle. How well do the two of you think this description fits what you have observed occurring between you?

Sharon and Wayne agreed that the therapist's observations were typical of their interactions. At this point, the therapist briefly discussed a number of related points with the partners, and collaborated with them in writing notes for their case file to remind all three of them to return to these topics in subsequent sessions. For example, the therapist drew Wayne's attention to the apparent inconsistency between his belief that Sharon had no interest in him as a person and his perception that she wanted more affection from him (as well as her statements in the session that she wanted him to talk with her more). The therapist also stressed the lack of clarity between the partners concerning their desires for affection and for sex, and what behavior each of them defined as affectionate or sexual. Concerning the latter issue, the therapist observed that Wayne felt threatened by Sharon's past sexual relationships, and that it seemed important to explore both his current sexual advances to her and his sensitivity to her rebuff of his advances in the context of his feelings about her past.

The exchange presented above is an example of how CBCT involves ongoing assessment, in which the therapist continually gathers information about the partners' behavioral patterns and cognitions about each other. Although the therapist is likely to identify some of the partners' major behavioral patterns, emotional responses, and cognitions about their relationship during the first session or two, it is our experience that more rich detail about their subjective experiences (especially more vulnerable feelings) is revealed over time, as the partners become more comfortable with the therapist.†

> †*This is an excellent point. Many cognitive-behavioral therapists attempt to gather information early during the assessment phase by using questionnaires or inventories designed to probe these aspects of the relationship (see Chapter 1 for a description of the instruments). In this case, however, the therapist, who was highly skilled, chose to weave the assessment effectively into the interview process. Typically, cognitive-behavioral therapists conduct both an initial assessment, which may include standardized questionnaires as well as a structured interview, and ongoing assessment during the entire course of treatment. Although straightforward questionnaires have an advantage of quickly surveying a wide range of topics that would require extensive interviewing, they may be intimidating to some clients, particularly at the beginning of treatment. For example, it seems likely that Wayne initially would have felt threatened by questionnaires (or even interview questions) that assessed vulnerable feelings (e.g., his insecurity about measuring up to Sharon's former lovers, his unease with physical affection). Consequently, therapists must use clinical judgment concerning the timing and modes of assessment. What is crucial is to form hypotheses from initial data, but to maintain an open mind and refine one's assessment on the basis of new information as therapy progresses.*

For example, during the session with Wayne and Sharon presented above, the therapist uncovered more information about the partners' attributions concerning each other's level of caring, as well as some of their selective perceptions (e.g., Wayne's view that Sharon had no interest in hearing about his thoughts and feelings). This example also illustrates the close link between assessment and intervention, wherein the therapist shares with the partners the information that he or she has gathered and helps them identify specific changes that each partner can work toward in order to develop more satisfying interactions. The sharing of information among the therapist and the members of the couple is also intended to facilitate a spirit of cooperation between the partners (in contrast to the adversarial stance with which many couples enter therapy), as well as an increase in each partner's empathy for the other's distress and disappointment. In the example above, the therapist attempted to increase mutual empathy when he drew Wayne's and Sharon's attention to the likelihood that they appeared to have a similar desire to feel more valued by each other.

Setting Treatment Goals and Structuring the Therapy

In CBCT, the therapist always has the option of meeting individually with each member of a couple, to gather information about individual history or personal concerns that each member might feel uneasy about discussing in a joint session. In our experience, this is most likely to be useful during the beginning stages of treatment, when many individuals experience considerable anxiety about allowing themselves to be vulnerable to potentially hurtful responses from their partners. In order to avoid having one or both partners divulge secrets to us in such sessions (which generally places a therapist in an awkward triangle with a couple), we discuss ground rules for any private sessions during the initial conjoint session. The position we take is that we do not want to be told secrets that cannot be shared; yet if there is an issue that one person would like to discuss in an individual session (early or later in therapy) in order to prepare to share it with his or her partner, we will be willing to do so. However, there is always a danger that one or both members of a couple will attempt to unbalance the therapy by repeatedly sharing private information with the therapist, and especially by resisting the therapist's goal of using separate sessions to prepare for sharing the information during conjoint sessions. We believe that it is important to catch such patterns as soon as possible, to reiterate the importance of keeping the therapist's relationships with the two partners balanced, and to actively discourage scheduling of individual sessions unless the clients demonstrate that they are using them to facilitate couple communication rather than to limit it.†

> † *This is a particularly cogent point, since the issue of secrets is so commonly encountered by therapists when dealing with couples. This rule should also apply to accepting individual telephone calls outside of therapy sessions, which can be equally destructive. In my opinion, addressing the aforementioned issues should also be made part of the ground rules. In fact, one technique that has proven to be effective is for a therapist to state that he or she will only accept telephone calls that are made in states of emergency and that are made by both partners simultaneously. This is usually quite effective in containing such random between-session calls.*

In the present case, the therapist hypothesized that each partner might have some individual sexual concerns, but he still decided to meet with the couple jointly unless it became evident that progress was impeded by such issues. Because there were no reported sexual dysfunctions, and Sharon's decreased sexual desire appeared to be linked to relationship problems, the therapist discussed his impression with the couple that working on the conflicts in their relationship could have positive effects on both the overall marriage and their sexual relationship. Sharon and Wayne both agreed with the therapist that the scope of their problems was broader than the sexual realm; together with the therapist, they generated a priority list of target issues for the therapy. The list included (1) learning better ways to discuss their disagreements, in order to replace their mutual criticism and with-drawal; (2) increasing their ability to find mutually acceptable solutions to problems in daily living, such as the division of household and child-rearing tasks, as well as the issue of financial strain and Sharon's employment plans; (3) decreasing the adversarial atmosphere that had developed in their relationship; and (4) restoring the sense of mutual caring, respect, and appreciation that they had experienced earlier in their relationship. The therapist stressed that a CBCT approach to achieving these goals would include attention to the specific behaviors occurring between the partners, as well as the manner in which each spouse interpreted those behaviors. He provided a brief description of the CBCT model (see Baucom & Epstein, 1990), and illustrated the concept of cognitive mediation by noting how the partners reported increased distress as they came to view each other's behavior as motivated by selfish concerns, in contrast to the mutual interest and support each person initially attributed to the other. The therapist also described the skills-oriented nature of CBCT. He explained how part of each session would involve practicing skills for communicating in a clear, constructive manner; for monitoring one's own emotional states and using them as cues to important issues that the couple needed to discuss; and for identifying and examining the validity or appropriateness of one's own cognitions about the relationship. Finally, he explained the importance of homework between sessions as the means for changing old relationship patterns and building more satisfying ways of relating to each other. He described how he would set aside some time at the end of each session for the three of them to collaborate on designing some homework that built on work done during the session, such as practicing communication skills.

Cognitive and Behavioral Interventions

In each therapy session, the therapist generally integrated interventions with cognitions and interventions with the couple's behavioral patterns, although in any one session there might be more of a focus on one or the other domain, depending on the needs of the couple. We have found that in the early sessions it is important to produce some positive behavior change, in order to counteract the partners' pessimism and passivity concerning change in long-standing negative patterns. Consequently, during the first session following the initial assessment, the therapist reviewed Wayne's and Sharon's own descriptions of their communication styles, and provided feedback about some patterns he had observed when they discussed their problems in front of him during the assessment. In particular, he noted that both members tended to engage in extended descriptions of problems, with each partner making many statements blaming the other. In addition, they frequently interrupted each other, and it was clear that their communication pattern made each partner increasingly angry as a discussion progressed, until one or both shifted to verbal and nonverbal withdrawal.†

> † *One technique that is particularly helpful with angry couples who tend to interrupt each other is the "pad and pencil" technique (Dattilio, 1996, in press). This technique involves providing each spouse with a pad and pencil and instructing the spouse to write down any automatic thoughts that occur while he or she is angry, instead of interrupting the other spouse while he or she is expressing thoughts and emotions, or giving a rendition of a story with which the other may disagree. In this manner, the potentially interrupting spouse is allowed to capture his or her thoughts or "hot cognitions" as well as the emotion, yet not to disrupt the flow of what the other is expressing. The therapist can later review the contents of each spouse's notes and intervene with cognitive restructuring, as the therapist, in this case, did so constructively.*

Sharon and Wayne indicated that this summary was a good description of their typical interactions. The therapist then introduced Guerney's (1977) communication guidelines, described the advantages of using them, and determined whether the couple felt motivated to practice the procedures in order to communicate more constructively. Wayne and Sharon were willing to apply the expressive and listening guidelines, first for discussing a relatively benign topic, and subsequently for sharing their feelings about the more conflictual issues in their relationship. The therapist emphasized that the goal of this form of communication was to understand each other, and that this did not require them to agree with each other.

At several points the therapist engaged in cognitive restructuring as the couple focused on practicing the communication skills in the office. For example, at one point Sharon was expressing the frustration that she typically felt when Wayne came home from work and paid little attention to her or Sarah. After Wayne listened to her and reflected her feelings to her satisfaction, they switched roles, and Wayne described how he felt very tense by the end of a work day and needed time to "decompress." As he was expressing himself, Sharon appeared angry and interrupted him, saying "All you can do is focus on yourself. Sarah and I are unimportant to you."

Generally, the therapist keeps a couple focused on following the communication guidelines, and he could have reminded Sharon not to interrupt but rather to wait until her turn to express those feelings to Wayne. On this occasion, he did remind Sharon about not interrupting, but then told the couple that one way to reduce one's urge to interrupt is to pay attention to one's thoughts that elicit anger and behaviors such as criticism. In this instance, the therapist intervened with Sharon's cognitions as follows:

THERAPIST: Sharon, could you describe the thoughts that ran through your mind as Wayne described his need to decompress after work?

SHARON: It was pretty much what I said to him. He just thinks about his needs and doesn't consider me or Sarah important.

THERAPIST: (*Addressing her attribution*) So when you see Wayne watching television or hear him talking about his stress, you tend to make an inference that his behavior reflects a valuing of himself rather than valuing you and Sarah?

SHARON: Yes. He's been that way for years.

THERAPIST: Well, the meaning that you attach to his behavior may be accurate, and I can see how you would be very upset if the person you hope values you a lot doesn't seem to do so. I also think it is important to check out whether the disturbing meaning that you attach to Wayne's behavior is the most accurate explanation, because there might be other explanations. If someone behaves a certain way because he or she doesn't care about you, it is hard to think of a way to change a lack of caring. However, perhaps the behavior is due to some other cause that is more changeable. I think it is important for the three of us to spend a few minutes exploring the cause or causes of Wayne's behavior, because your thoughts about his not caring often make it difficult for you to listen to him when using the communication skills. Wayne, I also have noticed some times you have difficulty listening to Sharon as well. This is something that we can explore in more detail. Sharon, what other possible reasons can you think of for Wayne's wanting to watch television and decompress, other than a lack of caring for you and Sarah?

SHARON: Well, he tells me that because he experiences a lot of stress at work, by the time he gets home he wants to shut it all out of his mind. He has said that he uses watching television as a way of getting his mind off what happened at work.

THERAPIST: What do you think about that? Does it seem like that could be what motivates his TV watching?

SHARON: Sure, but I also have plenty of stress to deal with, and I wouldn't choose watching television as the main thing to do if I had been away from my family all day. I'd want to spend time with them as a way to forget about work.

WAYNE: I *do* look forward to coming home and seeing you and Sarah. I'd rather spend time with the two of you any day, rather than put up with the junk I have to deal with at the office. How can you make it sound like I come home and it's no big deal to see you?

SHARON: If it's such a big deal to see Sarah and me, then why do you end up in front of the TV so fast?

THERAPIST: OK. This is starting to sound like the kind of argument about Wayne's television watching that the two of you said tends to occur at home. Does it seem like it to you?

SHARON: Yes, it's a lot like this.

WAYNE: Yes. And to tell you the truth, the more I get this kind of flak from her when I get home, the less I look forward to getting home.

THERAPIST: Well, Sharon, my impression of what you were saying was that you have a hard time fitting together Wayne's statement that he looks forward to seeing you and Sarah and his behavior of walking into the house and fairly quickly turning on the television. It seems that this combination doesn't make sense to you.

SHARON: That's right. What he says and what he does don't match.

THERAPIST: Wayne, it looks like Sharon has two conflicting perceptions, based on what you say and what she sees you doing when you get home. I got the impression that the two things fit together more easily for you than for her. Can you explain some more about what goes on for you when you get home, and explain to Sharon what your view is about how watching television and your statements about caring for her fit together?

WAYNE: OK. When I get home, I've already been trying to forget about work, and I usually try to do that by listening to the radio in the car as I'm driving home. That works a little, but dealing with the traffic doesn't allow me to relax much, and I still find myself thinking about problems that came up during the day. The way my mind works is that I need to completely zone out for a while in order to calm down.

THERAPIST: Can you describe what "zone out" means and how you try to do it?

WAYNE: It means focusing my mind on something that has no importance in my life. I watch what's on television, but actually only partly pay attention. I'm almost thinking about nothing. The last thing I want to think about is work. When Sharon comes in and gives me a hard time about watching TV, the first thing I think is "Oh, brother, first I have to put up with crap at work, and now I have to put up with it at home."

THERAPIST: What's you picture of what you'd really like an evening at home to be like?

WAYNE: I'd like to come home, get a warm greeting from my wife and daughter, zone out for a while so my thoughts of work are gone, and then spend time with them.

THERAPIST: Sharon, do you think it is plausible that the behavior you typically see reflects Wayne's attempt to create a boundary between his stressful work and his home life, protecting his home life from interference from work?

SHARON: Yes, I can see that as a possibility, but he sure isn't doing it well, because he gets so zoned out that he doesn't even respond to me when I ask him questions while he's watching television.

THERAPIST: So you are making a distinction between what might be a positive intention on Wayne's part, versus how he's going about trying to carry out that intention?

SHARON: Yes, but "talk is cheap," and it doesn't make me feel important when I see him staring at the television.

THERAPIST: Wayne, Sharon is considering the possibility that your intention to spend good evening time with her and Sarah is positive, but she finds that the specific way you have been trying to accomplish this leaves her feeling distance between the two of you. The difference between a person's intentions and how effectively he or she carries out those intentions can be significant. What do you think about the possibility that the way in which you are trying to act on your positive intentions to shut out work and have good family time is giving Sharon the wrong impression?

WAYNE: Yes, I can see how that could happen. I wish she could just see that I care.

THERAPIST: Well, perhaps if the two of you work on having discussions like this one, where you listen closely to the thoughts and feelings that each other is expressing, and avoid the exchanges of criticism that you have tended to engage in, it may become easier for both of you to have more understanding of the other person. We have done some work on communication skills here, and we can do more of that. However, what do you think about experimenting with some changes in how you try to separate work from your home life, to see if you can accomplish your goal but at the same time give Sharon more direct evidence that you are glad to see her and want to share life with her?

WAYNE: That seems OK. What I'm concerned about is if that means I have to walk in the door and get into big discussions. I really don't want to have to tell about my day, because that's what I've been trying to forget.

THERAPIST: Is that what you tend to experience when you walk in the door—that Sharon wants you to get involved in big discussions?

WAYNE: She seems very interested in talking, and she usually asks about my day.

SHARON: Well, I'm glad to see you home, and I'm checking to see how you are doing.

WAYNE: Yeah, but I don't want to think about how I'm doing. That just makes me think about the work day, and I want to leave it behind. You just don't seem to get it!

THERAPIST: *(Intervening quickly, because it appeared that Sharon was about to respond defensively)* Wayne, I can see that what you really want to do when you get home is forget about work, and that you don't want Sharon to ask you questions that start you thinking about it. However, I want to make sure that you heard the reason Sharon described what motivates her to ask those questions. A few minutes ago we were making an important distinction between *your* positive intentions about enjoying evening time at home with your family and your way of trying to accomplish that, which apparently hasn't been effective in conveying to Sharon how important she is to you. Well, now it seems important to check on whether there is a difference between *Sharon's* intentions and the way in which she tries to accomplish her goal. First, what did you hear her say her intention or goal is?

WAYNE: She said she's glad to see me and wants to check to see if I'm OK.

THERAPIST: Sharon, does that describe the intentions that you expressed a minute ago?

SHARON: Yes.

THERAPIST: Wayne, do Sharon's intentions toward you at such times seem to be positive or negative? Remember, separate her intentions from how her way of trying to carry them out affects you at the time.

WAYNE: She seems to have positive intentions toward me. She's concerned about how I'm doing after a day at work.

THERAPIST: OK. In what other ways might Sharon show those positive intentions when you walk in the door, which would help you accomplish *your* positive intention of distancing yourself from work and spending quality time with her and Sarah?

WAYNE: It would be good if she greeted me in a friendly way, but didn't ask me about my day.

THERAPIST: Sharon, does that seem like a reasonable approach, and one that you would be willing to try?

SHARON: Yes, I could do that. I'm just concerned that he'll give me a quick hello and go off to the television.

THERAPIST: Let's go back to the difference between Wayne's intentions and his way of carrying them out. A few minutes ago you said that you could see that he could have a positive goal of protecting his home life from the stresses of his work, but you also said that his way of shutting out thoughts of work tends to shut you out too. What could Wayne do when he walks in the door that could accomplish his goal of shutting out work, but still would make you feel like he is connecting with you and Sarah?

SHARON: I guess he could give each of us a good greeting and ask about *our* days. If he really needs to zone out in front of the TV, I think I could tolerate that better if he *said* that was what he needed to do and told me how long he plans to do it. I'll just leave him alone. However, I can't make Sarah leave him alone. She wants to see her daddy and just doesn't understand.

THERAPIST: Wayne, first, how does Sharon's idea about how you and she could behave when you get home sound to you?

WAYNE: It sounds a lot better than what goes on now.

THERAPIST: But what about Sarah? Sharon seems to be saying that Sarah isn't able to make the type of distinction between your intentions and your behavior that you and Sharon are making, and that Sarah is unlikely to understand your need to be alone with the TV for a while. What might you be able to do to meet Sarah's needs as well as your own?

WAYNE: I was thinking that Sharon could keep her out of the room while I'm watching TV, but I really don't want Sarah to feel like I don't want her around. Actually, I think that if I listen to her tell me about her day and show me the toys she's playing with, after a while she'll probably get bored sitting in front of the TV with me, and she'll go back to playing by herself. I think I can show her I'm interested in her, but also get some time by myself.

THERAPIST: Sharon, what do you think about Wayne's idea?

SHARON: I don't want to be responsible for keeping Sarah away from him, and I think it's important for him to spend some time with her. I think he's right that if she gets a chance to talk with him and he shows some real interest, she'll go off on her own after a while and he'll have his time alone.

THERAPIST: I think the two of you have come up with some good ideas that allow each person to carry out his or her positive intentions and also meet the needs of the other person. You are taking into account the fact that one's positive intentions aren't always carried out in the most effective manner, and that communicating with each other can help clarify intentions and produce ways of carrying them out that are satisfying to both of you.

The therapist used this approach to reduce each partner's defensiveness, to challenge negative attributions about each partner's intentions and feelings toward the other, and to initiate problem-solving communication so the couple could develop a new, mutually acceptable way for each person to carry out positive intentions. The therapist frequently shifted his attention back and forth between the partners, keeping each individual's attention on his or her own cognitions, as well as on behavioral changes that he or she could make in order to change the couple's typical pattern of reciprocal negative exchanges. This is also an example of how the therapist combined cognitive restructuring with problem solving in a relatively unstructured manner, rather than focusing on them separately in treatment modules. It is important that the therapist teach the couple the specific steps in the use of skills such as problem solving, but we have found that integrating cognitive, behavioral, and affective interventions within CBCT sessions often allows the clinician to address the interplay among those factors in couple interactions.†

> † *This is an excellent example of the essence of the cognitive-behavioral approach, as well as how it is integrated with other modalities, such as problem solving and communication training.*

It is also important to note that the excerpt above cannot capture all of the complexities that a therapist must consider in working with this or any other couple, including the possibility that an individual's attributions about a partner's negative intentions may be accurate. We want to emphasize the value of taking an empirical approach to each couple, exploring the extent to which each partner's behavioral patterns, cognitions, and emotions contribute to distressing interactions. Cognitive restructuring involves a variety of strategies that help each partner take as objective a view of his or her own cognitions as possible. At times, the therapist coaches partners to broaden their views by considering alternative explanations for events, examining whatever data are available for judging the relative plausibility of the alternatives. The therapist also encourages partners to devise and carry out "behavioral experiments" in which they set up the conditions to test their expectancies about each other's responses. For example, the therapist noted that Sharon was skeptical that Wayne could or would demonstrate his avowed positive intentions by behaving differently when he arrived home from work, whereas Wayne felt certain that he would do it. The therapist "challenged" the spouses to test out their expectancies, noting that regardless of the results of the experiment, it would provide important information for the two of them in learning to solve their problems. In fact, the experiment was successful for Wayne and Sharon, giving them some new hope about their ability to relate to each other in more satisfying ways.

The therapist used cognitive restructuring to deal with a number of other factors involved in the partners' chronic anger toward each other. For example, Wayne's standards about sexuality, which led him to be upset with Sharon's level of sexual activity before they met, were addressed in terms of his own conservative family upbringing. The therapist's Socratic questioning also uncovered Wayne's related standard that "I must be more experienced sexually than my partner or I'm not a real man," as well as his assumption that Sharon and other women don't respect less experienced sexual partners. It also became clear that Wayne's earlier experience of having his first wife leave him because of his depression contributed to his expectancies about being judged by Sharon. He revealed his tendency to assume that Sharon compared his lovemaking to that of former partners while they were having sex. Sharon had an opportunity in the therapy session to tell him that she found sex with him very pleasurable when they were on good terms with each other, and that she thought about him rather than others when they were together.

Similarly, the therapist helped the partners explore their different standards for gender roles, particularly regarding the division of household and child-rearing tasks. Viewed in the context of each person's family-of-origin experiences, their differences were understandable to both partners. The therapist then guided Sharon and Wayne in using problem solving skills to devise and implement solutions concerning the division of tasks that both partners found acceptable. In conjunction with the problem solving, the therapist coached each partner in considering the advantages and disadvantages of his or her personal standards for gender role behaviors. For example, Wayne concluded that his belief that women should be more responsible for household tasks had the advantage of reducing one form of work stress in his life, but had the disadvantages of giving more work to Sharon and of contributing to her impression that home life was a low priority of his. As described earlier, Wayne was motivated to become more involved with chores and child rearing as he and Sharon developed more positive attributions about each other's motives and initiated mutually supportive behaviors. Thus, although therapists from various theoretical orientations would help such a couple negotiate a more equitable division of labor, the cognitive-behavioral therapist facilitates the collaborative process by directly addressing cognitions that have maintained the status quo and the couple's adversarial approach to their differences. Thus, Wayne was able to see that his gender role standard concerning division of household tasks probably developed from observing his own parents' relationship, but that Sharon was not unreasonable in wanting more involvement on his part. In turn, when Sharon heard Wayne describe how he valued their family life but needed a way of decompressing from his work stress, she was able to challenge her assumption (which had been reinforced by her previous relationships) that men had little interest in investing time and energy in developing intimacy.

The couple's conflicts about Sharon's employment status were also addressed with a combination of cognitive restructuring (focused on the partners' negative attributions about each other's behavior) and problem solving (focused on resolving differences in their standards about how long Sharon would continue to stay at home with Sarah). Throughout this process, the therapist coached the spouses in applying cognitive restructuring and problem-solving skills increasingly on their own. Thus, the therapist's level of activity in sessions decreased gradually as the partners became proficient in using cognitive-behavioral strategies for identifying and challenging their cognitions, as well as for communicating effectively and negotiating solutions to problems.

Overall, the therapist worked on shifting Wayne's and Sharon's conceptualization to one of reciprocity and circular causality for their sexual and other problems, helping them see how each individual's negative cognitions and behavior contributed to a cycle of distressing negative exchanges. As the partners increasingly took personal responsibility for behaving toward each other in constructive ways and challenging their own negative attributions, expectancies, and other cognitions about each other, they reported (and the therapist observed during sessions) considerable improvement in their relationship.

CONCLUSIONS

A cognitive-behavioral couples therapist actively engages a couple in a collaborative effort with him or her to identify and modify specific cognitions, behaviors, and emotions that contribute to conflict and distress. Conjoint sessions afford opportunities for the therapist to observe and probe for these factors as the partners interact with each other. The educational, skills-oriented aspects of CBCT are well suited for producing constructive changes that help build couples' optimism about their relationships, and for working effectively in a relatively brief time frame. CBCT has a major focus on a couple's current relationship functioning, but it takes into account the couple's history together, as well as each person's individual history in significant relationships. CBCT pays significant attention to a couple's current, repetitive interaction patterns; the influences of the partners' personal histories (as these have shaped their standards, assumptions, and other cognitions, as well as their communication skills); and specific relationship themes, such as boundaries, control, and investment. Consequently, there is great potential for integrating CBCT with other theoretical orientations to couple therapy that share some or all of those characteristics.

REFERENCES

Baucom, D. H., & Epstein, N. (1990). *Cognitive-behavioral marital therapy.* New York: Brunner/Mazel.

Baucom, D. H., Epstein, N., & Rankin, L. A. (1995). Cognitive aspects of cognitive-behavioral marital therapy. In N. S. Jacobson & A. S. Gurman (Eds.), *Clinical handbook of couple therapy* (pp. 65–90). New York: Guilford Press.

Baucom, D. H., Epstein, N., Rankin, L. A., & Burnett, C. K. (1996a). Understanding and treating marital distress from a cognitive-behavioral orientation. In K. S. Dobson & K. D. Craig (Eds.), *Advances in cognitive-behavioral therapy* (pp. 210–236). Thousand Oaks, CA: Sage.

Baucom, D. H., Epstein, N., Rankin, L. A., & Burnett, C. K. (1996b). Assessing relationship standards: The Inventory of Specific Relationship Standards. *Journal of Family Psychology, 10,* 72–88.

Christensen, A. (1988). Dysfunctional interaction patterns in couples. In P. Noller & M. A. Fitzpatrick (Eds.), *Perspectives on marital interaction* (pp. 31–52). Clevedon, England: Multilingual Matters.

Dattilio, F. M. (1996). *Cognitive therapy with couples: The initial phase of treatment* [Videotape]. Sarasota, FL: Professional Resource Exchange.

Dattilio, F. M. (in press). Pad and pencil techniques. In R. E. Watts (Ed.), *Favorite counseling techniques with couples and families.* Leesburg, VA: American Counseling Association.

Dattilio, F. M., & Padesky, C. A. (1990). *Cognitive therapy with couples.* Sarasota, FL: Professional Resource Exchange.

Epstein, N., & Baucom D. H. (1989). Cognitive-behavioral marital therapy. In A. Freeman, K. M. Simon, L. E. Beutler, & H. Arkowitz (Eds.), *Comprehensive handbook of cognitive therapy* (pp. 491–513). New York: Plenum Press.

Epstein, N., & Baucom, D. H. (1993). Cognitive factors in marital disturbance. In K. S. Dobson & P. C. Kendall (Eds.), *Psychopathology and cognition* (pp. 351–385). San Diego: Academic Press.

Fincham, F. D., Bradbury, T. N., & Scott, C. K. (1990). Cognition in marriage. In F. D. Fincham & T. N. Bradbury (Eds.), *The psychology of marriage* (pp. 118–149). New York: Guilford Press.

Gottman, J. M. (1993a). *What predicts divorce?: The relationship between marital processes and marital outcomes.* Hillsdale, NJ: Erlbaum.

Gottman, J. M. (1993b). The roles of conflict engagement, escalation, and avoidance in marital interaction: A longitudinal view of five types of couples. *Journal of Consulting and Clinical Psychology, 61,* 6–15.

Guerney, B. G., Jr. (1977). *Relationship enhancement.* San Francisco: Jossey-Bass.

Jacobson, N. S., Follette, W. C., Revenstorf, D., Baucom, D. H., Hahlweg, K., & Margolin, G. (1984). Variability in outcome and clinical significance of behavioral marital therapy: A reanalysis of outcome data. *Journal of Consulting and Clinical Psychology, 52,* 497–504.

Jacobson, N. S., & Margolin, G. (1979). *Marital therapy: Strategies based on social learning and behavior exchange principles.* New York: Brunner/Mazel.

Liberman, R. (1970). Behavioral approaches to family and couple therapy. *American Journal of Orthopsychiatry, 40,* 106–118.

O'Leary, K. D., & Turkewitz, H. (1978). Marital therapy from a behavioral perspective. In T. J. Paolino & B. S. McCrady (Eds.), *Marriage and marital therapy: Psychoanalytic, behavioral and systems theory perspectives* (pp. 240–297). New York: Brunner/Mazel.

Stuart, R. B. (1969). Operant interpersonal treatment for marital discord. *Journal of Consulting and Clinical Psychology, 33,* 675–682.

Stuart, R. B. (1980). *Helping couples change: A social learning approach to marital therapy.* New York: Guilford Press.

Thibaut, J. W., & Kelley, H. H. (1959). *The social psychology of groups.* New York: Wiley.

Weiss, R. L., & Heyman, R. E. (1990). Observation of marital interaction. In F. D. Fincham & T. N. Bradbury (Eds.), *The psychology of marriage* (pp. 87–117). New York: Guilford Press.

Weiss, R. L., Hops, H., & Patterson, G. R. (1973). A framework for conceptualizing marital conflict, a technology for altering it, some data for evaluating it. In L. A. Hamerlynck, L. C. Handy, & E. J. Mash (Eds.), *Behavior change: Methodology, concepts and practice* (pp. 309–342). Champaign, IL: Research Press.

SUGGESTED READINGS

Baucom, D. H., & Epstein, N. (1990). *Cognitive-behavioral marital therapy.* New York: Brunner/Mazel.

Baucom, D. H., Epstein, N., & Rankin, L. A. (1995). Cognitive aspects of cognitive-behavioral marital therapy. In N. S. Jacobson & A. S. Gurman (Eds.), *Clinical handbook of couple therapy* (pp. 65–90). New York: Guilford Press.

Dattilio, F. M., & Padesky, C. A. (1990). *Cognitive therapy with couples.* Sarasota, FL: Professional Resource Exchange.

Epstein, N., & Schlesinger, S. E. (1994). Couples problems. In F. M. Dattilio & A. Freeman (Eds.), *Cognitive-behavioral strategies in crisis intervention* (pp. 258–277). New York: Guilford Press.

Notarius, C., & Markman, H. (1993). *We can work it out: Making sense of marital conflict.* New York: Putnam.

Chapter 3

Cognitive-Behavioral Family Therapy

FRANK M. DATTILIO

Sometimes families find their way into therapy via circuitous routes. In most cases, all members of an immediate family will come together for the initial visit; however, on occasion, one or both parents may come first to discuss the need for such therapy and to interview the therapist prior to agreeing to muster the entire family in for a group session. It may also be that certain family members are resistant to or have misgivings about submitting to therapy. This was the case with Ruth's family. Ruth was a middle-aged woman who had undergone individual psychotherapy in order to address her panic attacks and the behavioral problems that she was experiencing with her children. Her individual therapist had referred her to me for family therapy, hoping to reduce some of the stress that Ruth was experiencing at home.

Ruth consulted me about her desire to address problems that she and her husband had been experiencing with their four children. She explained to me that her husband, John, had planned to attend this consultation, but he was called to work at the last minute. Ruth decided to keep the appointment by coming alone.

During the initial interview, Ruth explained that several of her children (particularly one of her daughters) were rebellious, and that the children blamed the problems in the family on Ruth herself. Ruth explained that she had been in individual therapy for the past year and was struggling with feelings of depression and experienced episodes of panic. As I gathered background information on this case, it struck me that perhaps Ruth's need to seek therapy for her panic attacks made her feel that she was the one to blame for the problems at home. If this were the case, she certainly wouldn't have been the first mother to assume that her children's problems were her fault. During this initial session, I explained to Ruth the philosophy behind family therapy, and emphasized how important it was for all members of the immediate family to attend each session from the outset. Ruth agreed, and said that she and her husband had planned to "round up the troops" and bring everyone in after the initial interview. Subsequently, we scheduled an appointment 1 week later for the entire family, much to the teenagers' chagrin.

Because cognitive-behavioral family therapists attempt to identify both distorted schemas and maladaptive behavior patterns in family interaction, the first order of business in any case is to meet with the entire immediate family. As a result of the little information I had gathered from Ruth about her and her husband's families of origin, I had some foundation for understanding the diverse philosophies that existed in each of their backgrounds, and some insight into the schemas that had filtered down into their current family dynamics and family schema. These conjectures would of course have to be tested as I continued to develop a conceptualization during the first few family sessions.

During the initial family visit, the cognitive-behavioral therapist asks all of the members of the family to describe their perceptions of the family and how things operate at home. As can be seen in the following excerpts from the first few sessions with Ruth's family, I try to get a clear understanding of the family members' individual perceptions, and then attempt to conceptualize a joint view of the "family schema." The next step is to explain how cognitive-behavioral therapy works, and then to begin to collaboratively identify cognitive distortions and erroneous thinking patterns that lead to dysfunction in the family members' interaction.

INITIAL FAMILY SESSION

DATTILIO: Well, first of all, I want to thank everyone for coming today, since I know that you all have your own schedules and this may not be everyone's top priority. I'm Dr. Dattilio, and I am a family therapist. Maybe we could just go around and get everybody's name and age?

ROB: My name's Rob, and I'm 17.

ADAM: I'm Adam. I'll be 15 next month.

SUSAN: Hi. I'm Susan, and I'm 13.

JENNIFER: *(Said nothing.)*

I decided to ignore Jennifer's hostile silence and address her reluctance to participate later.

DATTILIO: OK, good. Ruth and John, have you explained why you decided to bring everyone to these meetings?

RUTH: Well, no, not really. We simply told them that we thought we needed to address some of the tension in our household.

DATTILIO: OK. Well, in essence that's what these sessions are designed to do, but we can also explore some other issues as well, particularly discontents that family members have with one another. Does that sound fair to everyone? *(Rob, Adam, and Susan nodded reluctantly.)*

JENNIFER: *(Interrupting)*It doesn't to me! I think this is bogus, and I really don't want to be here.

DATTILIO: So why did you agree to come?

JENNIFER: I didn't. I was forced.

RUTH: Oh, Jennifer, come on now!

JOHN: You were not forced. We need to be here as a family.

JENNIFER: I don't care. I don't want to be here. I don't even want to be part of this stupid family.

DATTILIO: I hear you, Jennifer, and I want you to know that I never expect individuals to come here against their will. So if you feel that strongly, you can leave, provided that your parents are OK with you being absent from the group. *(Long pause)*

At this point, I became intrigued with what was going on with this family. It struck me that there might be a shred of truth to what Jennifer said—that maybe the children were forced to come. I decided to test this notion by calling Jennifer's bluff right in front of the entire family. Surprisingly, no one flinched. I expected some type of reaction from the parents, but they remained inquisitively silent. Their passive response told me a great deal about their need to relinquish their own authority.

JENNIFER: Well, so what do I do, just leave now?

DATTILIO: Yes, if you wish.

JENNIFER: So where do I go?

DATTILIO: Well, that's really up to you, Jennifer.

JENNIFER: Well, that's dumb. I'm not going to just sit outside in the car, bored! This is so stupid!

DATTILIO: OK, you're welcome to stay. But I'm interested in hearing why you don't want to be here. What turns you off about this whole idea?

JENNIFER: Because this is all bull, and it's not my problem, it's Mom's. *(She glared at her mother.)*

DATTILIO: Hmm. I wonder whether anyone else sees things the way Jennifer does? *(Brief pause)*

JOHN: I don't. I think we all have some issues here that need to be discussed, besides Mom. But Mom does have her problems, I'll agree with that.

DATTILIO: OK. Anyone else have an opinion? *(No one said anything. John glanced at Ruth, while she looked around at the kids.)*

Already in a few short moments, it was obvious that tension was coming from somewhere in this system, and that it was being manifested through Jennifer. I also found it interesting that these children were so careful with their words, except of course for Jennifer.

ROB: I'd like to say something—I think our family definitely has some major problems. Everyone is, like . . . all over the place, and there's no sense of, how would you say . . . ?

DATTILIO: Family unity?

ROB: Yeah! Sort of. I mean, like, Dad is sort of off in his own world—no offense, Dad—and Mom is doing her thing and trying to do for everyone else . . . it's sort of nuts.

DATTILIO: So I'm hearing you say that things at home are somewhat chaotic at times and you're bothered by this?

ROB: Yes, but not "at times" . . . *a lot* of the time.

DATTILIO: OK, but I want to get back to Jennifer's statement about how Mom makes her problems everyone else's. Does that seem true? Do you all feel the same way Jennifer does?

JOHN: No, I'm having a problem with Jennifer's statement. Ruth and Jennifer have really been locking horns lately, and Jennifer will often take advantage every chance she can to blame her mother, or anyone else for that matter, except of course herself.

JENNIFER: I do not! Get real, Dad!

DATTILIO: John, in addition to your concerns about Jennifer, you sound a bit protective of your wife.

JOHN: Well, sure, but that's the way I really see it.

DATTILIO: OK, but is there any agreement with any of what the kids are saying?

JOHN: Maybe some—I mean, look, Ruth has some problems. She's had a really rough upbringing, so I sort of see our roles as being supportive to her and just not giving her a hard time.

These were interesting precedents that were being set, particularly John's apparent reluctance to challenge his wife. Thus far, Ruth had chosen to say very little. Of course, I didn't expect that John would go against his wife, but I was curious to see how he would handle Jennifer's accusation that Ruth was the one with the problem.

DATTILIO: It seems to me that this is somewhat how your family has functioned for a long time until recently. Is that true?

JENNIFER: Yeah, until I screwed everything up, right? Right, Mom?

RUTH: *(Beginning to cry)* Oh, Jennifer, stop!

ADAM: I think Jennifer's problem is that she wants to grow up, and Mom won't let her, and that's why she's mad at Mom.

SUSAN: I sort of agree. Mom is starting to do the same with me.

JOHN: Do what?

SUSAN: Uh-oh! Danger! I'd better shut up. *(Everyone laughed.)*

DATTILIO: No, that's OK, Susan. Say what you feel. I want you to be open and honest here.

SUSAN: Well, she's starting to be kind of overprotective with me like she has been with Jen.

JENNIFER: Yeah, and it's only with the girls. She's not like that so much with Adam and Rob.

DATTILIO: Ruth, how do you respond to what you're hearing? You've been sort of quiet.

RUTH: Well, I don't know. I have to be honest—this is hard for me to listen to.

DATTILIO: I'm sure that it is.

RUTH: I don't know. I feel like I just want to keep everyone from all of this hurt.

DATTILIO: OK, so you're protective of the girls. John is protective of you. Who's protective of Rob, Adam, and Dad?

ROB: Rob, Adam, and Dad. *(Everyone laughed.)*

DATTILIO: Ah, so the men take care of themselves. That's interesting.

I was being very polite here. The fact of the matter was that protection appeared to be essential for survival in this family. The reason, however, still wasn't clear to me at this point.

JOHN: Well, sure. That's the way it was with both mine and Ruth's family when we were growing up. Everyone sort of protected each other in both of our families.

DATTILIO: So I guess it would be fair to say that, in a way, protecting each other is carried down from your respective families of origin.

At this point, I began to explore in more detail Ruth's and John's family backgrounds, with particular emphasis on the roles that their respective parents played. I did so in front of the entire family, so that the children would be exposed to the evolution of the family schema (see Figure 3.1).

Ruth, who was an only child, explained that she came from an extremely rigid family. She described her father as the "ruler" and her mother as playing a very passive role. Her parents were religious. Her father was particularly demanding of Ruth. She could never do anything right in his eyes, which didn't exactly do wonders for her self-esteem.

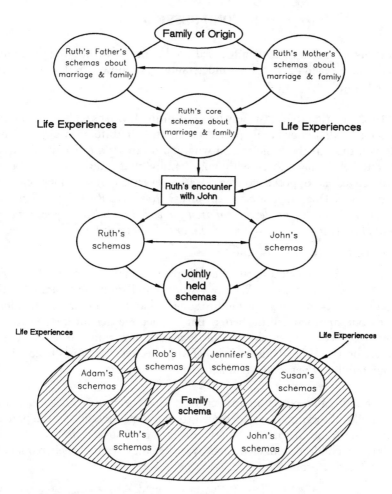

FIGURE 3.1. Ruth's family's schemas. From Dattilio (1996). Copyright 1996 by Brooks/Cole. Reprinted by permission.

John came from a vastly different background. His father had died of congenital heart failure when John was 2. He was raised by his mother and two older sisters, whom he grew to be very protective of over the years. In fact, John was always told by his sisters that he was the man of the house and that he had to take care of his mother. Although this was a dubious honor, he took it on without question.

The remainder of this session was devoted to gathering additional details about Ruth's and John's earlier years. At the end of the session, the family was invited to return for a second session about a week later. John and Ruth readily accepted. Three of the children agreed reluctantly. Jennifer once again said nothing.

SECOND SESSION

It was my intention to remain focused on the idea of identifying the family schema and reaching a better understanding of how this family system worked.

DATTILIO: During our last session, I identified what's called a "family schema"—that your family protects each other in different ways. So what do you think is the basic reason why you do this? In other words, what is the belief that exists with your family that causes you to be so protective, as opposed to the idea of everyone just taking care of themselves? Does anyone have any ideas? *(John and Ruth glanced at each other sardonically, while the children appeared distracted by extraneous thoughts. It was as though no one wanted to speak.)*

RUTH: Is it bad that we do this?

DATTILIO: Well, not necessarily. But the pattern that evolved in the family has caused some conflict. What we need to do is to begin to address this, and maybe even change or modify some behaviors so that you get along with one another a little better. But . . . let me get an answer to my question, because I think that this is a very important question. Again, where do you believe this basic belief of protectiveness comes from within your family? *(Everyone remained silent.)*

I didn't really expect an answer here. This was more of a statement of what I was observing; it was designed to put some pressure on the parents to examine some of their own motives. In fact, I suspect that one of the reasons the children remained silent was that they wanted their parents to answer for this protectiveness.

JOHN: Well, I guess as the father, I feel to blame for some of it. While I support Ruth, I've also kind of dumped on her by not taking more of an active role with the kids. I said that my father wasn't around when I was growing up, so I've always felt somewhat lost in my role, and I have to kind of improvise at times. Therefore, I sort of duck out, so to speak, but then feel guilty when the kids jump all over Ruth. So then I kind of become protective. I don't know, it's weird.

DATTILIO: It sounds as though, as a result of Ruth's upbringing, she's felt compelled to assume all the responsibility for the family, perhaps in part to compensate for you. So there may be several family beliefs that are distorted to some degree, as well as individual distortions regarding your roles in the family. Does that sound possible?

ADAM: What do you mean, "distortions"?

DATTILIO: Good question, Adam. Let me explain.

I explained and reviewed the 10 common distortions listed below, so that the family members could begin to formulate some understanding of what a cognitive distortion is. Using specific examples along with some humor that relates to family members can help personalize these concepts; it also alleviates some of the boredom that can accompany this type of didactic procedure. I passed out sheets listing the 10 distortions for the family members to follow as a guideline. I also attempted to show them how this belief system of protectiveness emerged from Ruth and John's family of origin. The distortions and the examples I used are as follows:

1. *Arbitrary inference.* Conclusions are drawn by family members in the absence of substantiating evidence. For example, when Rob returns home a half hour late for his curfew, he is judged by the family as having been "up to no good."

2. *Selective abstraction.* Information is taken out of context; certain details are highlighted while other are ignored. For example, John fails to answer Adam's greeting the first thing in the morning, and Adam concludes, "Dad must be angry at me."

3. *Overgeneralization.* An isolated incident or two is allowed to serve as a representation of similar situations everywhere, related or unrelated. For example, because John and the kids have left food out from time to time, Ruth develops the belief that her family is wasteful and that they take everything, including her, for granted.

4. *Magnification and minimization.* Something is perceived as having greater or lesser significance than is appropriate. For example, John demands that the children wash their hands before eating, but he fails to do this himself. When confronted by the children, he minimizes his failure by saying, "Well, I don't do it very often—so I'm excused."

5. *Personalization.* External events are attributed to oneself when insufficient evidence exits to reach such conclusion. For example, Jennifer

blames herself for her parents' repeated arguments, stating, "Perhaps I should have never been born."

6. *Dichotomous thinking.* An experience is identified as either all or nothing—a complete success or a total failure. For example, after an incident in which Adam becomes involved in trouble at school, John and Ruth conclude, "We failed as disciplinarians."

7. *Labeling and mislabeling.* Imperfections and mistakes made in the past are allowed to serve as stereotypes for all future behaviors. For example, Ruth and John have failed to follow through on a promise on one occasion, and are consequently regarded by the children as being unreliable.

8. *Tunnel vision.* Individuals see only what they want to see or what fits their current state of mind. For example, John holds on to the rigid belief that the man is the "head of the household," because this is the way he imagined a father to be when he was growing up.

9. *Biased explanations.* A polarized type of thinking develops during times of distress, in which there is an automatic assumption that another family member holds a negative ulterior motive. For example, John and the children distrust Ruth because she's reluctant to disclose to them what she's been discussing in her private therapy.

10. *Mind reading.* One person "magically" knows what another person is thinking. For example, Ruth is certain that the children view her as a failure because she's unable to stand up for herself and demand what she wants.

DATTILIO: OK, so let's see if we can identify some of the distortions that each of you engage in.

ROB: Oh! I have one that Mom does big time.

DATTILIO: All right, let's hear it.

ROB: I'm not sure which one this is, but, like, if we're out past curfew, she freaks out and starts accusing us of being up to no good—like we're guilty until proven innocent.

DATTILIO: That's an arbitrary inference, and one that you may perceive Mom as doing. Do any of the other family members engage in the same distortion?

ADAM: Yeah, Jen does!

JENNIFER: I do not, dweeb!

ADAM: Yes, you do.

SUSAN: You do, Jen. You're just like Mom.

DATTILIO: OK, look, guys, we're just trying to identify cognitive distortions that we all engage in from time to time. This isn't meant to be a jousting match. Also, we want to identify those distortions that you engage in yourselves more than those you see in other family members.

JOHN: All right! I have one about myself, as much as I hate to admit it. I sometimes get annoyed when my decisions are questioned. I guess I equate compliance from the kids with respect, yet I tend to dump a lot of responsibility onto Ruth.

At this point, I was attempting to uncover some of the family members' individual schemas, and also to identify cognitive distortions after explaining some of the basic principles of the cognitive-behavioral approach. The members of this particular family were rather bright, so, not surprisingly, they picked up on things rather quickly.

In therapy with a family like this one, the next step after identifying these distortions is to teach the family members to begin to question and weigh the evidence that supports the internal statements they make to themselves, and (ideally) to challenge any erroneously based assumptions. This approach assumes a more didactic posture in the early stages, not only to familiarize the family with the model, but also to provide some structure at the outset. The trick here is to try to introduce the model in a creative way, so as to not bore the family with theories. Therefore, conveying this information is sometimes done in a playful manner, using jokes and making a potentially heavy situation more lively. Most importantly, this process of education helps family members cut through some of the bickering and blaming by providing them with tools and allowing them to become students of their own behavior. In fact, one of the techniques used is to assign spouses or family members a pad of paper and a pencil, so that they can capture their automatic thoughts on paper during the course of their interaction at home (Dattilio, in press).

DATTILIO: All right John, that's a good one—so some of your beliefs, and one that you are choosing to identify as being based on a distortion, is that "the boss should never be questioned." It's a matter of "Do as I say, not as I do."

JOHN: Yeah, I guess. Boy, that sounds awful when someone else actually says it.

DATTILIO: Well, let's address that. Let's just analyze it for a moment and see if we can challenge some of the basic tenets of that belief. Now, do you have any idea why you believe this way—that the man should be the boss and his decisions should go unquestioned?

JOHN: Well, I don't know. I know I didn't get that from my father, so I guess, as I said before, I was left to sort of improvise as to what the father's roles should be. I also think that Ruthie's father had something to do with it early on. When we were first married, he used to . . . sort of . . . drill me.

DATTILIO: Drill you?

JOHN: Yeah, you know, like take me aside and give me his advice about how I need to act as the man of the house. Also, well, this may sound odd, but I kind of got the impression that this was what Ruthie was more comfortable with. You know, like she kind of—oh, I forget the word that you guys use all of the time. It's a popular term.

DATTILIO: Enabled it?

JOHN: Yes, enabled, that's it! She enabled me to be that way, I guess. I mean, in other words, that she kind of leans on me more than I lean on her, because she knows that I am used to it from the way I grew up.

DATTILIO: I see. So do you believe that you may enable Ruth with certain things that you do, and perhaps you both enable the children?

JOHN: I don't know. I never really thought about it that way.

DATTILIO: Might this be tied to the schema of taking care of each other? How does this all relate?

ROB: Well, I was thinking about that for a while when you were talking to Dad, and I think that we're like a pack of wolves that sort of just look out for one another casually, and if one of us is in need, somebody will step in—but we never talk about it openly otherwise.

What an interesting metaphor! It didn't actually strike me until later that there was a great deal of symbolism embedded in such a statement. The fact that caretaking was such a pronounced dynamic with this family, but that Rob chose the examples of wolves, also suggested a sense of primitive aggression that might be existing on a deeper level. Wolves are animals that are protective of one another, yet certainly capable of protecting themselves as well. The fact that this statement came from the oldest male child, who was in the process of challenging his father's authority, was another interesting aspect.

DATTILIO: OK, but how does this cause conflict?

ROB: I'm not sure!

SUSAN: I think that maybe the conflict comes when one person has one expectation and the other has a different expectation, and it's never communicated. We just sort of . . .

DATTILIO: Mind-read.

SUSAN: Yeah, whatever.

DATTILIO: OK, that's another distortion.

ADAM: Wow, we're one distorted family. Cool! *(Everyone laughed.)*

DATTILIO: Well, yes, we all have our distortions, but every family does.

RUTH: *(In jest)* I don't know, it makes us sound like we're the Addams Family or something. *(Everyone laughed again.)*

I smiled, too, as the family attempted to bolster some cohesion through levity. At the same time, I was desperately trying to understand the family dynamics and the way each member viewed his or her own life and the family's situation. I was also concerned about Ruth's passivity and lack of involvement in this discussion of cognitive distortions, particularly in light of the fact that she was the one to initiate therapy.

In the next session, I attempted to introduce slowly the idea of restructuring some of the family thinking style in order to facilitate change. Before the second session ended, however, I suggested that as a homework assignment, the family members should think about the various cognitive distortions we discussed and how these might apply to themselves. I also asked them to think a little about all that had unfolded in the first two sessions.

THIRD SESSION

One important issue that Susan mentioned in the second session was the idea of expectations. This was something I came back to later in the treatment process. The notion of the violation of expectations is one of the main areas of focus in the cognitive-behavioral model.

DATTILIO: Well, I'm glad to see everyone back. *(Jennifer smirked.)*

JOHN: I guess you could say that the kids have had a slight change of heart.

DATTILIO: Really?

JOHN: No. Actually, I simply told them that they had no choice and they had to attend.

DATTILIO: Well, this is something that I would like to address—particularly your forcefulness, John, and how that affects the family. *(To the children)* How do you guys feel about this?

ROB: I don't know. I kind of like coming now.

DATTILIO: Jennifer, what about you? *(She simply shrugged.)*

JOHN: Jennifer doesn't like you. She thinks you're making things worse.

DATTILIO: Is that true, Jen?

JENNIFER: *(To John)* I didn't say that! You're such a dork!

JOHN: Well, you said something like that.

JENNIFER: I said, "I don't care if things get worse"—oh, just forget it! I hate this.

DATTILIO: I'm wondering if this is an example of some of the distortions that we were discussing during the last session. The distortions that come as a result of misreading one another.

JENNIFER: No, just forget it. I'm not saying anything.

Jennifer answered my question by shutting down. John's misperception of Jennifer's statement was exactly the type of distortion and miscommunication that had apparently been causing conflict in this family. At this point, it was crucial to back off because of Jennifer's volatility. I didn't want to push her at this point, since I was pleased that she was even consenting to remain in the room, as reluctant as she was.

DATTILIO: I think it might be important for us to take a look at some of the distortions that you frequently engage in, now that we have identified a few of them, and see whether or not we may be able to challenge them—particularly those distortions that may interfere the most with your family dynamics. John, would you be willing to volunteer so that I can demonstrate?

JOHN: Sure.

I decided to use the father as an example here, since I noticed that the children were beginning to look at him during the brief moments of silence. I also felt that this might take the pressure off the other family members for a bit, and that it might be a good prelude to eventually addressing the issues of his relationship with the children.

DATTILIO: OK, you said, as I recall, that one of your beliefs as a father is that "The boss should never be questioned"—something to that effect. Is that correct?

JOHN: Yes.

DATTILIO: OK. Now how well do you believe that statement can be substantiated? In other words, is it based on any sound rule of thumb or theory of parenting?

JOHN: I don't know. It's just something I've come to believe, I guess.

DATTILIO: OK, so there's no substantiating evidence. It's merely conjecture. So, is it possible that it might be based on misinformation?

JOHN: Possibly—eh, I'm not sure what you mean when you say "misinformation."

DATTILIO: Wrong or incorrect. In other words, what do we know about the effect of this principle? What kind of results have you gotten from it thus far?

JOHN: Well, not too good. In fact, no one obeys it, and I'm sort of scoffed at by my kids for believing it.

DATTILIO: Scoffed at?

JOHN: Yeah! *(Beginning to chuckle)* Like the other day, when I was attempting to assert myself and Rob started making fun of me.

DATTILIO: How?

JOHN: He flexed his muscles and folded his arms Indian-style and mocked me. Then he challenged me by saying that I was being unreasonable.

DATTILIO: How did you interpret Rob saying that?

JOHN: That I'd better forget the tough guy approach and try more to reason with them instead.

DATTILIO: So perhaps it may not be the most effective approach, or maybe it needs some modification and you don't have to abandon the idea completely. I mean, respect is important, but to expect that no one will ever question what you say or do, particularly as the kids grow older, is perhaps a bit unreasonable.

JOHN: Yeah, I see your point. But then how do I get it out of my head? I mean, it's sort of ingrained there.

DATTILIO: Good question. Cognitive therapy utilizes a lot of homework assignments. Challenging negative self-statements, or what we call "automatic thoughts," takes practice. One way to do this is writing the alternative statement out each time you experience a negative thought statement or cognitive distortion. So what I would like you to do is to take a piece of paper and write across the top of the page several headings. Then draw a line down the side of each heading to make columns, like this. *(I took a piece of paper and demonstrated as follows:)*

Situation or event	Automatic thought	Cognitive distortion	Emotion	Challenging self-statement	Alternative response

Then each time a situation occurs where you have a negative automatic thought, write it down. Use the extreme left-hand column to record the situation in which you had the thought. In the next column, list exactly what the thought was. Next, try to attempt to identify what type of distortion you were engaging in. You can refer to the sheet I gave you last session. After that, note the emotional responses that accompanied it, and then try to challenge that thought or belief by weighing the evidence in favor of it. Finally, you might want to write down an alternative response, using any new information that you may have gathered.

ROB: Hey, Dad, do you want to borrow my laptop computer? *(Everyone laughed.)*

DATTILIO: *(To Rob)* You certainly are the comedian in the family, Rob, aren't you?

ROB: Yeah, I try!

DATTILIO: OK, John, does that make sense to you?

JOHN: Yes, but could we run through it once more so that I'm sure I have it right? It's a little confusing.

DATTILIO: Certainly. Let's try an example.

JOHN: Something happened last week with Adam where he came in a little past curfew. I said something to him about him being 5 minutes late and pushing the limits, and he started to challenge my authority by attempting to minimize what he did, saying that it had only been 5 minutes and that it was no big deal.

DATTILIO: OK, so let's get everything down on paper.

Situation or event	Automatic thought	Cognitive distortion
Adam arrives home 5 minutes late for curfew.	He's defying me. He doesn't respect my position. If I don't punish him, I'll be a lousy father.	Arbitrary inference, dichotomous thinking, personalization
Emotion	Challenging self-statement	Alternative response
Upset, angry	Just because he comes home 5 minutes beyond his curfew doesn't mean that it is aimed directly at me. It also doesn't mean that he is intending to defy me—kids just test the limits sometime.	I could talk to him about it rather than jump to conclusions and punish him. Perhaps he just honestly lost track of time or is being careless. He may be more receptive if I try this approach.

DATTILIO: That's excellent, John. Do you all see how we can attempt to restructure some of our thinking? Dad did a real nice job with that.

ROB: Yeah, but what if Adam really was defying Dad? I mean, how do we know what Dad is saying to himself is correct?

ADAM: Gee, thanks, Rob!

ROB: Don't mention it.

DATTILIO: Good question, Rob. We gather information to support our alternative beliefs, and so one of the things that Dad could do is, like he said on the sheet, to talk to Adam about what his reasons were for arriving home late. This is something he might want to do, but later on or even during the next day, after things settle down a bit between Dad and Adam. This could be applied to all of us at one time or the other, as you recognize yourselves engaging in distorted thinking. We want to begin to examine our mode of thinking and really question the validity of what we tell ourselves. This may make a monumental difference in how we interact with one another. It also forces us to slow things down a bit, so that we can really begin to examine what we say to ourselves. This is one of the reasons that we put it down on paper. Hopefully, in time you will be able to do this mentally without always writing it out.

SUBSEQUENT THERAPY

From this point, I continued to monitor the family members in challenging their belief statements in the fashion demonstrated above. During this process, feelings and emotions were also addressed, as well as communication skills and problem solving strategies.

The educational component continued as I oriented them to the many assumptions that families operate under, according to the cognitive-behavioral model. These assumptions, originally formulated by Schwebel and Fine (1994), are outlined below in modified form.

Assumption 1: Individuals seek to maintain balance in their environment in order to fulfill their needs and wants. They try to understand their environment and how they can function most effectively in it. As they gather data about how the family works, they use the information to guide their behavior and to aid in building and refining family-related cognitions. This process lends itself to the development of each individual's personal theory (PT) of family life and family relationships (Schwebel & Fine, 1994, p. 41). This PT shapes how the individual thinks and perceives, and serves as the central organizer to the mass of life events that he or she is exposed to (internally to and externally from the family unit).

Assumption 2: Individual members' cognitions affect virtually every aspect of family life. These are determined by five categories of cognitive variables identified by Baucom, Epstein, Sayers, and Sher (1989):

   a. Selective attention (what is noticed).
   b. Attributions (how individuals explain why any given event occurs).

    c. Expectancies (what individuals predict will occur in the short-, middle-, or long-term future).

    d. Assumptions (individuals' perceptions about how the world works).

    e. Standards (how individuals think the world should be).

Assumption 3: Certain "obstacles" block healthy family functioning. The roots of these "obstacles" lie within individual family members' PTs—specifically, the cognitions in the PTs.

Assumption 4: Family members need to become more aware of their family-related cognitions—how these cognitions affect them in certain situations, when they cause distress, and how to replace unhealthy ones with healthy ones.

These four assumptions serve as guides for a cognitive-behavioral therapist's intervention with a family, and may be modified to suit the specific situation or the level of problem at hand. With these assumptions as guidelines, the therapist attempts to enter the family's world and to help the family members, in a collaborative fashion, identify areas of dysfunction and institute the restructuring process.

Regular homework assignments were also employed in order to aid the members of Ruth's family in learning to challenge their distorted thoughts more spontaneously. At times during the session, I would walk each family member through the specific technique of challenging distortions, in order to insure its correct use. In addition, the use of behavioral techniques, such as the reassignment of family members' roles and responsibilities, became an integral part of the treatment regimen in this particular case. Hence, with the change and modification of dysfunctional thinking and behavior, family interactions became less conflictual, and the family members could begin to reshape their roles. The emphasis here, however, was on the fact that cognition must change through a restructuring process in order for emotion and behavior to change. The following is an example from the sixth session:

DATTILIO: Jennifer, I'd like to talk more about the concerns you voiced during a previous session regarding your mother's relationship with you. You said that you feel that your mother is too controlling and barely gives you a chance to breathe at times.

JENNIFER: Yeah, and I can't stand it. She keeps telling me that it's because she wants to get closer to me, when in actuality she's pushing me further away.

DATTILIO: Ruth, do you hear what your daughter is saying?

RUTH: Yes, I hear what she's saying, but I don't believe that's what she really wants. She needs me in her life more than she realizes. She's just confused.

JENNIFER: Oh, brother! Just because you think I *should* need you doesn't mean that I *do* need you. Get real, Mom. The only thing that I am confused about is why you're acting like a jerk!

JOHN: Settle down, Jennifer.

DATTILIO: Ruth, I'm beginning to think you may need Jennifer to need you maybe more than she actually does. Is that possible?

RUTH: *(Beginning to cry)* I don't know—I just know that I want to be closer to her.

JOHN: Could I interrupt?

DATTILIO: Certainly.

JOHN: It's real important to Ruth to know that she's special to everyone in the family, especially the kids. So she's kind of protective like this because it reassures her that she is doing the right thing. You know, being a concerned parent and all that.

DATTILIO: Ruth, I'd like to hear from you. Is what John said accurate?

RUTH: I guess—I don't know. I sometimes feel like no one needs me in this house. Like if I died, it wouldn't matter.

SUSAN: Mom, it's not that no one needs you; it's just that we all need you in a different way than you think we do. You are special to us. You're our mom. No one can ever replace that role *(beginning to cry)*.

DATTILIO: Ruth, I wonder whether or not we need to reexamine some of our thinking about roles in the family, particularly how each of you perceive them.

RUTH: What do you mean?

DATTILIO: Well, you seem to have this set idea of what your role should be with the kids, and theirs is something much different. But perhaps we need to all change some of our perceptions in order to fit the respective needs that we each have.

ROB: Ah, I'm sorry, Dr. Dattilio, I'm kind of out to lunch here. I have no clue what you are talking about.

DATTILIO: OK, let me say it this way: Jennifer wants Mom in her life, but in a way that allows her to be her own person. From what I gather from Jennifer, she wants to be the one to approach Mom, not the other way around. It's more comfortable for her that way. Mom, on the other hand, has a different perception of being close to Jennifer. Her view involves being more aggressive in her attempt to be close with Jennifer. The more aggressive she is, the more Jennifer pushes her away; hence the more Mom exerts additional effort to get close, the more they alienate each other—and so on and so forth.

JOHN: So you're saying it's a no-win situation. I mean, if both of them stand their ground.

DATTILIO: Well, yes, essentially. Unless they change their behavior, or, more importantly, unless they change their thinking, they will eventually just alienate each other completely.

RUTH: OK, so how do we do that [i.e., change our thinking]?

DATTILIO: I'm glad you asked. It's much like what John did with regard to Adam, only it's a bit more involved because it has to do with certain assumptions and expectations. And also, both of you must take the responsibility to give in a little, and not always wait for the other person to change first. The key is to challenge some of these assumptions by introducing alternative views for consideration. For example, Ruth, what is your assumption about why Jennifer doesn't want you to be so close to her?

RUTH: My assumption? You mean what I think?

DATTILIO: Yes.

RUTH: Well, I guess I just assume that she feels she doesn't need me because she's all grown up—at age 15! When the fact is that she isn't mature yet, and she still needs her mother's guidance.

DATTILIO: OK, now where does that belief come from?

RUTH: Oh, I don't know. I guess this type of thinking is what I was exposed to when I was growing up. We actually had little to say about our relationship with our parents. You just always assumed that Mom and Dad were right. I never questioned it. In fact, that's still the way it is today between me and my parents.

This was an example of Ruth's operating from a schema that evolved from her family of origin. More importantly, however, it appeared that Ruth was actually struggling with the same issue that Jennifer was. I recalled that during the very first interview I had had with Ruth months earlier, she mentioned that her individual therapist had made the connection between her panic attacks and her own sense of struggle as she was attempting to pull away from her parents as an adult. Ruth had tried many years before to emancipate herself from her parents during her own adolescent years and failed. I wondered whether or not Ruth's resistance to Jennifer's strivings for independence was actually a projection of her own failed attempts.

DATTILIO: OK, so this is your schema, so to speak—that offspring don't question their parents' motives; they just trust that they are doing the right thing. Now Jennifer is operating from a totally different schema. Jennifer, what is your perception or schema about your parents' involvement in your life?

JENNIFER: Well, they're always telling me to grow up and take responsibility, but they don't even let me! When Mom keeps nosing in on my life, I get crazy. I can't stand it.

DATTILIO: What goes through your mind?

JENNIFER: What do you mean?

DATTILIO: Would you be more specific about the private talk that you have with yourself when Mom "noses in" on your life?

JENNIFER: I told you, it makes me crazy.

DATTILIO: Well, that's more of an emotion. What I want to know is specifically what things you tell yourself about this situation that makes you crazy.

JENNIFER: I don't know. I guess just that she doesn't trust me and still thinks of me like a child.

DATTILIO: Now how else does that make you feel, other than crazy? Can you be more specific?

JENNIFER: I guess it bums me out a little.

DATTILIO: You mean, depresses you?

JENNIFER: Yeah, sort of. I feel down about myself.

DATTILIO: Then you get crazy?

JENNIFER: Yeah, really.

DATTILIO: Ruth, what thoughts do you have about what Jennifer's saying?

RUTH: Well, it doesn't make me happy to think that I depress my daughter.

DATTILIO: Well, I don't know that you actually depress your daughter. What she feels is more a result of what she tells herself. So what needs to change here is a combination of things. Mom may want to consider modifying her approach to Jennifer, which can be done by restructuring some of her thinking as well as making behavioral modifications. Also, the same may be considered for Jennifer, provided that both of you are agreeable to this. *(Both Ruth and Jennifer nodded affirmatively.)*

RUTH: I want to do what I can to make things better. I realize that I do a lot of things wrong, but sometimes I don't feel that I can help myself.

DATTILIO: Well, let's see what we can do. Now, Jennifer, is it possible that there might be some distortion in the way you view your mother's behavior, and more so her intentions in attempting to be close with you?

JENNIFER: I don't think so. I pretty much see what I see.

DATTILIO: Well, but I'm asking you to just consider for a moment that your view, regardless of its basic accuracy, may be slightly distorted by certain things, like your anger and your need for privacy. Things like that. That perhaps Mom's intention isn't so much to rob you of your individuality or keep you a child, but to just share in your life.

JENNIFER: I don't know. Maybe . . .

DATTILIO: All right, well, I want you to think about it. Now here's an important question. What evidence would you need to see as proof of that? That her intention is actually positive towards your genuine growth?

JENNIFER: That she just back off a little.

DATTILIO: So a change in her behavior would tell you that she really cared.

JENNIFER: Well, yeah!

DATTILIO: OK, so if her behavior would change, if she were to back off, how would that change how you think and feel about her and the situation?

JENNIFER: Well, I wouldn't mind talking to her about some things, when I'm ready. At least I could breathe some.

DATTILIO: OK, Ruth, now with that new information about how Jennifer sees the situation and how she feels, does that provide you with any motivation to make modifications in your perception and behavior?

RUTH: Yes, some. I mean, the thing that struck me most is hearing that she gets depressed *(beginning to sob)*. I've been through that, and I don't want that for her.

DATTILIO: OK, so you see that it's important for you to modify your thoughts and behavior, at least to the point that it may free Jennifer up to feel a bit more at ease to talk to you or possibly to confide in you.

RUTH: OK, but I don't know how to deal with these thoughts and emotions that I have about being a neglectful parent.

DATTILIO: Well, we can use the same procedure that we used with John several sessions back. The fact that our thoughts have a significant impact on how we feel and behave is very important. What we tell ourselves is crucial. What will be important to keep in mind, Ruth, is what information Jennifer provided to you about the situation. Use this to modify your thinking about your effectiveness in providing Jennifer with what she needs to grow up. In essence, you need to restructure your thinking, incorporating this new information and assimilating it into your general thinking style. In this way, it may not only help to ease your emotions about the circumstance, but change your behavioral interaction as well! Jennifer, you'll need to do a similar thing in order to do your part in establishing harmony between yourself and Mom.

From this point on, I continued to explore some of the specific underlying issues with family members—Ruth in particular, who attempted to overcompensate with her children for some of what she missed out on in her relationship with her own mother during her upbringing. This kind of exploration is a very important aspect of the cognitive-behavioral approach, and one that is often misunderstood by professionals. So often, a parent's struggle with a child is reflective of a conflict that the parent never resolved during his or her own upbringing. A common yet poignant example is that of individuals who grew up with few material goods and attempt to compensate during their adult lives by buying their children everything. Consequently, the deprived children within them become envious of their own offspring, instead of deriving a sense of fulfillment as anticipated. This conflict is often played out in a fierce competition between parents and children, causing confusion for the offspring—and understandably so.

Freud said that dreams are the window to the unconscious mind. For cognitive-behavioral therapists, schemas are the window through which people view themselves, their world, and their future. Cognitive-behavioral therapists often focus on the early childhood schemas that play a significant role in the conflict of an individual's immediate family. It seemed very likely that the emotional deprivation Ruth had experienced in her own upbringing was playing a major role in her difficulty with Jennifer. Perhaps Ruth wasn't finished dealing with her own mother, and Jennifer's assertion of her own independence represented something that Ruth never felt strong enough to do herself.

The continuation of therapy involved similar restructuring of cognitions among family members, along with altering their overall behavioral style of interaction. Some aspects of the joint family schema were also later addressed, along with the correction of distortions that family members had developed about one another. Such issues as power and control within the family were addressed, along with a redefining of family roles and boundary issues. The emotions of family members were also discussed in the context of distorted thinking and behaviors.

CONCLUSION

Ruth's family continued in treatment with me for another 6 months, for a total of 20 sessions. The family members continued to have their problems, but in general they reported that the harmony in the household had increased. I subsequently continued to work with John and Ruth on some marital issues, while Ruth herself continued with her individual therapy. John and Ruth had a number of strengths in their relationship that were an asset to treatment, such as their ability to be sensitive to each other and their level of commitment. John had a tendency to want to rescue Ruth, which she perceived as being controlling. This also stripped her of her independence, which contributed to her low level of self-esteem. As this issue was addressed, both became aware of the need for change. This allowed Ruth to become less dependent on John; it also had a profound effect on Ruth's role with the children.

We terminated treatment approximately 6 months later. I had occasion to bump into John approximately 1 year later while I was doing Christmas shopping. He greeted me like an old friend and gave me an update on the family's situation. Ruth was finishing up her individual therapy and was now getting along much better with Jennifer. Rob had gone off to college, and Susan and Adam—well, they continued to argue like brother and sister. In the brief minutes that John shared this update with me, he seemed content. As we parted, he thanked me while crossing his fingers, and said he'd call if they ever needed me again.

ACKNOWLEDGMENT

Portions of the case of Ruth and her family are adapted from Dattilio (1996). Copyright 1996 by Brooks/Cole Publishing Company. Adapted by permission.

REFERENCES

Baucom, D. H., Epstein, N., Sayers, S., & Sher, T. G. (1989). The role of cognitions in marital relationships: Definitional, methodological, and conceptual issues. *Journal of Consulting and Clinical Psychology, 57*, 31–38.

Dattilio, F. M. (1996). A cognitive-behavioral approach to family therapy with Ruth. In G. Corey (Ed.), *Case approaches to counseling and psychotherapy* (4th ed., pp. 282–298). Pacific Grove, CA: Brooks/Cole.

Dattilio, F. M. (in press). Pad and pencil techniques. In R. E. Watts (Ed.), *Favorite counseling techniques with couples and families.* Leesberg, VA: American Counseling Association.

Schwebel, A. I., & Fine, M. A. (1994). *Understanding and helping families: A cognitive-behavioral approach.* Hillsdale, NJ: Erlbaum.

SUGGESTED READINGS

Dattilio, F. M. (1997). Family therapy. In R. L. Leahy (Ed.), *Practicing cognitive therapy: A guide to interventions* (pp. 409–450). Northvale, NJ: Jason Aronson.

Dattilio, F. M. (1993). Cognitive therapy with couples and families. *The Family Journal, 1*(1), 51–65.

Dattilio, F. M. (1994). Families in crisis. In F. M. Dattilio & A. Freeman (Eds.), *Cognitive-behavioral strategies in crisis intervention* (pp. 278–301). New York: Guilford Press.

Dattilio, F. M., & Padesky, C. A. (1990). *Cognitive therapy with couples.* Sarasota, FL: Professional Resource Exchange.

Ellis, A. (1991). Rational–emotive family therapy. In A. M. Horne & M. M. Ohlsen (Eds.), *Family counseling and therapy* (pp. 302–328). Itasca, IL: Peacock.

Epstein, N., Schlesinger, S., & Dryden, W. (Eds.). (1988). *Cognitive-behavior therapy with families.* New York: Brunner/Mazel.

Schwebel, A. I., & Fine, M. A. (1994). *Understanding and helping families: A cognitive-behavioral approach.* Hillsdale, NJ: Erlbaum.

Chapter 4

Behavioral Family Therapy

MARION S. FORGATCH
GERALD R. PATTERSON

In the early 1920s, child guidance clinics were established in the United States to treat delinquent children. The assumption was that treatments based on dynamic psychiatry could be used to provide what was missing for such a child (e.g., the introduction of a relationship with a therapist would lead to increased self-control). The evaluation of thousands of hours spent in clinics across the country led to the conclusion that these treatments don't work for antisocial children (Levitt, 1957, 1971). Out-of-control children do have poor relationships with their parents; they are angry; and they do fail in school and lack self-esteem. However, it has become clear that these are secondary products of an ongoing process, not the causes of delinquency. The child guidance approach was a case of the wrong model and the wrong treatment for these children and their families. Aggression in children and adolescents is a behavioral problem, not a mental health problem. The cause lies in the social environment, not in the minds of the youngsters.

CONTINGENT PARENTS

Over the last decade, reviewers have consistently noted that parent training therapy (PTT) is the only treatment program for conduct problems that produces replicated results in well-controlled studies using objective measures of outcome (Greenwood, Model, Rydell, & Chiesa, 1996; Kazdin, 1987; Lipsey, 1992; Patterson, Dishion, & Chamberlain, 1993). In PTT, parents are taught effective family management practices that reduce their children's antisocial behavior. The changes in parent and child behavior are accompanied by commensurate changes in the youngsters' negative emotions and attributions.

The PTT approach assumes that the core problem lies in the social environment that supports deviant behaviors, not in a child. A child's difficult temperament or a family's stressful living conditions (e.g., social disadvantage, parental psychopathology, family structure transitions) are assumed to have an impact on the youngster's adjustment problems by disrupting parenting practices. Support for this mediational model has been demonstrated in a number of samples at the Oregon Social Learning Center (OSLC) (Bank, Forgatch, Patterson, & Fetrow, 1993; Larzelere & Patterson, 1990; Patterson, Reid, & Dishion, 1992) and at other sites as well (Conger, Patterson, & Ge, 1995; Laub & Sampson, 1988). Presumably, children can survive harsh living conditions as long as their parents maintain adequate levels of discipline, monitoring, family problem solving, and encouragement for prosocial development.

The theoretical underpinnings of the PTT approach grew out of field studies carried out in the homes of conduct problem children, beginning in the mid-1960s. Findings from these studies indicated that the parents of these aggressive children tended to provide inconsistent or inappropriate consequences for their children's behavior (Hawkins, Peterson, Schweid, & Bijou, 1966; Patterson & Brodsky, 1966; Wahler, 1968). Direct observations of family interactions revealed mutual anger, contempt, rejection, and low self-esteem as commonly occurring states for both parents and their children. In addition, the trained eye could detect that these parents seldom supported prosocial behaviors, such as cooperative play with siblings. The salience of already low levels of positive reinforcement was further diminished because they took place in conflict-ridden contexts. Conflicts between these children and other family members occurred about once every 3 minutes.

Children are literally trained to be aggressive during episodes of conflict with family members (Patterson, 1980; Snyder, Edwards, McGraw, Kilgore, & Holton, 1994; Snyder & Patterson, 1995). In normal families, coercive counterattacks *and* prosocial reactions (e.g., humor) appear to terminate conflicts. In problem families, *only* coercive counterattacks by the target children seem to work, especially those that involve an escalation to higher levels of aversive behavior (Patterson, 1980; Snyder et al., 1994). Parents of antisocial children ignore prosocial behavior and tend to be ineffective in their use of punishment. Periodically, they explode and physically assault their children. In nonproblem families, prosocial behaviors are reinforced frequently, and parents consistently set limits on deviant behavior. As children enter school, the family training is supplemented with rich schedules of both positive and negative reinforcement provided by peers and teachers. Positive reinforcement for aggressive behavior has been found in naturalistic studies of preschoolers (Patterson, Littman, & Bricker, 1967) and adolescents (Dishion, Patterson, & Griesler, 1994).

Parents of conduct problem children fail to teach their children reasonable levels of compliance. An observational study of six cultures showed that from the Bantu in the tropical rain forest of Africa to the suburban family in the United States, societies require about 70% compliance from their toddlers (Whiting & Whiting, 1975). A set of programmatic studies in the state of Georgia showed that families of young aggressive children fail to come even close to this level (Forehand, Wells, & Sturgis, 1978; Roberts & Powers, 1988, 1990; Snyder & Brown, 1983).

These field studies led directly to treatment procedures in which parents learn to teach compliance and alter payoffs for aggression in the home. The family management skills necessary to accomplish this include contingent support for prosocial behavior, effective discipline practices, family problem solving, and appropriate supervision. Parents also learn ways to limit their children's "street time" and involvement with deviant peers. A common positive side effect of these changes is an improvement in the quality of the parent–child relationship. The family management skills have been detailed in a set of books for parents and mental health professionals (Forgatch & Patterson, 1989; Patterson & Forgatch, 1987). A treatment study (Patterson & Forgatch, 1995) showed that PTT applied to preadolescent children significantly reduced future arrests and out-of-home placements when monitoring, discipline, and problem-solving practices were improved. Data from several treatment studies show that generally, the earlier the intervention, the better the outcome (Dishion & Patterson, 1992)

WHY DOESN'T TREATMENT WORK ALL THE TIME?

Once we naively believed that parents of conduct problem children simply lacked information about effective child rearing. Clinical experience soon suggested that this may be the case for some families with mild problems or very young children, but that information alone is not enough to help families with a mix of skill deficits, parental pathology, difficult living circumstances, and strong negative emotions. A conservative evaluation of treatment outcome for an extended series of families treated at OSLC showed that only about 50% to 60% of the youngsters were deviant at baseline and in the normal range at termination (Dishion & Patterson, 1992). After treating several hundred families with acting-out children, we became convinced of the need to study why it is so difficult to produce change.

We developed coding systems to describe therapist and client behaviors observed during treatment sessions, and embarked on a series of studies of therapy process (Patterson & Chamberlain, 1988; Patterson & Forgatch,

1985; Stoolmiller, Duncan, Bank, & Patterson, 1993). It seemed paradoxical that families seeking advice frequently responded to suggestions for change with "I can't" or "I won't" (Patterson & Forgatch, 1985). The observations of family therapy sessions revealed that predictors of these resistant responses came from antecedent therapist behaviors and family characteristics.

As we studied therapy tapes, it became apparent that therapists' attempts to intervene constituted a key source of resistance. When therapists suggested ways to change, resistance rose to 12% for "I can't" and a smaller proportion for "I won't" comments (Patterson & Chamberlain, 1988). In general, about 6% of the parents' total behavior during treatment was coded as resistant. There was a paradox that quickly became evident: No matter how gently social learning procedures were presented, intervention seemed to increase resistance. We (Patterson & Forgatch, 1985) analyzed therapy sequences and found that therapist behavior plays a powerful role in eliciting resistance. Therapist support, questioning, and facilitative behaviors were associated with resistance levels below the base rate for a given family. Teaching and confrontational behaviors, however, were correlated with resistance above the base rate. This suggested that therapists could reduce resistance if they simply refrained from teaching or confronting their clients, but presumably this would be accompanied by little or no change in parent or child behavior. We see changing parent contingencies for child behavior as the hard core of the intervention—a necessary condition.

Certain qualities that families bring into treatment are associated with failure to change. Family factors, such as parental pathology, social disadvantage, and high levels of stress, are directly correlated with resistance at all stages of treatment (Patterson & Chamberlain, 1994). The more of this sort of baggage a family brings into treatment, the more difficult it is to help the family members change.

WHAT'S NEXT?

Much work is needed to increase the success of PTT for children's antisocial behavior. One approach has been to add enhancement components that deal with common problems inherent in families with out-of-control children. Dadds, Schwartz, and Sanders (1987), for example, tested the addition of a marital component to PTT. In that study, a sample of families with child behavior problems was recruited in which half of the families were also experiencing marital problems. Families were matched on marital problems and assigned to parent training alone or to parent training plus partner support training. Both groups had improved parenting and significant reductions in child behavior problems at termination. At a 6-month follow-up, however, the child outcome improvements were lost for families in which the couples were maritally distressed and received parent training alone. Maritally distressed families that received the enhanced parent training maintained their positive outcomes.

Another goal for the improvement of the PTT approach will be to identify and study "soft" clinical skills that reduce parent and child resistance to change. Strategic approaches have found their way into many of our cases, as illustrated in the case study presented in this chapter. For now, we are applying such techniques on a case-by-case basis, learning what works and what does not. We consider clinical trials as necessary pilot studies for our next round of empirical analyses—an illustration of the "clinical science vortex" described by Forgatch (1991).

In summary, we think that enhancements to the PTT program and the study of clinical skills are necessary but not sufficient conditions for bringing about change in families with out-of-control children. The rest of this chapter describes one such experience.

"I CAN'T BECAUSE SHE WON'T": CASE EXAMPLE

The parents had divorced recently, and pieces of the family were still falling into place—at least from the perspective of Tina, a preadolescent girl referred to OSLC for treatment of out-of-control behavior. At school, Tina was in the program for gifted and talented youngsters; her basic ability and academic performance were well above average. She was at risk of being dropped from the program, however, because of behavior problems that included noncompliance, tantrums, and verbal and physical aggression toward peers. At home, Tina was noncompliant, destructive, and physically aggressive toward her younger sister, Suzie.

Mrs. S. was a well-educated woman who had been a homemaker for the past 7 years. After several years of working as a professional, she had resigned from her career following the birth of their second child. Suzie was born with a medical disability that required multiple surgeries during infancy. Now that Suzie was well and the parents were divorced, Mrs. S. needed work, but her credentials were out of date. Her new status as a single mother was overwhelming; now this proud, independent person was receiving welfare.

At intake, Mrs. S. explained that she'd neglected Tina after Suzie's birth because of the younger child's health problems. Mr. S. had taken over Tina's care, leading to what Tina described as a close and special relationship. But with the divorce, Mr. S. had pretty much dropped out of the family's life. Mrs. S. described him (in Tina's presence) as a selfish jerk who'd never cared much about his children. We suspect that before the separation, it was the father who could more effectively manage this high-energy, difficult little girl. The fact that Mrs. S. was currently depressed meant that she was also essentially noncontingent, neither encouraging Tina's prosocial behavior nor following through in her discipline efforts. In therapy, the mother made high rates of "I can't" statements—a type of helpless response that characterizes depressed single mothers.

Treatment would require wresting power from Tina and placing it more appropriately in the hands of her mother. However, this would take some work, because Tina was a virtuoso of temper tantrums. When things didn't go her way, she rapidly escalated from verbal noncompliance and grotesque facial expressions to screaming fits that included kicking, breaking things, beating with her fists, and swearing at the top of her lungs. One time when she was told to turn off the garden hose, Tina instead turned it full blast through the open kitchen window onto her mother's face. Such outrageous behavior led Mrs. S. to believe that she could do nothing to manage her child's behavior.

Suzie played her own role in this family misadventure. On the surface, she appeared to be the innocent victim of her sister's venom. However, Suzie often silently initiated the sibling conflicts with a hostile gesture or grimace. These actions elicited a highly predictable and vociferous response from her sister, which earned a reprimand for Tina and a sympathetic hug for Suzie from Mom. By the way, our observational studies show that much of the training for coercion in general and for hitting in particular is actually provided by siblings (Patterson & Reid, 1984). The reactions of siblings and parents make unique contributions to training for coercion.

The social learning intervention teaches parents a set of family management practices designed to encourage children's prosocial behavior and to discourage the deviant behavior that brings them to treatment. Parents learn to do this gradually, with skills taught in sequence. First, parents are helped to pinpoint their youngsters' positive and problematic behaviors in terms of specific actions that are readily observable. Compliance and noncompliance are preferred behaviors to target for change. After a week of keeping track of their children's target behaviors, parents are introduced to the concept of teaching prosocial behavior through contingent encouragement with incentive charts.

Contingent encouragement promotes positive relationships between parents and children. Children earn rewards while they learn prosocial skills. They value the incentives acquired through good behavior, and their self-esteem tends to grow with their successes and their parents' positive attention. Chores are broken down into several steps that are clearly defined, with points provided for each step. The parents define components of a given chore and determine how many points will be awarded. The number of points may reflect either the difficulty of the behavior or the value a parent places on it. Compliance is typically part of the chart, with 1 point given each time the child minds the parent or does what is requested. Initially, we attempt to keep the incentive program as simple as possible, with a total of 10 points possible and the child needing 6 or 7 points to earn a daily reward. Parents and children generate a menu of appropriate daily rewards, with parents having the final say about what is included on the chart.

Rewards tend to come in categories that include food, special time with a parent, household resources, privileges, and things that cost money. The details of the reward system are carefully negotiated to fit within the family's resources and values. Items used as rewards are changed regularly, to keep things current and interesting. When a child learns a given chore or behavior, the chart is altered to include something new. As youngsters grow older and have more responsibilities, families often shift from incentive charts to chore lists that indicate how allowances will be earned. The details of these arrangements are negotiated during weekly family problem-solving meetings. Each task is given a monetary value, and as a child completes a job, it is checked off the list or marked on the calendar. Allowance is paid weekly at a prespecified time, with money given for work completed along with a good deal of praise and approval. Parents tend to like this approach because it is similar to the experience of a job in the real world. Children like the incentives, and there is often a nice honeymoon until someone reports, "The chart doesn't work!"

The next step in the program typically involves the introduction of a discipline technique that is to be used contingent on a specific behavior. For preadolescent youngsters, we prefer time out. There are several varieties of time out currently in use. At OSLC, time out begins with removal to a boring place for 5 minutes. When a child refuses (as children usually do), a parent calmly adds time minute by minute, up to a 10-minute maximum. Then, if the child continues to refuse, a prearranged privilege is removed and the parent disengages from the situation. After several trials, the child learns that compliance earns points toward a reward and noncompliance earns time out. When parents are consistent, children quickly learn to go to time out for 5 minutes rather than to lose a privilege for up to 1 hour.

Another component in the intervention is training in family problem solving. This is a complex set of skills that includes communication, negotiation, and contracting. Families are encouraged to meet weekly to discuss important issues, such as the alteration of house rules, the negotiation of rights and responsibilities, and the planning of fun family events. Agreements made during these meetings are written down (including details such as who will do what, when they will do it, and positive and negative consequences for various actions), and signatures are obtained from all participants. Families are guided in the use of these problem-solving techniques to discuss and resolve new issues and conflicts that arise in later sessions.

In subsequent sessions, parents are taught strategies for monitoring their children when they are at school or elsewhere in the community. This includes networking with parents of their children's peers, making appropriate contact with the leaders of extracurricular activities, and staying in touch with teachers and other relevant school personnel. When needed, a school program is set up to improve communication between teachers and parents, to promote regular home study, and to provide sanctions at home for problem behavior at school. More recently, interventions have been added to the program to improve children's peer relations and to regulate negative emotions.

Each week there is a home practice assignment, in which procedures taught in the therapy session are to be used at home and discussed during the next session. During the week, the therapist calls the parents to check on the homework assignment, to discuss ways of managing difficulties, and to encourage success. Midweek calls provide important support for parents' efforts to carry out their homework and to alter strategies that aren't quite working. Procedures have to be tailored to each family. Brief calls to families between sessions enable therapists to prevent failures with early intervention.

In keeping with the usual approach, the first home practice assignment for Mrs. S. was to keep track of Tina's compliance and noncompliance for an hour each day on a chart provided by the therapist. The results of this assignment indicated that Tina complied about 40% of the time. "Non-problem" children tend to mind their parents about 70%.

The next step taught Mrs. S. to make effective requests that would increase the likelihood of compliance. Effective requests have the following characteristics: They are short and polite; are made in physical proximity to the child; are phrased as statements, not questions; and ask for only one behavior at a time. An example of an effective request would be "Tina, please hang up your coat now," as opposed to "Would you like to hang up your coat?" or "What's your coat doing there?"

The assignment that accompanies this session asks parents to track the quality of their requests and to continue tracking their child's compliance and noncompliance for an hour each day. Mrs. S. had several problems to overcome in the way that she made requests. She was extremely verbal, and her requests were often embedded in a thick cloud of words. Part of her assignment was to make requests in 10 words or less. Another problem was that her mild-mannered style was easily ignored by Tina. To counter this, Mrs. S. practiced using more powerful but nonthreatening body postures and speaking more firmly when making requests.

The incentive chart had been introduced as a tool to teach Tina prosocial skills that would help build her self-esteem. Mrs. S. liked this positive approach for encouraging Tina's development, and there was little resistance to this aspect of the program. Tina's chore was to take care of the family cat. Her incentive chart is shown in Figure 4.1.

"Cat care" was broken down into five steps that could earn a total of 6 points. All but one step earned a single point. Removing "poop" to the compost pile received 2 points, because this was a particularly unpleasant aspect of the job. Good chore descriptions include a time by which the chore is to be completed, which in this case earned an additional point. Neatness also

Incentive Chart

Name T_{INA} **Week** $Nov\ 12-19$

Review time _After Dinner Dishes_

	Point value	Mon	Tue	Wed	Thu	Fri	Sat	Sun
Activity: CAT CARE	6							
Step 1 FooD in FooD Bowl	1							
Step 2 WATER in WATER Bowl	1							
Step 3 Poop to compost	2							
Step 4 DoNe by 9 AM	1							
Step 5 DoNe NeATLy	1							
Cooperation Doing as asked. Starting within 10 seconds	1 each							
Daily total								

#Points needed for incentive   6

Incentive given each day							

Incentives

1. _Popsicle_   4. _____
2. _20 MiN GAme w MoM (alone)_   5. _____
3. _STAy up 30 MiN later_   6. _____

FIGURE 4.1. Incentive chart.

was given a value, because this was a serious problem for Tina. Families differ on the number of points possible for compliance, but most agree that any child can earn 4 or 5 points in a given day. On a given day, Tina could earn 10 points if she completed her chore and complied at least four times. To earn a daily reward, Tina required a total of 6 points, which allowed her a few mistakes without losing the incentive. Tina's reward menu included food, time with Mom, and use of household resources (e.g., access to Mom's makeup, choice of an extra TV program). Typically, she earned her reward 4 days a week, which both she and her mother agreed was significant progress.

Once the encouragement side of the program is working well, discipline strategies are introduced. The therapist met separately with Mrs. S. to introduce the concept of time out. After Mrs. S. watched a videotape showing how the procedure takes place, they discussed her concerns. When the therapist asked what would present the most trouble, Mrs. S. admitted that it would be a temptation to use lectures rather than time out. Some parents think that a good lecture is far better than a punishment. This was particularly true of Mrs. S., who used each episode of misbehavior as an opportunity to embark on a lengthy explanation about why one should or shouldn't engage in certain behavior. The only problem with this approach was that Tina didn't listen, and the lectures had no impact on her behavior. Grounding runs a close second to lecturing as an ineffective punishment, because the interval is often too long ("You're grounded for 2 months!") and parents give in to pleas for clemency.

Although Mrs. S. agreed that time out was a good idea, she was somewhat intimidated by her daughter. The therapist explained that the secret to success was having a set of backup privileges that could be withheld when Tina refused to go to time out. The privilege is removed for short periods of time, usually between 30 minutes and 1 hour. Common backup privileges include favorite toys, sports equipment, playing with a friend, stereo or radio use, telephone time, playing outside, and TV time. The most important aspect of a backup privilege is that the parent must be willing to withhold it and able to enforce its removal. This, of course, was a problem for Mrs. S., who said that there was nothing she could control. The therapist described how other parents manage this problem. Some parents lock up toys or equipment in closets, in the trunk of the car, or at a neighbor's house. Other parents have several potential privileges to remove and don't announce which one will be withheld until the item is secured.

Mrs. S. was advised not to use time out until backup privileges could be put in place. The home practice assignment was to continue use of the incentive chart and to identify some consequences for time-out refusal. Given the mother's anticipated response of "I can't," the therapist framed the assignment in a paradoxical manner: "This is probably a silly assignment, because, as you say, Tina controls everything in the family. Nevertheless, we may be missing one or two resources you've overlooked, so I'm going to ask you to identify one thing that Tina values that you do control." Paradoxical assignments put the therapist in a no-lose situation. If the mother fails, it was predicted; if she succeeds, the treatment can proceed.†

> †Paradoxical assignment is an interesting and effective technique when used appropriately in family therapy. The therapist did an excellent job of introducing this technique at a time that was most appropriate. There has been some argument in the professional literature as to whether this is actually considered a cognitive or

> *behavioral technique. Much of this may depend on the manner in which it works. As the reader can see, the technique worked nicely, and the mother produced two privileges that the child could control. Timing is crucial when this technique is used, since it may backfire if introduced at an inappropriate time.*

Mrs. S. came to the next session with two privileges she could control: Tina's bike (which could be locked in a neighbor's garage) and her bedside radio. This made it possible to move on to the use of time out at home. In preparation, the therapist and Mrs. S. carried out several time-out role plays. Sometimes Mrs. S. was asked to play Tina, sometimes herself. Sometimes they played out the scene correctly; at other times they purposely made mistakes, to demonstrate how this would interfere with the effectiveness of time out. After Mrs. S. began to feel secure in her role-play use of time out,† they invited Tina into the session to describe how things would be changing in the coming week. The explanation went something like the following:

> † *The use of paradoxical assignment was also quickly reinforced with the technique of role playing for the use of time-out procedures. This clearly helped to strengthen the mother's feelings of security, thus affecting her schema of functioning in a successful manner with her child.*

THERAPIST: *(Looking over the incentive chart and talking to Tina)* I see that you're minding your mom about 50% of the time now. That's a little better than when we started out. Good job!

TINA: *(Smiling and rubbing her hands together excitedly)* I like Popsicles!

THERAPIST: What's your favorite kind?

TINA: Orange.

THERAPIST: So you're getting about 4 points a day for minding.

TINA: *(Talking to the therapist about her mother)* Yeah, but sometimes *she* forgets, so *I* mark the points down. Then she gets really mad at me, but it's all her fault 'cause she doesn't write them down.

THERAPIST: We'll talk about that later. Right now I want to tell you about something new your mom's gonna do when you don't mind. She's going to send you to time out. Do you know what time out is?

TINA: They do it at school.

THERAPIST: At home, your mom's going to use it in a special way to help you learn to mind better. *(To Mom)* Do you want to tell her how it will go?

MOM: Sure. *(Turning to Tina)* From now on, when I ask you to do something, if you don't do it right away, I'm going to say, "Tina, that's not minding. Go to time out!"

TINA: Instead of saying "Go to hell"?

MOM: *(Sighing, shaking her head sadly, and whining)* Tiiinnnaa!

Mrs. S. reacted as she had a thousand times before, with a whimper and a whine. This was part of the pattern of interaction between mother and daughter that interfered with effective parenting. When Tina taunted her mother, Mrs. S. took the bait. In part, the mother's negative emotions created the problem. Sadness and defeat could be seen in her facial expression as she whined her disapproval. When Tina responded aggressively, it elicited a fearful reaction, which told Tina she could win the showdown. In PTT there is a heavy emphasis on teaching parents to stay focused on their goal, to remain calm, and to use neutral affect.

THERAPIST: *(Deflecting the incipient dispute between Mom and Tina, and continuing the explanation to Tina)* Time out is going to be in the bathroom. It lasts for 5 minutes if you go the first time your mother tells you. But if you argue or you don't go right away, you'll have minutes added, up to 10. If you don't go by 10, you'll lose a privilege.

TINA: I don't care.

This is a classic ploy used by many well-trained oppositional children. A variant of this theme is to say "I like it in time out," which is analogous to refusing to cry when spanked. For many parents, this buttresses their conviction that nothing they do will have an impact! Notice, however, that the therapist stayed focused on the agenda.

THERAPIST: Let's practice. Let's pretend I'm your mom. I'm going to tell you to put your coat on that chair *(pointing to chair)*. Please, don't do it. Then I'm going to tell you to go to time out. For now, time out is in the hall, just outside that door.

They practiced time out, first with the therapist as Mom, and then with Mom assuming her role. For the purpose of the role play, Tina was sometimes instructed to cooperate and at other times instructed not to cooperate. This familiarized both parent and child with several time-out principles: labeling behavior and invoking time out, adding minutes up to 10, removing a privilege, and staying calm throughout. Time-out role plays with wrong-way and right-way scenarios can be fun and instructional for parent and child. They also tend to reduce parental fears about unanticipated events at the same time they teach the child to behave appropriately.

The first week all went well, and everyone was encouraged. Tina earned rewards for good behavior 5 out of 7 days, and Mrs. S. was using time out successfully. However, one night the therapist received a telephone call at home from Mrs. S., who sounded quite desperate. The background noise was filled with screams and shouts; Tina was in a full-scale tantrum. Mrs. S. explained that she had sent Tina to time out, and Tina had subsequently destroyed the bathroom. Now she was up in her room having the tantrum of the century. Therapists can sometimes exert control over children by telephone in a way that seems quite magical. With a series of firm but quiet directives to calm down, breathe deeply, and go to bed, the therapist was able to get Tina to bed. An appointment was set up with the family for the next day. Meetings held immediately after a critical event can have maximal impact. The scene is still fresh in everyone's mind, with little time for distortions to develop. Furthermore, quick interventions prevent grudges from developing.

During the session, the therapist met separately with the mother and the child. Tina was asked about her feelings during out-of-control sieges. Tina explained that these were scary times for her. When they happened at school, they were especially embarrassing, and the kids would make fun of her and call her names. At home, they made everyone unhappy and caused a lot of trouble. Tina agreed that she needed to learn ways to calm herself down. With Mrs. S., the therapist was understanding of how difficult it is to change old patterns of behavior, but also pointed out that if the mother didn't take control while Tina was still a preadolescent, it could be impossible when she became a teenager. With both mother and child newly motivated to make time out work for them, the therapist brought them together and asked them to demonstrate exactly what had happened, so they could practice ways to avoid similar problems in the future. This led them into a reenactment of the previous night's explosion, which was videotaped.

Reenactments are a means for specifically retraining parents in effective handling of situations that have overwhelmed them in the past. Having them replay a troublesome scenario also evokes some of the negative affect that contributes to the problem.

THERAPIST: Try to be realistic, and do and say just what you did last night. *(To Mom)* You must have told her to go to time out? *(To Tina)* And you must have refused?

TINA: Yeah, I refused.

THERAPIST: *(To Mom)* Why don't you tell her to go to time out now? *(To Tina)* And you get yourself all riled up. But if you get riled up, will you be able to stop yourself later when I ask you to?†

> †*At this particular juncture, the therapist might have wanted to extend herself a bit to inquire into the specific thoughts that were passing through the child's mind as she was becoming "riled up."*

> *Perhaps her answer might have been that she was not thinking of anything in particular. However, sometimes "hot cognitions" accompany such behavior, and these can provide a therapist with a clue into a child's schemas at that moment. This line of inquiry might also have been applied to Tina's mother as well, and later used as a means to prompt the child into sharing her thoughts. The idea would have been to identify any erroneously based automatic thoughts and help the child begin a process of cognitive correction.*

TINA: Yeah, probably. I'll just act, and then I'll just stop.

THERAPIST: OK, good. As you act, I'll interrupt you both and ask some questions.

Asking whether Tina could regain control of herself set the stage for Tina's cooperation later on, should the reenactment get out of control. Tina's ability to control her behavior in session could also be expanded to an ability to control herself outside of the session.

MOM: At the same time this happened, I was trying to put Suzie to bed.

THERAPIST: Should we call Suzie in and have her be in this reenactment?

MOM: No, the big problem was with Tina. *(She turned to Tina, and, getting into role, explained:)* So you were hassling Suzie, pretty much, right?

TINA: *(Giggling)* Yeah.

MOM: And I said, "Go get ready for bed." *(Moving toward Tina)* OK, Tina, it's time now.

TINA: *(Putting her hands on her hips, sticking out her chin, and shouting)* NO!!

MOM: *(Softly)* It's late, though. It's time.

TINA: *(Shouting)* I don't care!

MOM: But you must go up.

TINA: I'm not going!

MOM: OK, that's time out. *(Tina made growling noises and swung both arms to pretend she was hitting her sister, all the while ignoring her mother. Mom approached Tina tentatively and took hold of her arms. Tina started hitting her. Mom disengaged and backed off.)* OK, now that's 6 minutes.

TINA: *(Growling and shadow-boxing)*

MOM: Seven minutes.

TINA: *(Still growling and swinging)* I don't care!

MOM: Eight minutes. *(She approached Tina, took hold of her by the shoulders, and started to move with her toward time out.)*

TINA: *(Yelling)* NOOOO!!

MOM: That's 9 minutes. And you'll lose your bike if you don't go now. *(She took Tina by the shoulders and gently pushed her toward time out.)*

TINA: NOOOO!!

MOM: Go in. You did go in at 9 minutes.

TINA: *(Pretending to go into time out and stand in the corner)*

MOM: *(Explaining now to the therapist)* I'm in the other room, and Tina is in the bathroom.

THERAPIST: *(To Tina)* OK, what are you doing in the bathroom?

TINA: *(Growling and pounding on the wall)*

THERAPIST: What are you doing with the toilet?

TINA: Suzie forgot to flush it. I flushed it and it went WHOOOSH!!! All over! It almost overflowed, and I tried to fix it.

MOM: And then what happened?

TINA: *(Screaming urgently while appearing to hold the toilet seat down)* MOOMMMMMMM!!!

MOM: *(Approaching and going in)* Tina was trying to hold the toilet seat down, and it was real crowded, so I told her, "Get out of the way, out of the way." *(She gently pushed Tina out of the room and stooped down, apparently trying to fix the toilet.)* And I got down and was fixing it, and you ran out, and what did you do?

TINA: I don't know.

MOM: You said, "You're in time out!"

TINA: *(Giggling in a silly way, pretending to slam the bathroom door, dancing around, and chanting)* Ha ha ha ha ha. You're in time out. Ha ha ha ha ha. You're in time out.

MOM: I was cleaning up, and then *(to Tina)* what did you do with the shovel?

TINA: I didn't do anything. Grabbed it, that's all. *(She pretended to grab a shovel, approaches the bathroom door while growling.)* Grrrrrrrr.

MOM: And I was cleaning up. What are you doing?

TINA: *(Pretending to bang on the door with the shovel)*

MOM: She's banging on the door with the shovel.

THERAPIST: *(To Tina)* While you're banging on the door with the shovel, tell me how you feel in your body.

TINA: *(Growling)* Mad.†

> † *The therapist chose here to focus on an affective level, which produced what one might expect—an emotion of anger. Perhaps more might have been gained by inquiring, "What thought is going through your head as you growl?" Focusing on the cognitive content is often a way to introduce a method for restructuring thought content without interfering with the process of emotion. It may also provide a therapist with a window into unrealistic or irrational belief processes, which can then be restructured through weighing alternatives.*

THERAPIST: Where do you feel mad the most?

TINA: In my hands.

The purpose of this interruption by the therapist was to gather information that would be used later in the session to help Tina with anger control. (The technique was first introduced to us by Robert Wahler during a workshop in Banff in 1981.)

THERAPIST: OK, go back to banging on the door with the shovel.

MOM: *(Approaching Tina and trying to stop her)* Tina, you can't bang on the door. Give me the shovel. Give me the shovel. *(The two of them struggled over the shovel.)* Give me the shovel before you break something. *(They continued to struggle. Tina was laughing hysterically. Mom got the shovel and tried to physically guide Tina upstairs to bed.)*

TINA: Give me that! Give me that! *(Giggling hysterically)*

MOM: That's pretty much how it went until I got her upstairs.

THERAPIST: Were you laughing or were you crying during all that, Tina? *(Silence)* Laughing or crying?

TINA: Uhhhhhhh. *(Nervously)* Crying. *(She was dancing around the room, all hyped up, shaking her hands.)*

THERAPIST: Are you all hyped up now?

TINA: *(Nodding)*

THERAPIST: I want you to sit down on the floor. Sit down on the floor. *(Tina sat down.)* Feel how your hands feel. Feel all that energy in your hands?

TINA: Yeah.

THERAPIST: Shake the energy out. *(Tina shook her hands vehemently.)* Close your eyes and breathe real deep. *(Tina did, but her body was obviously very tense. The therapist went over to Tina and got on the floor with her, placing her hands gently on her arms and showing her what to do.)*

As you breathe in, the energy goes up your fingers, up your arms, into your shoulders. Breathe out and the energy goes down your arms and out your fingers. *(Slowly the therapist had Tina breathe in and breathe out, directing the energy up and down her arms with her hands. After four or five sets of breaths, Tina appeared relaxed.)* Now how do you feel?

TINA: Better.

THERAPIST: Calmer?

TINA: Yeah.

THERAPIST: It's easy to be calm now 'cause it's not the real thing.

TINA: I wouldn't still be mad.

THERAPIST: Instead of letting your body run away with you, you need to take charge of your body. It's hard to take charge unless you sit down and . . .

TINA: Relax.

THERAPIST: Right. Relax yourself.

Teaching Tina to regulate her own out-of-control behavior was an effort to prevent explosions and reduce the "I won'ts" that drove her mother's "I can'ts."

MOM: When she starts to get out of control, she gets a demonic look on her face. She just changes.

TINA: Like . . . I get all . . . *(She growled, scrunched up her face, and started flailing her arms and legs around.)*

THERAPIST: *(Getting up and walking over to the camera)* OK, I'm going to zero in on your face.

TINA: *(Making a variety of silly faces)*

THERAPIST: Give me your most demonic expression.

TINA: *(Making a silly face)*

THERAPIST: Out of control.

TINA: *(Growling, throwing her body around, baring her teeth)*

THERAPIST: Are you really out of control?

TINA: *(Nodding and continuing)*

THERAPIST: OK, now calm yourself.

TINA: *(Trying, but very tense)*

THERAPIST: *(Quietly)* Really calm yourself. Breathe deeply. Inhale and feel the energy go up your arms. Now exhale. Inhale. Exhale.

TINA: *(Obviously starting to relax)*

THERAPIST: Look up now and give me a sweet smile.

TINA: *(Trying, but it's silly)*

THERAPIST: Oh, that's silly.

TINA: *(Improving her smile)*

THERAPIST: That's nice!

TINA: *(Embarrassed, but continuing to smiling sweetly)*

THERAPIST: Want to see yourself on TV now?

TINA: *(Jumping up, excited to do so)* Yeah!

This session was a turning point in the case. Tina and her mother were now working together instead of at odds. Portions of the reenactment videotape were used in separate meetings with Mrs. S. and Tina. In the sessions between Mrs. S. and the therapist, the two brainstormed and role-played ways to prevent such problems and to intervene more effectively when they did take place. With Tina, the focus was on relaxation training and social skills with peers. There were also some sessions with Tina and Suzie together, teaching the sisters to play more cooperatively.

At about the midpoint of the treatment, the therapy focused on the mother's depression. Unfortunately, aggressive children don't give their parents much respite, even when it is sorely needed, and the parent training had to continue. Mrs. S. complained that she was too overwhelmed to do the kind of parenting it takes to raise a girl like Tina (i.e., the parenting procedures introduced in the intervention). The therapist responded paradoxically, telling her that in fact, Mrs. S. should *not* use incentive charts or time out. She should just go back to the way things were when Tina ran the family. Mrs. S.'s response was predictable: *"I can't!"* she exclaimed. *"I could never regain control if I give it up now!"* That moved the session into a problem-solving mode aimed toward figuring out how Mrs. S. could parent, given her low energy level. Gradually, Mrs. S.'s mood lifted; the parent training was completed; and after 17 sessions the family was able to terminate.†

> † *This is an excellent example of how a straight behavioral technique was able to lift a depressed mood and enable a weary mother to find strength to go on. Unfortunately, this isn't always the case; at times, the use of cognitive interventions may be useful in dealing with distorted perceptions such as those experienced by the mother in this situation. It would be interesting to investigate whether the mother's depression was a familiar pattern and whether this was her way of shutting out or sabotaging progress in treatment. A cognitive-oriented*

approach might have investigated more into the thoughts and perceptions of the mother, in order to insure that such a pattern would not become a future entity. Such techniques as cognitive restructuring of automatic thoughts and distortions might have been helpful.

The short-term outcome for this case was positive. Tina was retained in the gifted and talented program at school. Data from the observations at home revealed significant reductions in Tina's aggressive behavior from baseline to termination. Reports by Mrs. S. and Tina's teacher also indicated a significant reduction on the Aggression scale of the Child Behavior Checklist (Achenbach & Edelbrock, 1983). The long-term outcome was less impressive, however. Approximately 2 years after termination, Tina went to live with her father, who had moved out of state. During the time she lived with her father, she had four documented police contacts—one for running away, one for menacing, and two for assaults. The charges were dropped on all four arrests, but they do indicate that the long-term outcome for this case was less than perfect. We have often thought that families who are successful with their treatment for children's behavior problems would benefit from regular "booster shots," particularly during critical transitions, such as change of custody or the transition into adolescence.†

† The authors have done a superb job of presenting a case in which the therapist utilized straight behavioral techniques. The addition of the cognitive strategies proposed might have served to fortify the effects of the behavioral strategies, and perhaps would have resulted in more of a likelihood of permanent behavior change.

AUTHORS' REPLY TO EDITOR'S COMMENTS

The core idea in PTT is that if parents change the contingencies, then the child's behavior will change. As these changes occur, there will be commensurate changes in emotions and in how family members feel about each other. As neobehaviorists, we can be convinced by empirical findings that we should add other components, such as anger control techniques or cognitive elements. Nearly 20 years ago, we were convinced that family therapy as it was being taught in Palo Alto by Sluzki, Watzlawick, and Weakland could be added to our standard parent training procedures. As this case study illustrates, we have actually put these procedures into practice as part of our standard treatment package. The fact that there are now at least two well-controlled studies demonstrating the utility of combining ideas from behavioral approaches and strategic family therapy convinces us that this is a good thing. The studies that relate to the issue of enhancing PTT are reviewed in the paper by Patterson et al. (1993).

On pages 97–98, 100, and 103, we find ourselves disagreeing with Dr.

Dattilio's comments. We realize that the primary assumption of a cognitive therapist is that to change behavior, one must change thoughts. However, in our 20 or 30 years of clinical experience, we find that the extent to which the therapist begins to delve into the myriad thoughts, recollections, and memories that a client might have about a given event actually slows the therapy down. It's a lot easier and perhaps a lot more fun for the therapist to do this, but we do not think it contributes directly to progress in the case. Again, it's a question of providing data to demonstrate that adding thought probes to PTT would speed up the process. The data we have collected suggest that as parents change their behavior and the problem behaviors of the child are reduced, thoughts also change, as do the angry feelings. The PTT movement is still strongly data-based. The fact that three different centers have been able to use random assignment designs and produce replicable results leads us to believe that being data-based is a healthy thing. So, in that spirit, it would be interesting to run some studies where we add thought probes to PTT to determine whether the addition of these new components speeds things up or (as we suspect) slows them down.

In summary, it may well be that the cognitive-behavioral techniques are compatible with our PTT model. Again, however, it is an empirical question, and the truth remains to be demonstrated.

ACKNOWLEDGMENTS

We would like to acknowledge the following grants from the National Institute of Mental Health, which provided support for the writing of this chapter: Grant Nos. R01 MH38318, R01 MH54703, and P50 MH46690, all from the Prevention and Behavioral Medicine Research Branch, Division of Epidemiology and Services Research.

REFERENCES

Achenbach, T. M., & Edelbrock, C. S. (1983). *Manual for the Child Behavior Checklist and the Revised Child Behavior Profile*. Burlington: University of Vermont, Department of Psychiatry.

Bank, L., Forgatch, M. S., Patterson, G. R., & Fetrow, R. A. (1993). Parenting practices of single mothers: Mediators of negative contextual factors. *Journal of Marriage and the Family, 55*, 371–384.

Conger, R. D., Patterson, G. R., & Ge, X. (1995). It takes two to replicate: A mediational model for the impact of parents' stress on adolescent adjustment. *Child Development, 66*, 80–97.

Dadds, M. R., Schwartz, S., & Sanders, M. R. (1987). Marital discord and treatment outcome in behavioral treatment of child conduct disorders. *Journal of Consulting and Clinical Psychology, 55*, 396–403.

Dishion, T. J., & Patterson, G. R. (1992). Age effects in parent training outcomes. *Behavior Therapy, 23*, 719–729.

Dishion, T. J., Patterson, G. R., & Griesler, P. C. (1994). Peer adaptation in the development of antisocial behavior: A confluence model. In L. R. Huesmann (Ed.), *Current perspectives on aggressive behavior* (pp. 61–95). New York: Plenum Press.

Forehand, R., Wells, K., & Sturgis, E. (1978). Predictors of child noncompliant behavior in the home. *Journal of Consulting and Clinical Psychology, 46,* 179.

Forgatch, M. S. (1991). The clinical science vortex: Developing a theory for antisocial behavior. In D. Pepler & K. H. Rubin (Eds.), *The development and treatment of childhood aggression* (pp. 291–315). Hillsdale, NJ: Erlbaum.

Forgatch, M. S., & Patterson, G. R. (1989). *Parents and adolescents living together: Vol. 2. Family problem solving.* Eugene, OR: Castalia.

Greenwood, P. W., Model, K. E., Rydell, C. P., & Chiesa, J. (1996). *Diverting children from a life of crime: Measuring costs and benefits* (0-8330-2383-7). Santa Monica: RAND prepared report for the University of California, Berkeley, James Irvine Foundation.

Hawkins, R. P., Peterson, R. F., Schweid, E., & Bijou, S. W. (1966). Behavior therapy in the home: Amelioration of problem parent–child relations with the parent in a therapeutic role. *Journal of Experimental Child Psychology, 4,* 99–107.

Kazdin, A. E. (1987). Treatment of antisocial behavior in children: Current status and future directions. *Psychological Bulletin, 102,* 187–203.

Larzelere, R. E., & Patterson, G. R. (1990). Parental management: Mediator of the effect of socioeconomic status on early delinquency. *Criminology, 28,* 301–324.

Laub, J. H., & Sampson, R. J. (1988). Unraveling families and delinquency: A reanalysis of the Gluecks' data. *Criminology, 26,* 355–380.

Levitt, E. E. (1957). Research on psychotherapy with children: An evaluation. *Journal of Consulting Psychology, 21,* 189–196.

Levitt, E. E. (1971). Research on psychotherapy with children. In A. E. Bergin & S. L. Garfield (Eds.), *Handbook of psychotherapy and behavior change* (pp. 474–494). New York: Wiley.

Lipsey, M. W. (1992). The effect of treatment on juvenile delinquents: Results from meta-analysis. In F. Losel, D. Bender, & T. Bliesener (Eds.), *Psychology and law: International perspectives* (pp. 131–143). New York: Walter de Gruyter.

Patterson, G. R. (1980). Mothers: The unacknowledged victims. *Monographs of the Society for Research in Child Development, 45*(5, Serial No. 186).

Patterson, G. R., & Brodsky, G. (1966). A behavior modification program for a child with multiple problem behaviors. *Journal of Child Psychology and Psychiatry, 7,* 277–295.

Patterson, G. R., & Chamberlain, P. (1988). Treatment process: A problem at three levels. In L. C. Wynne (Ed.), *State of the art in family therapy research: Controversies and recommendations* (pp. 189–223). New York: Family Process Press.

Patterson, G. R., & Chamberlain, P. (1994). A functional analysis of resistance during parent training therapy. *Clinical Psychology: Science and Practice, 1*(1), 53–70.

Patterson, G. R., Dishion, T. J., & Chamberlain, P. (1993). Outcomes and methodological issues relating to treatment of antisocial children. In T. R. Giles (Ed.), *Effective psychotherapy: A handbook of comparative research* (pp. 43–88). New York: Plenum Press.

Patterson, G. R., & Forgatch, M. S. (1985). Therapist behavior as a determinant for client resistance: A paradox for the behavior modified. *Journal of Consulting and Clinical Psychology, 5,* 237–262.

Patterson, G. R., & Forgatch, M. S. (1987). *Parents and adolescents living together: Vol. 1. The basics.* Eugene, OR: Castalia.

Patterson, G. R., & Forgatch, M. S. (1995). Predicting future clinical adjustment from treatment outcome and process variables. *Psychological Assessment, 7,* 275–285.

Patterson, G. R., Littman, R. A., & Bricker, W. (1967). Assertive behavior in children: A step towards a theory of aggression. *Monographs of the Society for Research in Child Development, 32*(Serial No. 5), 1–43.

Patterson, G. R., & Reid, J. B. (1984). Social interactional processes within the family: The study of moment-by-moment family transactions in which human social development is embedded. *Journal of Applied Developmental Psychology, 5,* 237–262.

Patterson, G. R., Reid, J. B., & Dishion, T. J. (1992). *A social interactional approach: Vol. 4. Antisocial boys.* Eugene, OR: Castalia.

Roberts, M. W., & Powers, S. W. (1988). The compliance test. *Behavioral Assessment, 10,* 375–398.

Roberts, M. W., & Powers, S. W. (1990). Adjusting chair timeout enforcement procedures for oppositional children. *Behavior Therapy, 21,* 257–271.

Snyder, J. J., & Brown, K. (1983). Oppositional behavior and noncompliance in preschool children: Environmental correlates and skill deficits. *Behavioral Assessment, 5,* 333–348.

Snyder, J. J., Edwards, P., McGraw, K., Kilgore, K., & Holton, A. (1994). Escalation and reinforcement in mother–child conflict: Social processes associated with the development of physical aggression. *Development and Psychopathology, 6,* 305–321.

Snyder, J. J., & Patterson, G. R. (1995). Individual differences in social aggression: A test of a reinforcement model of socialization in the natural environment. *Behavior Therapy, 26,* 371–391.

Stoolmiller, M., Duncan, T. E., Bank, L., & Patterson, G. R. (1993). Some problems and solutions in the study of change: Significant patterns of client resistance. *Journal of Consulting and Clinical Psychology, 61,* 920–928.

Wahler, R. G. (1968). *Behavior therapy for oppositional children: Love is not enough.* Paper presented at the meeting of the Southeastern Psychological Association, Atlanta, GA.

Whiting, B. B., & Whiting, J. M. (1975). *Children of six cultures.* Cambridge, MA: Harvard University Press.

SUGGESTED READINGS

Forgatch, M. S., & Knutson, N. M. (in press). Prevention science vortex: Linking basic and applied research. In H. Liddle, G. Diamond, R. Levant, & J. Bray (Eds.), *Family psychology intervention science.* Washington, DC: American Psychological Association.

Forgatch, M. S., & Patterson, G. R. (1989). *Parents and adolescents living together: Vol. 2. Family problem solving.* Eugene, OR: Castalia.

Patterson, G. R., & Chamberlain, P. (1994). A functional analysis of resistance during parent training therapy. *Journal of Clinical Psychology: Science and Practice, 1*(1), 53–70.

Patterson, G. R., & Forgatch, M. S. (1987). *Parents and adolescents living together. Vol. 1. The basics.* Eugene, OR: Castalia.

Patterson, G. R., & Forgatch, M. S. (1995). Predicting future clinical adjustment from treatment outcome and process variables. *Psychological Assessment, 7*(3), 275–285.

Chapter 5

Structural Family Therapy

SALVADOR MINUCHIN
MICHAEL P. NICHOLS

The first thing to understand about how couples are structured is that some measure of complementarity is the defining principle of every relationship. In any partnership, one person's behavior is yoked to the other's. This simple statement has profound implications: It means that a couple's actions aren't independent; they're codetermined, subject to reciprocal forces that support or polarize. It also challenges the cherished belief in one's own Self—that good old free-willed, autonomous island of a Self everyone likes to think of themselves as.

Couple therapy seems to go against logic. What members of a couple want isn't help but vindication. They want to tell the world how unfair their partner is, how insensitive, and how difficult it is to live with such a person. At other times, they want absolution: "It's my drinking, my depression, my temper." Complaints are presented in individual terms: the accusatory "She this," "He that," or the penitent "It's me." They come to therapy to settle accounts. But, to the family therapist, they're both wrong. It's not him; it's not her—it's the structural patterns that make them a family, a system of interconnected lives governed by strict but unspoken rules (Minuchin & Nichols, 1993).

When structural family therapists begin to analyze such destructive patterns of interaction, part of what we do is disentangle individuals from their automatic yoked reactions. We help them discover their individuality, their power, and their responsibility. It's paradoxical: By helping people understand their contexts, we empower them to take responsibility for their choices and change (Minuchin & Fishman, 1981).

In this chapter, we describe a case that illustrates our use of these principles. Although we have written the chapter together, Dr. Minuchin served as the therapist for this case, and thus he is the "I" in what follows.

FIRST SESSION

"Marital problems." That's what he said. He was Philip Lockwood, a neuropsychologist on the staff of a prominent hospital. A mutual friend had given him my number. He apologized profusely for calling me at home, saying he knew how busy I must be, but he wanted to see me as soon as possible. As a matter of fact, I'd been expecting his call. The friend who recommended me had called and said that he was afraid the Lockwoods were on the verge of divorce. I told Dr. Lockwood I'd been expecting to hear from him, and offered him an appointment that he accepted immediately.

The Lockwoods were waiting in my reception room when I arrived just before 9 A.M.. Philip Lockwood was a tall, handsome man, elegantly groomed and carefully dressed. His short curly hair was still black, but his meticulously trimmed beard was flecked with white. He introduced himself and shook hands. Then he introduced his wife, Lauren. She took my hand but didn't shake it. She spoke with a refined Southern accent. Lauren Lockwood had the natural ease of a woman who knows she's beautiful but is no longer self-conscious about it.

I invited them into my office, and Philip sat down on the couch, crossed his legs, and clasped his hands around one knee. Lauren started toward the couch, but then moved to the chair next to it.

I asked who wanted to begin, looking automatically at Lauren. She turned to her husband and said, "Why don't you start?" That surprised me. Usually when couples come for therapy, wives start in with their list of grievances, while their husbands sit back in the dock and wait to defend themselves.

"Well, we've been married 20 years," Philip began. "I'm 50, Lauren is 42, and we have one child. We met in Zambia, when I was in the Peace Corps—we both were. I thought what we were doing was important. That we could make a difference. Lauren seemed to feel the same way. She seemed to believe in the same things I did—back then."

I glanced at Lauren. She seemed prepared to sit and listen patiently, so I listened too, nodding occasionally, waiting for him to get to the "marital problems." He spoke at great, windy length, making sure I got all the facts right. He talked about going to graduate school. He talked about his career and eventually about their son, Jeffrey, now 12. He talked about how they'd waited so long because they didn't want to bring a child into the world until they were secure enough to support him. I glanced at Lauren, and she nodded, accepting this statement of the facts.

Philip went on talking, still not getting to those marital problems. He'd been talking nearly 15 minutes. I was struck by the orderly march of his narrative, his emphasis on himself, his love of complicated phrases. Absent from his arid account was any sense of the affection and desire that can keep two people together for 20 years, or of the frustration and bitterness that can make it a trial.

I looked again at Lauren, wondering when, if ever, she would challenge his version of events. But she seemed content to sit and listen, silent, lovely, composed.

Finally, as Philip approached the present, he touched on what brought them to see me. "Over the years we've had some basic differences of opinion—which . . . we aren't always able to communicate in a civilized manner."

"*Communicate?*" All at once, Lauren was blazing. "Why don't you tell him how you communicate!" She turned to me. "He hit me and knocked me down! He broke my collarbone! And it wasn't the first time, either."

I waited to hear more, but she fell silent. The anger she'd been holding back suddenly erupted, and then, just as suddenly as it began, it was over.

"I didn't mean to hurt her," Philip muttered. He was sullen, clearly embarrassed, but not quite contrite. "She keeps harping and harping at me. I never get a break. Sometimes she makes me so mad I don't know what I'm doing, and that's the truth." I've heard that complaint many times. It's what some psychologists call "pleading violence": "Please stop making me hurt you."

I turned to Lauren, giving her the floor. Now I heard a very different story of the marriage. Lauren's account was more about the relationship and feelings.

"When we were in Africa, I looked up to him." Calmer now, she spoke quietly. "He seemed so mature, so sure of himself. Of course he was 8 years older. Then again, it was a special time. I'll be honest: I joined the Peace Corps mainly because I wanted to live abroad for a few years. I wasn't all that idealistic. Philip really believed in what we were doing. I really admired that. He made me feel important, too." She paused.

"But from the day we were married, everything revolved around him. It was *his* PhD, *his* career. Things were fine as long as everything went his way. As long as I was the good little wife, he was happy. I put him through graduate school. I typed his papers; I did all the housework; and when he wanted to throw parties for the department, I did that too. All he ever thought about was himself. He'd come home whining about how hard everything was or how someone hurt his feelings, and I was supposed to hold his hand."

Philip shot her a look of pure hate, but she continued. "Then we had Jeffrey. And I did everything for him, too. If Philip condescended to change a diaper or take the baby for a walk, he expected to be showered with praise."

I listened, as I usually do in a first interview—trying to hear, beneath the content of what they were saying, the desires and fears that kept them from hearing each other. Lauren's presentation puzzled me. Her anger seemed to switch on and off. When she listened to Philip, she seemed totally receptive. When she did finally speak, she showed only her anger and none of the hurt and longing behind it. And Philip listened about as well as most people do when they feel attacked.

Their story was common enough. A perfectly decent, somewhat insecure, somewhat self-centered man had married a beautiful and intelligent woman. She had many attractive traits, none more attractive than how good she made him feel about himself. A perfectly decent, somewhat insecure 22-year-old woman, with little sense of herself other than as someone who was attractive to men, had married a serious man who adored her. What could be more natural?

Like most couples, they'd learned to cope with conflict through a combination of distance and compromise. Lauren had done most of the accommodating. This seemed natural to both of them. Philip had his career; his struggle was to make it in the larger world. Lauren had the relationship; her struggle was to make it work.

The first crack in the structure of their relationship came when Philip started putting more into his doctoral studies and less into the relationship. In marrying Philip, Lauren forsook any prior existence of her own and stepped into her husband's life. She moved from Charleston to New York to be with Philip, giving up friends and familiar surroundings. But as Philip began spending long hours at school, his interests increasingly excluded her. When she complained or asked for more attention, he'd react as though she'd broken the rules: "Why have you become so demanding?" As far as he was concerned, she'd changed.

He'd come home tired. (He'd come home late.) He wanted to rest. (She wanted to talk.) He'd turn on the television. She'd make some crack, "You're so selfish," and he'd respond, "You're such a baby." They traded insults, but neither could bear the heat of the other's anger and so they'd back off, smoking and sputtering until they cooled down. After a day or two they'd resume as before, with the unresolved issues between them forgotten for the moment.

Then something happened that upset the whole balance of the relationship. When Jeffrey was old enough for day care, Lauren went back to school and got an MBA—"with Philip's full support," she emphasized. Lauren was amazed at how well she did in graduate school. She'd never thought of herself as particularly intelligent, and so it came as a real surprise to discover that she was able to grasp economics with so little trouble and that she had a real flair for analysis. After completing her degree, she landed a job in a management consulting firm. There, her unused energy, charm, and ability to analyze complex management structures propelled her to a full partnership in less than 5 years.

If the first crack in the harmonious structure of the marriage occurred when Philip started putting his career first and Lauren second, the real rupture came when her success made her no longer dependent on him. Now, she said, she was making more money than Philip. (She shot him a look.) After Lauren started working and the balance of the relationship shifted, their arguments took on a different quality. Philip felt the threat of her independence much more powerfully than her previous complaints of neglect. And now when Philip started in on her, instead of backing off, Lauren snapped back at him. That's when the hitting started.

As Lauren told her side of the story, her face hardened in rage and pain. When she first mentioned the hitting, Philip looked away, ashamed. But as she went on and on, I could see him getting angrier and angrier. Lauren said that she was afraid: "I don't know if I can stay in this marriage." She glanced at Philip, then dropped her eyes.

I said to them, "I'm sorry, but I don't work with primitive people." Philip looked down. Lauren looked hurt. I let that sink in for a minute. "Therapy is a privilege. People who hit people are too primitive to take advantage of it. They don't have enough self-control." My words were hard. In this volatile situation I didn't want to be understanding; I wanted to be in control.

Lauren looked at her husband. She looked at a stone wall.

I continued, "I will, however, offer you a consultation on one condition. I'll see you for six sessions. At the end of that time, I'll give you my recommendation as to whether you should separate or seek therapy to stay together. But I must have your absolute assurance that there will be no hitting during this period."

Grateful for this chance to prove himself, Philip said, "Don't worry, it will be all right."

"It's not *it* I'm worried about," I said bluntly. "It's *you*. If you even start to lose your temper, leave the room. Go for a walk. Go in the kitchen and break a dish. But cool down. And Lauren, if there is any hitting, or if you even think there might be, I want you to call me at once."

"I will," she said.

I ended the session with a question. I told them that they seemed to have become inflexible with each other. Their success in other areas of their lives indicated that there had to be more to them than I was seeing here. Why had they become so intolerant and unforgiving with each other? "Maybe you can begin to think about what you two do to trigger this reactive emotionality in each other."

They left, and I sat alone in my office. In agreeing to see Lauren and Philip together, I knew I was taking a risk, and I was aware of the alternatives. I was taking the chance of seeing them together, because I believe that this is the best way to get at the sequence of events that triggers violence. But I also knew that I had to structure the sessions carefully and take a directive stance. With violent couples I remain distant, controlling the nature of the communication even while we explore patterns of interaction.

I knew that I would have to stop the spiraling escalation of emotions. With most families I encourage dialogue between family members right from the beginning, as a way of exploring how people talk together and of exposing the structure of their relationships. In violent families, however, I discourage interaction. I tell couples that until they can have a dialogue with more light than heat, they should take turns, each talking to me without interruption. I do everything I can to slow them down and make them think. I encourage them to be specific, using concrete details as an antidote to emotionality.†

> †*Already, in the initial session, Dr. Minuchin addressed the issue of physical abuse and solicited a promise from the husband that there would be no more hitting. Although this was a prudent move, it ran the risk of setting Philip up to fail by providing him with little in the way of strategies to curtail a behavior that was apparently already rather strongly ingrained. The therapist could have addressed this issue in a bit more structured form by providing Philip with some specific strategies for dealing with his anger. Minuchin made a good move in directing Philip to extricate himself from a tense situation at the point at which his anger began to swell; however, the additional techniques of deep breathing and cognitively restructuring his thoughts could also have served as excellent diffusing agents to prevent any future altercations (Dattilio & Padesky, 1990).*

This isn't my natural way of working. It's something I learned from Murray Bowen 20 years ago. "Don't tell me how you feel," he said to a violent couple. "Tell me what you think."†

> †*I couldn't have stated this better myself. To the cognitive-behavioral therapist, thought content during emotionally charged situations is paramount.*

SECOND SESSION

To my considerable surprise, Philip and Lauren were very late for the second session. He walked in alone 25 minutes late. While we waited for Lauren, I asked Philip to explain why they weren't together.

"We were waiting for the subway, and she suddenly announced that she wasn't going to ride on the subway with me. She was going to take a cab. She's always doing things like that. Maybe she decided not to come, or maybe she had trouble finding a cab."

Three minutes later Lauren arrived, red-faced and out of breath. She gave Philip a withering look, and he glared back. Before their anger erupted in the usual barrage of recriminations, I said, "Please tell me exactly what happened this morning, from the time you got up. I want a very detailed account, from each of you, one at a time." This couple seemed to operate at two speeds: idle and out of control.

Philip spoke first. "I got up at 5, as I always do, so that I could do my exercises and my meditation. I knew Lauren wouldn't get up until about 6:30, as usual, and that I'd have plenty of time to dress and get ready, so I thought I had time to finish the book I was reading—Henri Bergson's *Introduction to Metaphysics*. Do you know it? It's the one where he talks about two different ways of knowing, the symbolic way of science and—"

"Oh, Christ, Philip, get on with it," Lauren cut in. "Nobody's interested in your—"

"Can't you keep your mouth shut for 2 minutes?" Philip was livid.

I stood up and said, "Please slow down." I also asked Philip to move his chair away from Lauren and closer to me, so that I could hear each of their versions without interruption.

After Philip had done his exercises and meditation, and while he was reading his Bergson, Lauren got up and made breakfast for Jeffrey. She got him out of bed, dressed, and into the kitchen, where she ate with him and got him off to school. She showered and dressed, but when she was ready to go she found that Philip was still reading "his stupid book."

She said, "I'm ready, let's go," and he said, "I just need to put my jacket on." But when he was dressed, she discovered that he still had to pack his briefcase. Lauren said, "Why don't you pack everything the night before instead of always making us late? If you would just think ahead 5 minutes, instead of leaving everything to the last minute—" "Oh, just shut up," he told her. "Go hail a cab; I'll be right there." She went, but by this time she was seething. Down on the street, Lauren couldn't find a cab. When Philip arrived they waited a few more minutes, but still no cabs. Then he said, "It's getting late. Let's take the subway." They walked to the train, but as they entered the station, Lauren said, "I can't ride that thing. My shoulder aches. I'm going to find a cab." And she left.

These people lacked both the capacity to see the other's perspective and the sympathy that allows tolerance of differences, so that every issue became a struggle for the survival of self. Every conflict became a conflagration, while they remained ignorant of the ways they provoked each other.†

---

†*Dr. Minuchin comments that Philip and Lauren "lacked both the capacity to see each other's perspective and the sympathy that allows tolerance of differences." A significant part of cognitive-behavioral*

> *therapy involves teaching partners and family members how to see the situation at hand from different perspectives by considering alternative explanations and utilizing a technique known as "reframing." Here, the use of the Dysfunctional Thought Record (see Chapter 1, Figure 1.3) might have been useful in urging Philip and Lauren to explore and weigh out alternative explanations—to attempt to view the situation from an alternative perspective. This could have encouraged them in a therapeutic way to relinquish some of the "struggle for the survival of self" that Minuchin accurately identified. This could also have offered them a selection of tools to which they could refer during crisis periods.*

Philip held Lauren entirely responsible for their being late. Even though he had gotten up an hour and a half before his wife, he still expected her to take charge of getting Jeffrey off to school and making sure that they got to their appointment on time. They were like the couples Mary Catherine Bateson describes, in which the wife is expected to respond to and manage multiple events in the family, while the husband remains focused on what for him is the "main event." I knew I would be challenging this structure.

One reason people react with alarm to applying a systems point of view to a case in which a man beats his wife is that such a viewpoint may be seen as denying the awful wrongness of physical violence and overlooking the need for strong steps to stop it. Cases in which a man batters a woman to bend her to his will generally do require restraint by separation, and often intervention by the police and judiciary; the priority is to protect the victim. But there are couples, like Philip and Lauren, who want to stay together but are locked in a cycle of mutual provocation that leads to violence.

In this case, my first priority would be to control Philip's attacks. But I would also challenge Lauren's sense of helplessness. For some reason, she seemed to think of herself as incapable; I would focus on her competence, supporting her ability to stand up for herself.

THIRD SESSION

By the third session I felt comfortable with Lauren and Philip, and I sensed that they trusted me. By staying with them in the face of their snarling and snapping in the two previous sessions, and remaining respectful of them, I'd given them hope. But I decided that they still weren't ready to talk together without slipping into attack and defense. Somehow the maturity they demonstrated as individuals got lost when they interacted as a couple.

I decided therefore to continue with the same format, asking each one consecutively to talk with me. When I do that, I always accept each person's perception of what the other does as correct, but I explain that I want them to learn to see their own behavior. "You're so focused on responding that you're blind to yourself," I explain. "I want you to look at your contribution."†

> † *This may have been an excellent point at which to begin to introduce the notion of schemas. As readers will recall from Chapter 1, a "schema" is a familiar pattern of ideas and a manner of thinking to which new experiences can be assimilated. Philip and Lauren had clearly developed schemas about themselves, each other, and their relationship. If the therapist had begun to facilitate the revelation of Philip's and Lauren's schemas in the therapy session, this might have shed light on their pattern of behaviors. This was also a point at which some additional homework assignments might have been utilized. The use of the Dysfunctional Thought Record, mentioned previously, would have helped Philip and Lauren to keep track of their automatic thoughts in a systematic fashion and to identify cognitive distortions, especially regarding their perceptions.*

I started with Lauren because something seemed to be happening with her. She was more involved and interested in the process, and she seemed more ready to look at her role in the couple's troubles. Besides, I wanted to keep Philip uncertain of my affiliation with him, as a way of keeping him alert and in control of himself.

"Lauren, I'm really interested in what you do to diminish each other. The way you make each other less than what you are. But I want to talk to you one at a time, until you can talk to each other without attacking." I kept my tone formal, almost pedagogical, as part of my message that there were rational solutions to their emotional quandaries.

"Well, I think he doesn't like what I do—"

"No, no," I said. "That's for him to say. Let him make his own complaints. What does he do that bothers you?"

"Oh, you want me to tell you what *he* does to me?"

"Yes."

"Well, he makes me just furious sometimes, the way he treats me."

"What does he do?"

"Everything centers on him. He expects me to listen to every little thing that goes on at the hospital, but he never asks me about my work. If I try to tell him something, he may listen for a minute, but that's all I get. I think he's jealous of the people I spend time with. He just can't stand it that I might have a life of my own."

"What do you want me to do?" Philip began.

"Philip, please," I said. Lauren glared at him.†

†*Sometimes the use of straight behavioral interventions alone is necessary. For example, Philip's propensity to interrupt his wife when she was talking could have been addressed by providing both of them with a pad and pencil and requesting that instead of orally interrupting, they record their automatic thoughts on paper so that they could return to them at a later point in the session (Dattilio, 1996, in press; Dattilio & Padesky, 1990). This technique is important for two reasons. First, it allows for the uninterrupted flow of conversation, while it also allows individuals to hold on to those "ripe automatic thoughts" that may be very important. Second, it sets a precedent for the mutual respect between partners and serves to diffuse anger in a productive manner. The technique is something that may be included in homework assignments as well.*

"Go on, Lauren," I said. "How does this jealousy make you feel? How do you two so quickly end in a rage?"

"I don't know. I just know he makes me crazy," Lauren said, packing into that one sentence a whole complex set of emotions—emotions that were unavailable to her because she condensed her hurt and longing and frustration into explosive outbursts. Philip never heard the hurt or the longing; all he knew was her anger.†

†*Thoughts are essential. A fine example of this is with this exchange, where Dr. Minuchin asked Lauren, "How does this jealousy make you feel?" Unfortunately, her answer was vague. If the question had been rephrased as "What thoughts are going through your mind right now?," the answer might have provided more clues to Lauren's schema about the entire ordeal, which would have led nicely to her feelings and emotions. If this question had met with difficulty, imagery could also have been used here to recall "hot cognitions" or emotions.*

I tried to explore with her what she did when Philip was unfair—when he was mean, when he was annoying, when he was cold, when he was jealous—in order to move her away from quixotic eruptions of anger and avoidance. Lauren needed a clearer idea of the sequence of events that took place between her and Philip, as well as a clearer idea of her own power. When I asked her how she reacted when she felt attacked, she said, "I try to avoid him. I answer abruptly. I go into my shell." All these responses were the responses of a frightened person, someone avoiding attack. Lauren couldn't see the alternatives available to her.

"Do you ever daydream about killing him?" I asked.

"Certainly not!" She was shocked.

"Haven't you ever thought of pushing him out the window or poisoning his coffee?"

Lauren flushed, shook her head, and said, "Oh, no, nothing like that." She didn't say anything else for a moment, and I didn't say anything. And then, looking embarrassed, she said, "Sometimes I have these dreams. He's been killed—run over by a car, or a sudden heart attack—and I wake up terrified. But it's never anything *I've* done. It just happens."

I laughed and asked her who she thought dreamed up her dreams. She looked thoughtful, and I turned to Philip.

"Tell me about some small incident that illustrates the conflicts between the two of you. A very small incident."

"Well, one thing comes to mind, but it was kind of silly."

"OK. Let's talk about that."

"Well, as I said, it was kind of stupid. I asked the cleaning lady to throw out some flowers that were starting to wilt. Lauren hit the ceiling. She said I was talking down to the woman. I just asked her to throw out some flowers, for Pete's sake! I can't do anything!" He seemed on the verge of tears. Here was the other side of Lauren's helplessness and fear: Philip's self-pity. "Regardless of what hoops I jump through to please her, nothing I ever do is right."

"Was your mother a queen?" I asked.

Philip looked startled. Then he said evenly, "A queen? She was Catherine the Great. Everybody did what she wanted. Us kids, even my father. Especially my father."

"That's fascinating," I said. Then I had an idea.

"Lauren," I said, "would you mind taking off your shoes and standing up on that chair?" She gave me a funny look, but no argument. She bent down, slipped off her stylish pumps, and stepped up gracefully.

"Tell me about your mother, Philip." He looked up at his wife, standing on the chair, and then he looked at me; he got the point. He described Catherine Lockwood as a tall, formidable woman. An elementary school principal. "She looked it, too. Absolute type casting. Heavy-set, long hair braided and coiled, unsmiling. She kept everything in order, in school and at home."

"Sounds grim," I said.

"Well, she was a good mother. She was always concerned, always ready to help. I owe her a lot." Philip glanced up at Lauren, smiling a little uncomfortably. Perched on a throne she didn't know she'd inherited, Lauren smiled back a little awkwardly, but she made no attempt to get down.

When I said that it was time to stop, Philip looked up and said, "I'm sorry," as though in talking about himself and his memories he'd been guilty of a forbidden act of self-indulgence. I knew he could talk a long time about his past. But the past was something I wanted to dip into only long enough to help him realize that—brought up as he was to see requests as royal commands—he was overreacting to his wife's needs.

"You know, I'm absolutely fascinated by the pair of you!" I said, rising to help Lauren down. "For a couple of intelligent people, you're playing the damnedest absurd drama I ever saw."

At this point I felt a sense of understanding with Lauren. She seemed able to examine her own motives and reactions, and ready to see new possibilities for relating to Philip. I didn't have the same sense of connection with Philip, but I felt that he and I were working toward it. I helped them gather their coats and briefcases, and Lauren thanked me with a smile. "What would we do without you?"

I smiled back, accepting her reliance on me as a step in the direction of coming to rely on herself. Perhaps her confidence in me would make her feel safe enough to explore new possibilities.

FOURTH SESSION

Five minutes after the next session was due to start, the phone rang. It was Lauren. "Can you tell me your exact address?" she asked sheepishly. She said she was one block away and would be there in 2 minutes. But it was Philip who arrived first, apparently unconcerned about being late. "Where's Lauren?" he asked.

"She just called. She'll be here any minute."

Quite a few minutes later, I heard Lauren open the outer door, but it was a few minutes more before she walked into the office—still a little out of breath, but her makeup perfect and every hair in place. "I'm sorry I'm late," she said. "I was only a block away when I called, but then somehow I walked west instead of east. It's so hard to find the numbers on these buildings. Before that I took the wrong subway. It wasn't until I got to 59th Street that I realized it was going uptown instead of downtown. I'm sorry."

Was Lauren late because she didn't really want to come? Was getting lost just an ordinary human mistake or a sign that she wasn't used to relying on herself? All these things might be true, but I decided to focus on the part of the truth that related to Lauren's underutilized competence.

"Lauren, you amaze me," I said. "Clearly you are a bright and capable woman. No one gets to be a partner in a consulting firm without talent and ability. Yet in many ways you present yourself as helpless. You get lost coming to the office. You put up with your husband's hitting you. Don't misunderstand me—I'm not excusing him. But Lauren, how can you be so competent and see yourself as so helpless?"

"Well, I suppose I grew up that way." She sat down, apparently not minding my calling her "helpless." As she went on, her vowels traveled south. "Where I grew up, in Charleston, girls weren't expected to be independent. My daddy always told me how pretty I was. I didn't do real well in school, but I was popular, and I guess he thought that was enough. When I got to be homecoming queen, that seemed like all the success anyone could want. It was the same at Clemson. I kind of majored in parties." She smiled, as though not doing well in school was something to be proud of, a feminine accomplishment.

I don't take histories at the beginning of therapy because the historical facts change, depending on context and on people's trust of the therapist. I let the facts emerge later, organically related to what's happening in therapy. Lauren's historical exploration at this point was related to how she learned to be helpless.†

> † *But had this history been taken earlier, at least a few initial clues might have been available for use in developing a conceptualization of Lauren's thought processes and belief systems, and of how these were linked to her emotions.*

Lauren had grown up petted and pampered by a doting father who loved her but didn't take her seriously. Later she learned to depend on the status that great beauty confers. Now, although she was still beautiful, she had ceased to rely on her looks or on her role as Dr. Lockwood's wife. She'd become an independent woman. But old habits die hard, and in many ways she still thought of herself as defined by her femininity and good looks. Homecoming queens don't need to know which subway to take, or how to defend themselves against a man's fists.

As Lauren talked about her well-bred Southern upbringing, I couldn't help thinking about Blanche DuBois's famous line from *A Streetcar Named Desire*: "I have always depended on the kindness of strangers." Like Blanche, Lauren seemed to take a strange, stubborn pride in being helpless. And like Blanche and many other women, Lauren paid a lot for this curious accomplishment.

Philip had been very silent. It occurred to me that I had just handed him some ammunition in his battle with Lauren, so I moved to involve him. Childhood might have set the stage for Lauren's dependence, but the roles in this marriage were mutually determined.

"Philip, do you like a woman who is a little bit helpless?" I asked. At that moment the radiator began to clank, and in jest I said, "Lauren, please make it stop doing that."

Lauren smiled, indulging my little joke. Just at that moment the noise stopped, and I said, "Thank you, Lauren," with a straight face.

"Why do you give me that power?" she asked in all seriousness.

We grow up, but in some ways we never do. Here, perhaps in response to the tension generated by their conflict, I had slipped back 60 years to childhood to make a silly joke. And then Lauren, perhaps in response to her own anxieties about the situation, had shed 30 years to become a credulous girl—willing to believe (or to pretend to believe) that I was serious, and that my remark must have some unfathomable meaning. Until she began to feel whole and worthwhile, she would continue to long for someone to look up to, someone to rely on.†

> † *This particular style was rather artful and clandestine, as Dr. Minuchin kept his intentions suppressed through his stylish manner. A cognitive-behavioral therapist might have been a bit more collaborative and direct with regard to Lauren's dependence and Philip's need to keep her dependent.*

"I don't mind when she asks me questions," Philip went on as if there had been no interruption. "At least then we're connected." His face darkened. "What I do mind is that when she doesn't want something, she ignores me. She pays more attention to her friends than she does to me."

I remembered Freud's famous remark that a patient is cured when the neurotic symptoms lift and the person returns to the normal miseries of everyday life. Now Philip's complaint sounded more like the normal miseries of an unhappy couple than the pathological extreme of violence.

"Talk with each other about that," I said. "I want to see how you two talk together."

Now that Philip and Lauren had explained their relationship to me, I wanted to see them demonstrate it by how they communicated. I'd waited this long because they were so volatile and reactive. Now, however, they seemed less defensive, and perhaps they could begin to listen to each other. Lauren's complaint was that Philip didn't take her seriously; his was that she didn't pay him enough attention. As they talked, I could see why.

"Well, let's see," Philip began. "You remember that article in *The New York Times Magazine* we were talking about the other day?"

"*You* were talking," she said. Lauren made this crack without bitterness, and Philip, who either didn't notice or chose to ignore it, went on. He talked about the article, and how he'd tried to explain it to her, and how she never got involved in these discussions. As far as he was concerned, it was her fault—some combination of reticence and deliberate withholding. "There's an unwillingness on her part to enter into dialogue," was his ponderous way of putting it.

Lauren answered in monosyllables. It was hard to tell whether she disagreed with Philip, or didn't fully understand him, or was simply bored. Her silence made him try harder to get through to her, until their "conversation" took on a familiar form: He talked, she listened. The less she said, the more pedantic and verbose he became. And the wordier he became, the more silent and sullen she grew. In less than 5 minutes, he'd become the kind of long-winded teacher who doesn't understand why his students don't participate in the discussion.

As Lauren sat there, trapped by Philip's verbosity and her own silence, both of them grew increasingly impatient. I could see the seeds of a scene to come. After a while she'd say something nasty. He'd retaliate, and pretty soon they'd end up in the kind of spiteful finger pointing that would escalate into a fight. Not wanting them to get anywhere near that point, I interrupted.

"Stop!" I said, and they both looked up, startled. "There's no flexibility in this dialogue. You're both still too invested in being right to listen to the other's perspective, or to change." I told them that we weren't getting anywhere, and ushered them brusquely out of the office.

I ended abruptly because I wanted to force them to recognize the signals of a loss of control. The possibility of further violence—even one more episode could destroy this marriage—made it imperative that each of them become alert to their intentions and aware of how they expressed them. Here spontaneity was dangerous. There are times in any relationship where distance and caution are necessary; for the Lockwoods, this was surely one of them.†

> † *Couples often present with anger that has been compounded over time. It is not unusual for this to be released during therapy sessions, as can be seen in this case with Philip and Lauren. Cognitive-behavioral therapists deal very differently with anger and take a focused approach in diffusing it. Once again, little was done at this point with Philip's and Lauren's automatic thoughts and their perceptions of each other. This would have been fertile ground for cognitive restructuring to occur, and its use outside of the session could have been suggested as well.*

FIFTH SESSION

The following week, when Lauren arrived on time but alone, I started with her alone. It gave me a chance to hear her individual perspective. But because I didn't want my understanding to come at the expense of helping the couple learn to understand each other, I planned to repeat what was said when Philip arrived.

Lauren was in an upbeat and hopeful mood. As usual, she was dressed for work the way some women would dress for dinner. She said that things had been "status quo," though communication had been better. Philip, she said, had been allowing her to talk—he was even listening. "It's been nice. In fact, we spent the whole weekend without any major blowups."

At that point Philip walked in, and I said that I was going to take a minute to tell him what Lauren had said. I told him that she'd said communication was better. He was allowing her to talk, and he was listening, and it was nice. Philip looked relieved, as if he'd just been told that he passed a test.

"But," Lauren put in, "I also said that things were status quo."

Philip looked wounded. He hadn't passed after all.

I jumped in before he could say anything. "Lauren, what happened just now?"

"Nothing. I just wanted Philip to know exactly what I said."

"Lauren, did you feel that I was siding with Philip? Or betraying your meaning? Are you afraid that if I rephrase what you say, Philip or I will use it against you? Why can't you trust me?"

This was a long reach, but I felt that Lauren might be able to see her experiences with her husband from a different perspective if she could see herself also being anxious and mistrustful with me. "I won't hurt you, Lauren. I'm on your side. I respect you, and I support you. How is it that you can't trust me? Does the world seem that dangerous to you?"

She was silent for a moment. "Well, I suppose that I grew up—"

"Don't tell me about your childhood. Childhood ends." I didn't want to hear about the past, where she learned helplessness; I wanted to hear about her career, where she unlearned it. "Tell me about your work. Your colleagues. What if I asked your partners to describe you? What would they say?" Surely she must think of herself as competent and powerful at work.†

> † *The past is important to cognitive-behavioral therapists for conceptualizing individuals' schemas. In this respect, I would have wanted to know what experiences had contributed to Lauren's view of herself, her world and her future. I might also have assigned her the task of gathering information about how others saw her, in order to test the validity of her conceptualization.*

"Well, I'm a people person. I don't really know that much about management. Most of my success comes from supporting other people. I know how to get along, how to flatter people, how to come out of a deal with everybody feeling like he's gotten something. You get along by going along, and—"†

> † *This supported the evidence of why Lauren continued to be a "pleaser." She believed that it was part of her success in life. If the therapist had used the "downward arrow" technique here, he might have found that Lauren would feel like a failure if she did not continue to be a pleaser.*

I stood up in mock despair. "Lauren, Lauren, Lauren! How can I wake you up?" I went over and knocked on her forehead. "Lauren, please wake up! You don't have to deny your competence." She looked at me, dismayed. Minimizing herself was something Lauren did so automatically that she had ceased to be aware of it.

Philip laughed out loud. I turned to him. "What about you, Philip? How was the week from your point of view?"

"Well, I believe the matrix of our communication is changing. I've been trying to accept Lauren's unavailability, her disengagement, as having to do with her, not necessarily as a negative response to my input." While I was still trying to digest that, Philip went on, saying, with his characteristic cloud of words, that he was learning to live with Lauren's silence. Lauren leaned forward, listening intently.

On and on he went, making an important point—that he was beginning to feel that the only way for them to live together was if he became resigned to Lauren's disinterest and distance. However, he spun this out in so many words, circling around his feelings, that the point was drowned in words—as was any real chance for Lauren to respond. She sat, meanwhile, listening with apparent interest, until I broke in.

"Lauren, at what point did you stop listening to Philip?"

Taken aback, she said, "What do you mean? I was listening."

"I don't think so. I didn't see the exact moment, but at some point you stopped listening. And so instead of a dialogue, there was a monologue. But this isn't just something he does. It's something that you—both of you—do together."

Philip stiffened slightly. Hearing himself accused of being pedantic was unpleasant but not, after all, unfamiliar. Lauren said, "Well, I guess I do tune him out sometimes. I know he needs to say what's on his mind. And I feel I owe it to him to listen. But I get so tired of his never offering to listen to me. Damn it!" Suddenly there were tears in her eyes. "It's always your lousy day. What about my day? Why can't you give me even a fraction of the attention—" And suddenly she stopped herself, as though by complaining she had somehow broken the rules.†

> † *Once again, to the therapist interested in cognitions, this would have been a favorable time to inquire into Lauren's automatic thoughts.*

Philip was astounded. Lauren's anger, stored up from long hours of one-sided conversation, seemed so extreme, so unfair to him. If she had something to say, why didn't she say it? Philip didn't lecture Lauren into silence, boredom, and finally fury because he sought to dominate. He'd been brought up to achieve and be interesting. She'd been brought up to attend and be interested. The two of them brought these roles into the marriage so naturally that neither had ever given them a thought. Hard as it was for either of them to change, it was twice as hard in the relationship, where mutual habits were reinforced by mutual expectations.

"You both want something you're not getting," I pointed out. "Attention. Genuine attention. That's not too much to ask of a marriage." I paused. "Now I'm going to give you some homework. I would like each of you to find some other way of getting what you want from each other.

Philip, your attempt to reach Lauren with words is pushing her away. Maybe words aren't the answer."

Philip made a helpless gesture. "What do you suggest?"

"I don't know," I said. "This is one of those things everybody has to do in his own way. But I do know that you—both of you—are more complex than you know. And, Lauren, you need to find words to express your point of view—and to interrupt Philip when he's giving one of his monologues." Lauren glanced at Philip. I went on, "I've suggested to Philip that he make an effort to stop dominating conversation between the two of you, but I doubt that he can change without your help."†

> † *Dr. Minuchin used homework in this session quite effectively. This is probably one of the strongest tools that couple therapists can utilize to facilitate change, since couples are very prone to becoming lax between sessions. Cognitive-behavioral therapists place great emphasis on the structure of homework assignments with couples, particularly during periods of intense change. In the dialogue below, Lauren asked for a couple of weeks between sessions. It is crucial from a cognitive-behavioral standpoint that when there is a longer gap than usual between sessions, the interim assignments be structured in order to facilitate change. The therapist might have worked collaboratively with this couple in selecting an assignment that would help them achieve their short-term goals in the interim weeks.*

Lauren smiled. "You don't think we can learn to do that in 1 week, do you?"

"I'm not asking you to *learn* anything. I'm only asking you to start doing something you're perfectly capable of doing."

"Well," Lauren said, "maybe it would be a good idea not to meet for a couple of weeks. That would give us a chance to practice."

I took this as a good sign. Most people think that therapy is something that happens in a therapist's office. Maybe therapy does, but change takes place at home. I agreed to see them again in 2 weeks.

SIXTH SESSION

Lauren arrived on time, without Philip. I gave her a questioning look, and she said calmly that Philip should be there in a few minutes. "He's never ready on time. But I decided that I didn't want to argue with him, and I didn't want to be late. So I told him I was leaving, and he should come when he was ready."

Lauren said this without any of the usual antagonism. She'd left on time and before Philip—not to provoke or antagonize him, but simply because it was time to go. It was a small declaration of independence.

"Well," she began as she sat down, "I've been working on your suggestion. I've been trying to be more honest with myself, accepting my competence, and my right to make demands."

Actually, that wasn't what I'd said. The task I'd given them was simple and concrete. But Lauren had gone beyond the specifics of my suggestion to work on the essential imbalance in the relationship. I nodded. It sounded good.

"I'm trying not to put up with his brutality," she went on. "I'll give you an example. Last Sunday I was sitting in the living room, relaxing for a minute with the *Times* in my lap. Philip came in and grabbed 'The Week in Review.' I said, 'Hey, I was just about to read that. You can have it when I'm done.' He looked surprised, but he gave it right back. I felt I'd done the right thing."

"Of course you did the right thing," I said. "But I'm surprised to hear you use the word "brutality" to describe Philip's taking the paper away form you."

"It all feels the same to me. Grabbing the newspaper, or going on and on forever, or slapping me—it's all part of the same thing. But I guess I don't have to put up with it. Any of it."†

> †*Here, Lauren was engaging in the cognitive distortions of "emotional reasoning" and "dichotomous thinking" in the sense that she viewed Philip's behaviors as "either–or" (see Chapter 1). It might have been helpful at this point for the therapist to cue Lauren in evaluating her own behavior and labeling her distortions without abandoning the major tenet of her concern. This could have aided her in tempering her response and consequently in soliciting a more cooperative response from her spouse.*

I thought that it wasn't the same thing—that in time she would have to make distinctions. But for the moment her progress seemed wonderful. So the thought remained silent.

"I've been working on the second task you gave me, too. You said I should start participating more in conversations with Philip. You said he needs me to be involved, and I have been. He's always reading highbrow stuff. I never used to know what he was talking about. But lately I've been reading what he reads, so I have some idea what he's talking about. Some of it's actually interesting."

At that moment Philip walked in. "Are you always late, Philip?" I asked. "Or is it only here?"

He looked offended. "Maybe the truth is I didn't feel like coming today. Last time we were here, you suggested that Lauren start speaking up more. What about me? It seems to me that you always pay more attention to her. What am I supposed to do?"

If at that moment Philip sounded like a rivalrous sibling, perhaps it was understandable. In this couple, where the partners got so little appreciation from each other, they were understandably jealous of any attention paid by anyone else. What Philip didn't seem to understand was that if Lauren started speaking up more, saying what was on her mind rather than just sitting there in bored silence when he talked, he'd gain a partner.†

> † *Although Dr. Minuchin handled this well, he could also have asked Philip to apply the same strategies requested of Lauren, and to weigh the evidence supporting the notion that he was being "left out."*

And then Philip got to what was really weighing on his mind. "Besides, I was afraid to hear what you would say today about us staying together or not. Lauren hasn't said a word. I have no idea how she feels."

Lauren cast me an urgent look, but I said nothing. For 15 minutes, she'd talked with me about how hard she was working to make her relationship with Philip better. What was amazing was that she had conveyed none of this commitment to Philip, and that he could be in such doubt about what was so clear: that Lauren was fighting hard to preserve the marriage.

"I know she's been making efforts to become more informed," Philip continued. "I appreciate that. And she's stood up to me a couple of times—showed me she thought I was being overbearing, when I didn't mean to be. And I think that's good. But the big question, our staying together . . ."

Characteristically, Philip then began to repeat his points. Lauren frowned, shook her head, and gave me a helpless look.

"Lauren, for heaven's sake," I interjected. "You clearly have something to say. Why don't you say it?"†

> † *Here, Dr. Minuchin encouraged Lauren to be assertive and say what was on her mind to Philip. He used verbal reinforcement with both of them to encourage a continual verbal exchange, which was very effective in this case. He might also have gone a step further, however, and attempted to uncover Lauren's schema behind why she remained so quiet—where she learned to be passive, and what core beliefs shaped and maintained this type of silent behavior. Unless a therapist uncovers such core beliefs, he or she runs the risk that the same patterns of behavior will return, and that not enough restructuring will occur to facilitate to incur permanent change. Behaviorists are also notorious for using assertiveness training techniques as strategies in communications with couples. This might have been addressed directly in some of the conjoint sessions or in individual therapy with Lauren's therapist. In any case, assertiveness certainly needed to be a focal point here.*

"Well, yes, I do. I have a lot of feelings about what he's saying. But he keeps talking. He'd just get mad if I interrupted him."

"I've told you a million times," Philip said peevishly, "if you have something to say, say it!"

"You could try asking me what I think. Just once in a while. Give me a chance to speak without having to interrupt you. As though you were interested in what I have to say."

Philip started to retort, but he caught himself. "But I *am* interested."

"Excellent, Philip. You too, Lauren. Go on talking."

They did, for the rest of the session. He was very clear about the problems her silence caused. She was very clear about his talkativeness. There were complaints. But somehow they got past blaming and accusations, and down to the place where the deep hurt resided. The complaints and the hurts were confined to words, and they were words that left room for each partner to listen to the other's point of view.

"This is really promising," I said. They turned to me. I think we all sensed it was time for the verdict.

"I promised you my opinion," I said. "I'm not going to try to tell you whether to stay married or not—that's up to you. What I can tell you is that the violence in your marriage is predictable, and if you want to, you can change that pattern. As a matter of fact, you've already begun to change. You both want the same thing from each other—a little understanding and a little respect. You haven't been getting it, and that's sad. But Philip, hitting your wife is not sad. It's unconscionable."

He looked down. Lauren looked away. I went on, "It must not continue. But I don't think it will. You know it's wrong, and you know you can control yourself. What's more, and maybe more important, I don't think Lauren will tolerate it any more." Lauren's eyes filled with tears. So did Philip's.

"You're not dangerous people," I continued. "You're destructive. I don't think there will be any danger if you decide you want to stay together. But I do think you may continue to be unhappy. That, I don't know."

"Well, I think we both want to change that," said Philip. "Don't we, Lauren?"

"Won't you help us?" she asked.

CONCLUSION

That was several years ago. There were no further incidents of violence. I continued to see them for several months, and, off and on, their son Jeffrey as well. Philip and Lauren's marriage was never going to be the match made in heaven they once hoped for in the unreason of love. But they did return to the "normal miseries of everyday life." To say that they still clashed in many ways, and in many ways disappointed each other, is to say no more than that they were married, and for a long time.

When Philip and Lauren first came to therapy, they both felt controlled and helpless, victims of each other's stubborn refusal to cooperate. As far as they were concerned, they had no choice in their ritual battles; each partner was only submitting to a fate that the other forced on him or her. It was their acceptance of themselves—not simply as victims, but as two people who had survived and had the power to make choices—that finally liberated them. The explosive quarrels that once ended in violence changed to occasional arguments that they both knew how to start and stop.†

> †*Salvador Minuchin, once again, has proven his artistic style as an effective therapist in working with what truly could have become a disastrous case. He blended his own style of insight orientation with a directive approach that is also commonly found among cognitive-behavioral therapists.*
>
> *Any therapist wishing to utilize the same style that Dr. Minuchin so clearly demonstrated with this case may find its effectiveness borne out in the results. The use of the aforementioned techniques in structuring the sessions, and the use of schema focus, may also prove to enhance the effectiveness of this approach.*
>
> *As a follow-up to the remaining sessions, I might have suggested the continuation of structured communication skills, as well as home-work assignments to reinforce their use. I would also have reviewed with persistence the use of reframing of automatic thoughts with both Philip and Lauren to insure more lasting change.*

AUTHORS' REPLY TO EDITOR'S COMMENTS

In emphasizing the common ground between his approach and ours, Dr. Dattilio underscores the fact that what therapists from different schools do is probably more alike than different. His endorsement of many of the interventions in this case shows a generous appreciation for a colleague's work. But in celebrating similarities, he may be blurring major differences between the cognitive-behavioral and structural approaches.

On page 113 (top), for example, Dr. Dattilio suggests that it might have been useful to provide Philip with more concrete strategies for controlling his anger. This suggestion implies that self-control is a skill that can be taught. We have a different perspective. We think that people change their behavior when they accept responsibility for it and then decide to do something about it. What holds people back from behaving more responsibly in relationships isn't that they don't know what to do. It's that they don't recognize—or accept—the need for them to face up to their own contribution to their problems.

There's also a technical point to be made about this intervention. Confronting Philip with the wrongfulness of his brutality, and holding *him* accountable, were designed to make it clear that he needed to take responsibility for his behavior. Shifting from pointing out the destructive consequences of his actions to making suggestions for how to act differently would have risked shifting the focus from the client to the therapist and to the usefulness or lack of usefulness of his advice.

On pages 114–115, Dr. Dattilio again suggests that it might have been helpful for the therapist to take a more active role in teaching the partners to improve their behavior—this time, to be more sensitive and tolerant of each other. On page 117 (top), he suggests techniques for helping them learn to stop interrupting each other; on page 122, he notes that a more directive and educational approach might have been taken when the partners lapsed back into their familiar destructive pattern. All of these suggestions underscore the cognitive-behaviorist's faith in the power of simple instruction to change the habits of a lifetime.

In contrast to those suggestions that imply taking over more, Dr. Dattilio also indicates a couple of places where he would have dug more. On page 127 (bottom), he suggests that it might have been useful to explore *why* Lauren didn't speak up, rather than just urging her to do so; on page 116, he uses the notion of uncovering "schemas" to suggest that each partner could have been helped to appreciate why the other one seemed to perpetuate unhelpful actions. These are excellent suggestions, both of which capture what makes the cognitive-behavioral approach such a distinct improvement over pure behaviorism—helping people confront the self-defeating points of view that keep them stuck.

ACKNOWLEDGMENT

The case of the Lockwoods is adapted from *Family Healing,* by Minuchin and Nichols (1993). Copyright 1993 by Salvador Minuchin and Michael P. Nichols. Adapted by permission of the authors and the Free Press, a division of Simon & Schuster, Inc.

REFERENCES

Dattilio, F. M. (1996). *Cognitive therapy with couples: The initial phase of treatment* [Videotape]. Sarasota, FL: Professional Resource Exchange.

Dattilio, F. M., & Padesky, C. A. (1990). *Cognitive therapy with couples.* Sarasota, FL: Professional Resource Exchange.

Minuchin, S., & Fishman, H. C. (1981). *Family therapy techniques.* Cambridge, MA: Harvard University Press.

Minuchin, S., & Nichols, M. P. (1993). *Family healing: Tales of hope and renewal from family therapy.* New York: Free Press.

SUGGESTED READINGS

Colapinto, J. (1988). The structural way. In H. A. Liddle, D. C. Breunlin, & R. C. Schwartz (Eds.), *Handbook of family therapy training and supervision.* New York: Guilford Press.

Minuchin, S. (1974). *Families and family therapy.* Cambridge, MA: Harvard University Press.

Minuchin, S. (1984). *Family kaleidoscope.* Cambridge, MA: Harvard University Press.

Minuchin, S., & Fishman, H. C. (1981). *Family therapy techniques.* Cambridge, MA: Harvard University Press.

Minuchin, S., & Nichols, M. P. (1993). *Family healing: Tales of hope and renewal from family therapy.* New York: Free Press.

Minuchin, S., Lee, W. Y., & Simon, G. M. (1996). *Mastering family therapy: Journeys of growth and transformation.* New York: Wiley.

Nichols, M. P., & Schwartz, R. C. (1998). *Family therapy: Concepts and methods* (4th ed.). Needham Heights, MA: Allyn & Bacon.

Chapter 6

Strategic Family Therapy

JAMES KEIM

The goals of this chapter are to present a case example of a highly effective and gentle intervention for oppositional behavior in children and adolescents; to demonstrate how a therapist of the Washington school of strategic therapy (founded by Jay Haley and Cloé Madanes) thinks and works; and to facilitate the volume editor's comparison of various types of therapy with cognitive approaches. Since its inception, strategic therapy has borrowed from and contributed to other approaches and disciplines. Our continued ability as therapists to learn from and share with others is dependent upon the maintenance of a common language of therapy. It is thus an honor to contribute to the work of Frank M. Dattilio, who is at the forefront of efforts to overcome barriers to such exchanges.

This chapter begins with a review of the individual definition of oppositional defiant disorder. An interactional definition of oppositional behavior is then presented. Through the presentation of a case study, a four-stage intervention for oppositional behavior is described. This intervention was developed by studying successful interventions for oppositional behavior and attempting to distill their commonalities. As the reader will recognize, this intervention borrows from the traditions of the Washington school of strategic therapy (Haley and Madanes); the traditions of the Brief Therapy Center of the Mental Research Institute (MRI) (Fisch, Weakland, and Watzlawick); and structural approaches (Minuchin, Fishman, and Montalvo). Observing the work of Cloé Madanes, Jay Haley, and Neil Schiff was especially helpful, as was hearing and reading the case of "The Aversive Adolescent" in the book *The Tactics of Change* (Fisch, Weakland, & Segal, 1982). The members of the Brief Therapy Center are fond of describing models of psychotherapy as "maps"; in other words, therapy theory proposes grand oversimplifications, which serve the pragmatic function of moving from one point to another. The present intervention for oppositional children is such a grand oversimplification. It works by focusing on just a few facets of oppositional behavior. The view of oppositional behavior described in this chapter oversimplifies and shrinks a complex terrain, for the pragmatic function of facilitating change in the context of therapy.

THE INDIVIDUAL DESCRIPTION
OF OPPOSITIONAL DEFIANT DISORDER

DSM-IV (American Psychiatric Association, 1994) describes oppositional/defiant disorder as a disturbance of at least 6 months during which at least four of the following are present: A child frequently loses his or her temper, frequently argues with adults, frequently defies adults or refuses to obey adult rules or requests, frequently does things on purpose that irritate other people, frequently blames others for his or her own misdeeds or mistakes, is frequently touchy or easily irritated by others, is frequently resentful and angry, and/or is frequently vindictive or spiteful.

One problem with the DSM-IV criteria is that the diagnosis must be changed if the behavior escalates to a major violation of the rights of others (the diagnosis then becomes one of conduct disorder). As many clinicians will agree, this is a rather unhelpful distinction, since the oppositionality—not the degree of acting out—is the salient feature of this problem (Loeber, Lahey, & Thomas, 1991). Oppositional behavior is best viewed in terms of degrees, the more serious of which involve major violations of rights of others. The interactional definition of oppositional behavior described below includes acting out that constitutes major violations of the rights of others.

MOVING TO THE INTERACTIONAL VIEW

The strategic clinician turns individual diagnosis into a systemic description. For the Washington school, the two most important tools for viewing a problem are the concepts of the "sequence of interaction" and the "hierarchy of interaction." Sequence and hierarchy are viewed as utilitarian constructs that encourage the clinician to focus on problem solving.

The Escalating Sequence of Oppositional Interaction:
Process versus Outcome Orientation

The sequence of interaction is simply a step-by-step description of a behavior; it focuses on what is happening between people. Strategic therapists view change in therapy as movement from an unsatisfactory sequence to a satisfactory one. In the therapy of oppositional behavior, change involves movement from an escalating sequence (where fighting escalates painfully and without resolution) to a resolution sequence (where the child is soothed by the adult).

The present intervention is based on the finding that it is helpful to focus on certain aspects of the sequence of oppositional behavior. The critical sequence of this intervention is as follows: *During a confrontation between a child and an authority figure, the child is primarily focused on the process of communication, while the adult is focused on the outcome.*

Neither process nor outcome orientations are by themselves problematic; the issue is the mismatch that occurs when one party in a confrontation is focused on outcome and the other on process. This difference in focus leads to painful escalations when confrontations arise. Writers such as Deborah Tannen (1990) and John Gray (1993) have described the painful escalations that occur in the context of male–female differences in process and outcome communication. These gender-related escalations have their counterpart in generational communication problems, of which oppositional interactions are a prime example.

During confrontation, the process-oriented child is especially focused on determining the timing of the confrontation and the content and direction of communication during the confrontation. At the same time, the adult in the confrontation tends to focus on determining the outcome of the confrontation. As the argument progresses and tensions become greater, the child tends to become increasingly focused on process, and the adult tends to become increasingly focused on outcome. This is the sequence of oppositional behavior that the present intervention focuses upon. Oppositional children often engage in arguments for the mere sake of arguing, as opposed to necessarily achieving any stated goal.

The Hierarchy of Oppositional Interaction

Oppositional behavior is best described as being characterized not only by a certain sequence of interaction (described above), but also by a certain hierarchy of interaction. In the context of this intervention, the concept of "hierarchy" describes the degree to which the parents and children interact in age- and role-appropriate ways (Minuchin, 1974; Haley, 1976). The Washington school doesn't view inadequate or dysfunctional hierarchy as *creating* problems; it is believed, however, that focusing on hierarchy is often helpful in *solving* problems.

The hierarchy of interaction of oppositional behavior is as follows. The children behave as if they have the authority of adults, not kids, and tend to argue with adults as if arguing with peers. In some cases of oppositional behavior, the adults often begin to behave less like parents and more like peers vying for power.

A child who claims an adult level of authority and argues with adults as if they were peers is described as a "high-hierarchy child." If a child isn't "high on the hierarchy," the situation wouldn't be described as oppositional and the present intervention would not be applied. At the Washington school, the concept of "low-hierarchy child" also exists; the low-hierarchy child feels powerless in relation to the parents. With a low-hierarchy child, therapy is designed to empower the young person to have more mature authority. With a high-hierarchy child, therapy is designed to empower the child to have more child-like functioning rather than adult authority.

The double-column list below depicts some issues that play a strong part in who is functioning as an adult in a social system. To the degree that children assume the roles described below, they tend to claim the authority of adults. To the degree that adults carry out the interpersonal tasks below in a benevolent fashion, and to the degree that there is balance between the "hard" and "soft" sides of hierarchy, adults tend to increase their benevolent ability to guide and protect children.

The "hard" side of hierarchy	*The "soft" side of hierarchy*
Who makes the rules	Who soothes whom
Who defines the punishments	Who provides reassurance to whom
Who carries out punishments	
Who tells whom what to do	Who protects whom
Who has final responsibility for making major decisions	Who has responsibility for expressing love, affection, and empathy
Who is responsible for making others feel safe and provided for in the environment	Who is the provider of good things and good times
	Who usually determines the mood of situations
	Who has the responsibility to listen to whom

When children perceive that their parents aren't fulfilling their responsibilities as described above, they tend to respond by assuming these responsibilities themselves and by seeking to meet their needs with others, especially peers. In order for a child to assume age-appropriate behavior, both the "hard" and "soft" sides of hierarchy need to be created by what is perceived as an adult generation.

DIRECTIVES

The intervention described below is typical of strategic family therapy, in that the therapist uses both "client-inspired" and "therapist-inspired" directives. A client-inspired directive occurs when the therapist asks the clients to develop an idea and then urges the clients to try it. A therapist-inspired directive occurs when the therapist develops an idea and encourages the clients to try it.

This intervention attempts to bring about change through an accumulation of small steps. As Jay Haley wrote:

> Two general approaches are thought of as appropriate: one is to induce a crisis in the family that unstabililzes the system so that the family must reform with different patterns; the other is to choose one aspect of the system and cause it to deviate. This deviation is encouraged and amplified until the system goes on a runaway course and must reorganize into a new set of patterns. (1973, p. 35)

Although strategic therapists of the Washington school employ both types of interventions, the method described in this chapter is of the latter, amplification-of-small change variety. This "start small, start slow" approach was originally described by Milton Erickson (see Haley, 1973) and is emphasized in the writings of the Brief Therapy Team of the MRI.

THE INTERVENTION

The stages of this intervention for oppositional behavior are as follows:

1. A collaborative reframing helps parents understand differences in adults' and children's perceptions of power; this moves the focus of the problem past the issue of who is to blame, and refocuses the parents' energy instead on resolving the problem in a new fashion.

2. The parents are coached to employ new information on the child's process orientation by resisting the child's attempts to draw them into confrontations. One goal is for the parents to determine their own mood, rather than allowing the child to manipulate it. Also addressed are any possible triangulations among the child, a parent, and a third party. In addition, issues related to improving the endurance and coping abilities of adults are addressed. Stage 2 focuses on what the MRI model describes as "not repeating what's already not working" (Watzlawick, Weakland, & Fisch, 1974).

3. Rules, rewards, and consequences are restructured to make them sensitive to the child's process orientation and to the parents' endurance. This stage includes setting limits, rules, and consequences, and putting them down on paper for the child to see; timing of "tagging" and giving consequences; nonconfrontational punishments; a two-tiered system of consequences; not pushing parents too hard initially in setting limits; making sure that there are regular, scheduled times for positive parent–child interaction, regardless of the child's behavior; and using rewards as shaping tools.

4. Parents are coached to soothe their oppositional child. Parents move from merely focusing on maintaining a loving attitude themselves (Stage 2) to actively attempting to soothe the child's pain and anger. Whether or not the parents succeed isn't as important as whether they try lovingly to soothe the child. It is in this stage that the "expected conversations" (this concept is defined later) start to flow more freely.

CONTRACTING FOR THERAPY

Mr. and Mrs. Smith (all names in this case history have been changed) knew they were in for a difficult time when they adopted five sisters through a private agency; the adoptive parents were told that the five had been raised partially on the city streets, and that the biological parents had had troubles with drugs. What the adoptive parents weren't told was that the birth father had murdered the children's mother. Even though the birth father was never charged with the murder, protective services removed the children from his custody not long after the mother's death, since the father, a drug addict, was severely neglecting them. Apparently the evidence fell short in allowing for a formal charge of homicide. After the intervention by social services, the children spent 2 years residing with their paternal grandparents in Canada. The grandparents then placed the children for adoption with Mr. and Mrs. Smith through a private agency. The adoptive parents had no children and were mild-mannered vegetarians with an interest in transcendental meditation. The children were charming and intelligent, but toughened by years of living on the streets.

The family was referred to the Family Therapy Institute of Washington, D.C., years after the simultaneous and open adoption of all five children. At the time of the first interview, Beth, the oldest, was 17 years of age. The second oldest was Shera, aged 10, followed by Cindy, aged 8, and twins, Melinda and Belinda, aged 6. The referral came from a community hospital, where Beth had been placed after she started abusing PCP and LSD and began to act in a bizarre manner, making irrational statements. The referral of the family to the Institute was in preparation for Beth's release from the hospital. When Beth was released from the drug treatment center, however, she did not return to the home of her adoptive parents; she decided that she would prefer instead to resume living with her biological grandparents in Canada. After Beth announced that she wasn't going to return home, the next oldest child, Shera, progressed from mildly oppositional behavior to outright defiance. Refusing to follow the directions of her adoptive parents or teachers, Shera became increasingly confrontational and angry. She seemed to enjoy going head to head in arguments with her parents and the school faculty. Punishments seemed to have no effect on her behavior. She also displayed an unnerving ability to enrage authority figures in her life. As a result, the parents decided to contact me for therapy to help them deal with Shera.

I began the first session by interviewing the entire Smith household (with the exception of Beth, who had just departed for Canada). The parents said that Shera was being nasty and disobedient at home. Shera was also so confrontational in the classroom that her teachers were insisting that she be transferred to a different school.

After meeting for 15 minutes with the entire household, I then met with Shera alone for an additional 10 minutes, during which time I questioned her about her life and performed some magic tricks with a coin (I wanted to make at least one part of the visit fun). I then met with Mr. and Mrs. Smith alone and asked for any details that they didn't want to (or hadn't wanted to) discuss in front of the children. I was disheartened to hear that one of Shera's teachers had said that she was "an evil seed." The parents were becoming increasingly afraid that Shera was turning into an evil person.

The parents were exhausted and at a complete loss as to how to handle Shera. Like most parents in oppositional situations who seek therapy, Mr. and Mrs. Smith said that they loved Shera but felt tremendous anger and resentment toward her. The Smiths were also heavily burdened with self-blame and suspected that the therapist was going to blame them for being bad parents.

Mr. and Mrs. Smith contracted with me during the initial session, first to work on the issue of Shera's extremely oppositional behavior, and then to work on other issues that the parents would decide on later. The ritual of the clients' "hiring" of the therapist provides necessary balance in the client–therapist relationship. Asking for help from a clinician puts the clinician in a "one-up" position; the formal "hiring" of the therapist by the clients equalizes the relationship by making the clinician the employee of the clients. This overt process of hiring and contracting also clarifies roles; the therapist is less likely to be viewed as behaving like a family member, and is thus less likely to inspire or foster transference.

In accepting the presenting problem as being Shera's oppositional behavior, I wasn't ignoring the other issues (trauma over the biological mother's death, the children's subsequent adoption, loss and separation issues, etc.). A strategic therapist organizes treatment around the issue that most strongly motivates the clients to seek help (Haley, 1973). Because of the interconnection of issues, I knew that I would have to eventually deal with the issues of loss, separation, and so forth through initially trying to resolve the presenting problem—Shera's oppositional behavior.

STAGE 1 OF THE INTERVENTION:
DEFINING THE PROBLEM IN AN EMPOWERING WAY

The first stage in the strategic intervention is defining the problem in a way that empowers both the clients and the therapist. In the case of the Smith

Family, was necessary to disavow unhelpful descriptions such as "evil seed" or "bad parenting." Meeting alone with the parents during the first interview, I explained that I agreed with them that Shera had oppositional tendencies. I said that at the Family Therapy Institute a four-step intervention that has been found to be very effective with oppositional children. The empowering thing about the intervention, I explained, is that it focuses on a difference in the way oppositional kids perceive confrontation. "Oppositional children don't view confrontation the same way you and I do," I shared with the parents.

The Smiths expressed great interest in this idea, and I continued to explain the differences between how parents and oppositional children view confrontation. "In order to meet the definition used at this clinic," I continued, "oppositional children must have two characteristics. They must be 'process-oriented' while their parents are 'outcome-oriented,' and during confrontation the children must approach adults more like equals . . . as if the children were arguing with peers as opposed to authority figures." I then explained the concepts of outcome and process orientation: "Children who are process-oriented tend to react to confrontation by tenaciously focusing on the process of communication rather than on the outcome. If the other party is instead focused on the outcome of the confrontation (outcome orientation), there can be terrible miscommunication."

To illustrate my point, I asked the Smiths to imagine that they had to go to the Internal Revenue Service for an audit of their tax return. They were also asked to imagine that the auditor was very polite and friendly. During the audit, would they be more concerned about whether or not they owe money (the outcome), or would they be more interested in the process of the audit? Mr. and Mrs. Smith, who looked at each other and smiled softly, both answered that they would care more about whether or not they owed money at the end of the meeting. "That," I noted, "is because you are, like most adults, outcome-oriented."

For the outcome-oriented parents, I explained, the goal of an argument is to determine the outcome of the discussion. For the process-oriented child, however, the goal is to control the process of the argument; the outcome is secondary. In other words, for a process-oriented child, the argument is about the argument; the child's perception is that the "winner" of the argument is the one who controls the process. The parents, who are trying to "win" the confrontation by determining the outcome of the argument, are extremely frustrated. They have a sense that they aren't "winning" but don't know why.

As a second example of process and outcome orientation, I asked the parents to think about the Japanese tea ceremony, with which they were familiar. The central part of the Japanese tea ceremony, Mrs. Smith explained, is the process of the ceremony. The goal of the tea ceremony isn't to get a cup of tea, Mrs. Smith assured me. I asked Mrs. Smith to think about how frustrated someone would be who was outcome-oriented and just wanted a quick cup of tea, but was being served in a 2-hour, process-oriented tea ceremony. Mrs. Smith just laughed. I then explained that this was an example of how frustrating it can be when one party in an argument is process-oriented and the other is outcome-oriented. This was the frustration that both they and Shera were feeling.

I assured the parents that there is nothing wrong with being process-oriented, but it is a perceptual style that requires a different approach. Parenting strategies that work with most outcome-oriented children don't work with process-oriented children. The problem with Shera might not have been improving, I explained, if the parents were doing what normally works with most children. When they heard that their child's behavior problems weren't proof of bad parenting, tension seemed to drain visibly from Mr. and Mrs. Smith. I'm always heartened by the relief parents express (or seem to feel) when they hear this explanation for oppositional behavior. The parents' relief comes from finding a practical explanation for their pain that doesn't blame them, but instead provides them with hope and inspiration for change.

I asked Mr. and Mrs. Smith whether, before the next session, they might be able to double-check my observation of process orientation by observing the degree to which Shera invested herself in negatively determining the three issues of process orientation. The Smiths were given a written description of process orientation (see Table 6.1) to take home with them. I noted that all children, to one degree or another, behave in the ways described in this table; therefore, the issue of frequency is important.

I also mentioned to the parents that many oppositional children at some point refuse to come to therapy, and I assured them that the intervention was designed to work without her cooperation or even, if necessary, her attendance. The parents were also told that they would be asked to attend at times without Shera. With the clarification of these points, the first interview with Mr. and Mrs. Smith ended.

The importance of parents' perceptions of blame cannot be overestimated. One of the central accomplishments of Stage 1 of this intervention is getting past the "who's to blame" discussions and moving along to the "what do we do about it" discussions. In my experience, most parents in oppositional situations assume that the therapist thinks they're at fault. When the therapist focuses on a difference in perceptual styles as being a practical and important part of the problem, the parents are usually able to get past the concern over who is to blame.†

> † *This is an excellent point. I wonder whether it would be effective to take this one step further. Perhaps if the therapist were to explore parents' schemas and automatic thoughts in more detail, it might be revealed that they anticipate the therapist's negative perception as a result of their own recriminations. More plainly stated, perhaps they are engaging in their own negative automatic self-statements based on distorted beliefs.*

TABLE 6.1. Three Aspects of Process Orientation

1. *Determining the timing of confrontations.*

   Is the timing of confrontations almost always chosen by the child?

   When the child initiates discussion at an inopportune time, are the parents usually unsuccessful in delaying discussion until a later time?

   Does the child usually allow the parents to initiate conversations about painful issues, or will the child only discuss such issues in conversations he or she initiates?

2. *Determining the content and direction of communication during confrontation.*

   The classic process-oriented discussion begins with an authority figure's approaching a child to discuss hypothetical issue A. The child responds instead by accusing the adult of hypothetical issue B. The adult then defends himself or herself against the child's accusation of issue B. In this example, the adult has initiated the content (issue A) and the direction (the adult is asking the child questions). However, the child quickly takes control of the conversation; the subject becomes issue B, and the direction becomes that of the child's asking the questions and the adult's engaging in self-defense. The child thus ended up determining the content and direction of the conversation.

3. *Determining the mood of the conversation during confrontation.*

   An adult and a child with two different moods enter a confrontation and tend to leave with the same mood. The critical issue is whether the adult takes on the child's mood or the child takes on the adult's mood.

Stage 1 of the intervention thus achieves the following:

a. The therapist interviews the entire family as well as meeting with the child alone and the parents alone.

b. The parents hire the therapist and complete a contract to work on the issue that is their greatest concern at the moment—the oppositional behavior of their child.

c. A collaborative reframing (a jointly accepted redefinition by parents and therapist) of the presenting problem occurs. There is a change from viewing the child as being evil or bad to viewing the child as perceiving confrontation in a different way than the parents and other authority figures perceive it.†

> † *This is another fine point to make early in treatment—one that may begin to prepare the parents for future reframing of their individual and joint cognitions about the child and the child's role in the family.*

d. The therapist helps the parents to move past the issue of who's to blame and to begin working on the issue of what to do about it.

e. It's made clear that although the therapist is providing the general framework for the intervention, the parents must provide most of the specific strategies for its implementation.

    f. The therapist describes to the parents the four steps of the intervention.

    g. The parents are assured that therapy can succeed with or without the cooperation of the child. The parents are also told that the child often refuses to come to therapy for a number of sessions, and that this refusal needn't be an impediment to progress.

STAGE 2: BEGINNING TO CHANGE THE INTERACTION AND TO RECHARGE THE ADULTS

The central part of Stage 2 was coaching Mr. and Mrs. Smith to avoid allowing Shera to determine their mood in a negative way. The parents were not yet asked to try to change the mood of the child, nor were the parents led to expect that Shera's behavior would improve at this stage. Stage 2, I was explained is directed only at responding differently to the child.

    Most of the coaching took place with only the parents present. A good part of the therapy hour was spent with the parents, and part of each hour was spent with Shera. Sometimes part of the hour was spent with both the parents and all the children. I met individually with Shera to find out more about her view of the problem, her family, and her peers, and to find out about third parties involved in the difficulties. In addition to collecting information, I joined with the child and encouraged her to have both patience and hope for improvement. I further tried to find out what needs she had that weren't being met by her parents. In Shera's case, a significant third party involved was a school counselor, and this was dealt with later. Although meeting with the child individually is helpful for gathering information and providing hope, it tends not to affect oppositional behavior. Oppositional behavior changes significantly only when relationships with central authority figures change.

Developing a Defense

With Mr. and Mrs. Smith, I reviewed the concept of process orientation, and emphasized that at this part of the intervention there would be one focus. This focus would be on preventing Shera from engaging negatively in the three aspects of process orientation—determining the timing of a confrontation, determining its content and direction, and most importantly determining the mood of the conversation.

    The parents were asked to describe three common confrontations representative of the sort of trouble that brought them to my office. After describing three typical arguments, Mr. and Mrs. Smith discussed what they usually tried when these confrontations occurred. They responded by stating that they simply attempted to ignore her. I remarked that their responses in those situations would work with most kids, but evidently not with process-oriented children. The Smiths and I then devised "process-sensitive" ways to cope with the three representative confrontations described. Process-sensitive ways of handling confrontations are those that don't allow the child to determine in a negative manner the timing, content/direction, or mood of confrontations.

Developing process-sensitive strategies is a collaborative process. At this stage the therapist guides the conversation and provides the framework, but the specific strategies should come from the parents. In practice, the therapist usually ends up giving a few suggestions, but does so with the understanding that the parents can try them until they come up with a better plan themselves. In hierarchical terms, part of what is occurring in Stage 2 is that the therapist is raising the level of the parents in relation to their child. This effort to anchor the parents in the role of adults is contradicted if the therapist treats the parents as if they are incompetent or unable to do what's necessary (Haley, 1976, 1980).

Gradually, Mr. and Mrs. Smith, with my coaching, developed a number of strategies aimed to help prevent Shera from determining the timing, content/direction, and mood of confrontations. To prevent Shera's determination of the timing of confrontations, the Smiths decided that when Shera started to argue with them, they would refuse to engage her; instead, Mr. and Mrs. Smith would try one of several strategies, including retreating to a different room. To prevent Shera's determination of the content and direction of communication during confrontations, the Smiths chose a practical experiment: They decided to try at times to write notes to Shera when it was necessary to convey punishments or other potentially explosive information.

I mentioned that this intervention required much tinkering, and that this set of strategies would be the first of several drafts. Mr. and Mrs. Smith were asked to try to use one of the strategies that they had devised on just one occasion before the next session. For some parents, asking them to use one jointly created strategy on one occasion over 1 or 2 weeks amounts to an optimistic request, while other parents come in having done it numerous times.

Something that was repeatedly emphasized with the Smiths was that the most important issue in changing Shera's behavior was preventing her from determining the mood of confrontations. The Smiths were asked what kind of mood they would like to have during confrontations with Shera. They said that they would like to remain calm, yet firm. I agreed that this was the most therapeutic attitude to take. In Stage 4 of this intervention, the parents would move from merely protecting and maintaining their own moods to actually soothing Shera.

Reinforcing the Parents' Marriage

It is often critical in Stage 2 to work on strengthening the parents' marriage. Some of the reasons for strengthening the marriage should be voiced to the parents, whereas others should not be mentioned, lest they be misinterpreted as blame. If the parents themselves suggest that marital tension has contributed to the child's problems, the therapist should respond with a neutral comment and move the parents to a problem-solving as opposed to a "who is to blame" discussion.

I addressed the issue of strengthening the marriage by reminding the Smiths that therapy places additional pressure on a marriage, and that they should balance this additional pressure with more individual and marital self-care. Mr. and Mrs. Smith were also asked to display appropriate, overt affection for each other in front of Shera. Affection between the parents emphasizes the different roles that children and parents occupy; it demonstrates that there is a special relationship between the parents that's different from the parents' relationship with their children. Mr. and Mrs. Smith were also asked to use affectionate gestures to help each other maintain control in emotional situations. Mr. and Mrs. Smith agreed that one partner's giving the other a kiss on the ear during a confrontation with a child would be a nice way of noting that the other was losing control of his or her mood. The parents practiced kissing in this manner in the session.†

> †*It would have been interesting to inquire whether or not Mr. and Mrs. Smith's schemas changed as a result of the behavioral exercises the therapist used with them. One of the basic tenets of behavior therapy is that a change in behavior will change patterns of belief.*

The present intervention ultimately works to the degree that parents are capable of soothing a child. It's common, however, for parents to start therapy in a state so burdened by anger, blame, and shame that they're unable to demonstrate much empathic behavior. Working to enrich the quality of the parents lives leaves the parents in a better position to give warmly and empathically to a child. Stage 2 starts improving the quality of the parents' lives by disengaging them from the disempowering and maddening strife and by working on structure, which gives the parents time to relate to each other as romantic figures rather than just as wardens of a difficult child.

Fishing for Triangles

From the systemic point of view, the attempted assumption of adult authority by the child is never a solitary enterprise. To succeed, the child must perceive that there are others who support his or her attempted undermining of grownups' authority. In the case of Shera, this role was inadvertently assumed by her school counselor. Shera went to the counselor one day to discuss her sadness at her biological father's having murdered her mother. The counselor was deeply touched by Shera's pain; at the child's request, she gave Shera permission to leave class at any time to come and talk about her pain. As a result, whenever Shera's teacher tried to discipline her, Shera would stand up and announce, "I've got to go to see the counselor." The teacher began to resent the counselor for interfering with her authority, whereas the counselor began to dislike the teacher for failing to have empathy for the child's pain. I visited the school after speaking by telephone to the principal, teacher, and counselor, and met with them as a group in order to mediate the situation. This triangulation was soon ended as a result of our meeting.

In Stage 2, therefore, the following steps are emphasized:

a. The therapist helps the parents disengage from the oppositional sequence by redirecting their focus to not allowing the child to determine the process of confrontation in a negative way. The parents' confidence in being able to help the child increases with every small success by not allowing the child to determine process in a negative way.

b. The therapist reinforces a healthy sense of entitlement to happiness in the parents' relationship, and helps them structure private time for communication and romance outside of the home.

c. Relationships that are contributing to the child's sense of having adult-like authority are found and detriangulated. School visits by the therapist are strongly recommended.

STAGE 3: RESTRUCTURING RULES AND CONSEQUENCES

In Stage 3, the therapy continues to work on the issues of Stage 2, but adds a new set of rules and consequences, sensitive to the three major issues of process orientation: the timing, content/direction, and mood of confrontations. Stage 2 usually starts a week after the reframing of Stage 1 has occurred, and Stage 3 usually begins 2 weeks after that. Ideally, Stage 3 starts after the parents grasp and begin to put into practice the concept of not allowing the child to determine their mood.

The discussions with Mr. and Mrs. Smith on rules and consequences emphasized two points. The first was lowering the anxiety involved in punishment, especially by separating in time the occurrence of misbehavior and the delivery of punishments. The second issue emphasized was developing a process-sensitive system of positive and negative consequences, complete with a two-tiered system of rules and consequences. Because parental endurance is a theme through this intervention, strong consideration was given to Mr. and Mrs. Smith's endurance in helping them with Stage 3.

Anxiety and Punishment

I described to Mr. and Mrs. Smith the relationship between anxiety and learning in oppositional kids. I informed the Smiths that most children learn better when, in contrast to their usual calm state, they are momentarily made just a little bit anxious. What's unusual about oppositional children, however, is that they tend to have extreme impairment of social perception and learning with a rise in anxiety. What's characteristic of an oppositional child is that when the child is anxious at the time of punishment, the connection between the child's own behavior and the consequences is often lost. In other words, I noted to the Smiths, "The more anxious Shera becomes, the less she'll connect her own behavior with your reaction." Shera tended to remember vividly her parents' reactions but not her own part in evoking their anger. The challenge, I shared with Mr. and Mrs. Smith, is to punish oppositional children with as little anxiety as possible.†

> † This was a great move, particularly since anxiety was likely to be what was truly fueling Shera's behaviors. It might also be helpful for a therapist to suggest some imagery to parents when attempting to lower their anxiety—for example, perhaps some relaxation exercises and imagery of reprimanding their children. Perhaps practicing this may make it more successful when parents attempt it in vivo.

Rules and Consequences

I then noted that process-oriented children need a process-sensitive set of rules and consequences, and that the Smiths might want to alter theirs to make their lives easier. I then asked Mr. and Mrs. Smith to write down a list of current rules and consequences. The Smiths' reply was typical of parents of a child with oppositional problems: They complained that there were no longer consistent rules or consequences available. Although such rules did exist in the past, they'd been abandoned for lack of effectiveness. The therapy session was then dedicated to drawing up *separate* lists of rules and punishments (these should not be placed on the same page). I told the Smiths that the reason for my suggesting the alteration of some existing rules and consequences wasn't that these rules were "wrong," but that they were for ordinary behavior, not oppositional behavior.

After Mr. and Mrs. Smith completed the separate lists of rules and of consequences, I asked them to divide consequences into "cooperative" and "noncooperative" punishments. A cooperative punishment is one that requires the cooperation of the child to be effective. For example, if a parent administers a punishment of having to rake leaves, the consequence isn't put into effect until the child cooperates by actually raking. A noncooperative punishment is one that doesn't require the cooperation of the child. An example of the latter would be a parent's withholding a child's allowance; the punishment is achieved without any need for the child's cooperation.

I shared with Mr. and Mrs. Smith that usually parents have access to only a few effective and practical noncooperative punishments, so it's best *not* to use them as a first response; rather, it's better to use noncooperative punishments to back up cooperative ones. The use of a noncooperative consequence to back up a cooperative consequence is called a "two-tiered" punishment system. There is a second consequence given until or unless the first consequence is completed. For example, with a cooperative punishment such as raking leaves, the parents add that until the leaves are raked, the television will remain locked in a closet.

Of prime importance is that the punishments devised should not be harder on the parents than on the child. Mr. and Mrs. Smith laughed at this; they'd often felt that their punishments were harder on them than on Shera. I mentioned that in order for this intervention to work, punishing Shera had to be relatively easy for them, or else they wouldn't have the endurance to be consistent. We set about redesigning the rules and consequences of the household to make them easier for the Smiths to employ. The rules and consequences were then redrawn to integrate a two-tiered system. Copies of the rules and consequences were then posted by Mr. and Mrs. Smith on either side of the refrigerator door.

The Size of Punishments

Early in Stage 3 of the intervention, it's wise to emphasize succeeding with the delivery of consequences over finding punishments that exactly fit the crime. Finding an exact punishment to fit the crime is a form of intellectual quicksand; many parents get stuck here and never proceed to any punishment at all. With adolescents and oppositional children of most ages, small, irritating punishments are sometimes more effective than large, dramatic ones (though the latter also have their place—see Jerome Price's book *Power and Compassion* [1996]). To help Mr. and Mrs. Smith understand this concept, I shared a personal story. When I was a teenager, I told them, I was hiking with a friend when we came upon a bull in a pasture. My friend got into the pasture and baited the bull into charging him. At the last moment, my friend jumped out of the bull's pen, and we thought that this was grandly amusing. Some minutes later we stopped for a snack, and a yellow jacket came to rest on my friend's backpack. My friend wouldn't go near the backpack until the wasp was gone . . . and this happened just minutes after he'd baited a bull. Sometimes a small, dramatic, but irritating punishment is more effective than a major confrontational one.

Punishment as a Crucial Moment

Giving a punishment is one of the most crucial moments in reversing oppositional behavior. Of central importance is that parents should announce punishments at a time when they feel calm and in control. A firm but empathic mood tends to empower the role of the parent most substantially in relation to the role of the child. If the child picks the timing of the confrontation, it's almost guaranteed to be at a moment when the parent is tired, in a rush to get somewhere, or otherwise distracted. If a parent has a domestic partner, I often recommend that punishments not be given out until both adults are at home and can discreetly coach each other to be calm and empathic while giving the punishment. If the parent doesn't have a partner, an adult friend or neighbor will do.

I asked the Smiths to experiment with something that other parents in similar situations have found very helpful. Sometimes the exact punishment for breaking a serious rule shouldn't be announced at the time of the bad behavior; it's sometimes better to "tag" significant bad behavior. "Tagging" is a parent's telling a child that the parent is aware of the bad behavior and will deal with it later. It's only appropriate to tag bad behavior if it seems to the adult that the child is purposefully provoking the adult, or if the adult isn't in the best of conditions to control his or her own mood in a confrontation. The announcing of a punishment is almost always a confrontation of sorts, and waiting to deliver the punishment prevents the child from determining the timing of this particular confrontation. Furthermore, delaying the announcement of the punishment allows the parent to pick the best moment in terms of his or her emotional endurance. Interestingly enough, an oppositional kid often seems to dwell more on a punishment before it's given than after; thus, delaying punishment can lend increased weight to consequences of behavior.

Balancing Positive and Negative Consequences

It's important when setting up negative consequences that they be balanced by positive ones that motivate good behavior. The existence of positive consequences helps both parents and child feel that the goal of the system is a benevolent one. With a volatile adolescent, it's sometimes a good idea to give punishments at a "balancing-of-accounts" meeting that includes giving both positive and negative consequences within the same discussion; the mixture of rewards prevents misinterpretation of the situation as "mean."

The Smiths were urged to use traditional positive reinforcements for good behavior. The parents began to use a system that had been helpful to them in the past, involving the administering of a star on a chart for a good day and a special prize for 7 good days in a row. Self-help books tend to be especially strong when it comes to helping parents with these sorts of positive reinforcement systems. The parents were to find or invent their own positive reinforcements.†

> † *Research has shown repeatedly that the use of positive reinforcement is extremely effective in behavior change, particularly with oppositional children.*

Scheduling Fun, Regardless of Behavior

It was also recommended that Mr. and Mrs. Smith set aside some special times with Shera and the other children that would occur, regardless of the children's behavior. I explained to the Smiths that part of the foundation of their authority was their role as providers of good things and good times. Parents in oppositional situations, in their efforts to keep up with punishment, frequently end up removing all opportunities to be the good-thing/good-time providers; this seriously undercuts their authority. It is thus of vital importance that regular parent–child fun be scheduled and that it never be interfered with by consequences or other events. I also noted that it's easier to maintain one's mood with a child if there has been some recent positive interaction. Moreover, for punishment to work, there needs to be some contrast between the state of being punished and the state of not being punished. Some children are punished so often that additional punishment has little or no impact.

The major steps of Stage 3 are thus the following:

a. The therapist introduces the idea that process orientation requires process-oriented rules, rewards, and punishments.
b. The parents are helped to create a new set of rules and consequences, with consequences being organized in a two-tiered system that links cooperative and noncooperative punishments.
c. The therapist emphasizes on the importance of the parents' controlling their mood during punishment.
d. The therapist also emphasized the need for a balance between positive and negative consequences, as well as the need for fun time between parents and child, regardless of the child's behavior.
e. The therapist must pay attention to parental endurance when designing rules and consequences. Consequences should not be hard on the parents.

STAGE 4: SOOTHING THE OPPOSITIONAL CHILD AND HAVING THE EXPECTED CONVERSATIONS

Stage 4 could be attempted only after Mr. and Mrs. Smith had increased their self-care to the extent that they could offer more emotional support to Shera. Another requirement was that the parents had to have recovered some confidence in their competence as parents, and thus to be secure enough to move beyond issues of blame and to focus on change.

Soothing the Child

The fourth stage moves the parents from merely focusing on maintaining a loving attitude themselves to actively attempting to change the child's mood from negative to positive. The focus is on how, in an oppositional situation, an adult and a child usually begin a confrontation with two different moods and come out with the same mood. The question is thus: Is the adult going to take on the child's mood, or is the child going to take on the adult's mood?

The challenge of soothing is that it's most effective when it's used both in calm moments *and* during the child's attempts at emotional "button pushing." In other words, a point at which the child is trying to provoke the parents is one of the most important times for the parent to soothe the child. Through the earlier steps of the intervention, Mr. and Mrs. Smith had become more secure in the notion that a large part of the power of parenting comes from the ability to help children moderate their moods. The Smiths were reminded, both through our discussions and through their own successes, that a big step in helping children moderate their own moods is refusing to allow them to negatively determine adults' moods. Weathering the child's worst provocations while maintaining an empathic but firm mood goes far in soothing the oppositional child.

More severe cases of oppositional behavior tend not to change dramatically until Stage 4, when the adults consciously work on soothing the child's mood. I worked with Mr. and Mrs. Smith and established a number of techniques that would facilitate change in order to alter Shera's mood from a negative, escalating, inappropriately powerful mood to a positive mood appropriate for her age.

One strategy of mood changing that sometimes works with young children who are only moderately oppositional and aren't experiencing much emotional pain is for parents to reinterpret oppositional behavior (back to the child) as being benevolent or playful. This is called "playful diversion." An example of diversion is turning the child's initiation of defiant behavior into a joke or game. The response to "I won't do that" may be that the parent tickles and kisses the child while mimicking the youngster in a playful way. The child will often go along with the game and pretend that he or she was actually just playing instead of really being defiant.

Having the Expected Conversations

Shera, however, had severe emotional pain that would have made playful diversion inappropriate. Beth—Shera's older sister, who had served as a maternal figure—was moving away, and the child had a traumatic history. What Shera needed wasn't diversion, but rather discussion of issues that were causing her great emotional pain. Critical to the understanding of severe oppositional behavior is why the expected conversations haven't taken place already.

One of the defining acts of parenting is soothing a child. According to the earlier list describing the "hard" and "soft" sides of hierarchy, soothing is one of the primary characteristics of the parental role. However, if a child is trying to function as an adult and trying to assume the authority of an adult, being soothed represents a step backward from adult-like functioning. Thus, to the degree that the child feels the need to function as an adult, the child will try to resist being soothed. This resistance is often manifested as an avoidance of discussions with parents that might result in soothing. Despite the efforts of her parents to discuss how Shera felt about her older sister's moving away, Shera refused to discuss the issue with them. Shera would complain about her sister's departure when her parents were talking to each other about other topics, but as soon as the parents directed their attention to Shera and her pain, she changed subjects or left the room.

The desire to be adult-like and to avoid being soothed is, however, balanced by a desire to be age-appropriate and to be soothed. Soothing entails more than just comforting behavior; it must also include discussions that one would expect to happen naturally between parent and child concerning the child's pains. Thus we have the concept of the "expected conversations"—the conversations that should be happening between loved ones but that, for one reason or another, aren't.

Transcript of a Session with Mr. and Mrs. Smith and Shera

The following transcript is from a videotaped session approximately seven interviews into the therapy. The goal of the session was for Mr. and Mrs. Smith to soothe Shera and to have the "expected conversation" with her. The topic of the expected conversation was Shera's pain over her older sister Beth's departure from the home to live with their biological father's parents in Canada. In the room were Mr. and Mrs. Smith (Mom and Dad), Shera, and the therapist (myself, Mr. Keim). The interview began with Mr. Smith's holding Shera on his knee and telling her that he and her mother would like to discuss how she felt about her sister's leaving.

SHERA: No, no!! Get off!! No! I want to see her. I don't want to be with you! 'Cause you ruin my life! Get off of me!

DAD: No, come here. Come here.

SHERA: NO!

MR. KEIM: Shera . . .

Shera immediately erupted and within a number of seconds left the room. However, she almost immediately returned. Shera simultaneously did and did not want to discuss her older sister's departure. Several minutes into the interview, I coached the parents by initiating discussions that were directly soothing to Shera: I complimented Shera's outfit. This is called "the bob-and-weave technique"—if a child won't allow direct soothing, the adults try indirect soothing by talking to one another about the child.

MR. KEIM: That's a pretty outfit.

MOM: I think it was a gift from the Gap.

MR. KEIM: Um-hm. I love children's clothes from the Gap.

MOM: Yeah. They're really fun.

DAD: So we were talking a bit about you before, but we thought we should talk with you while you're here. And, um, you've told us a number of times, and it's—it's clear from what you've said that you're upset a little bit because Beth's leaving now and she won't be in the family, at least at home. And, um, I thought you might want to say something about how you feel.

There was a long silence. Shera would talk when not spoken to, but would not talk when directly addressed. This was an example of Shera's determination of the content and direction of communication. Mrs. Smith then broke the silence with more indirect soothing.

MOM: Shera gave me a wonderful massage last night.

MR. KEIM: Did she?

MOM: Yeah. She wanted me to come into her bed, and I went into her bed, and she gave me a really nice massage. She's very good at that.

SHERA: Next time I'll be sure to kill you.

MR. KEIM, DAD, MOM: Mmmm.

MOM: I know she's feeling mad.

DAD: I—I think we know that you don't mean those things when you say them.

SHERA: Ph! Ahhhhhh!

DAD: We know that you're upset.

Before therapy, Mrs. Smith had reacted to Shera's threats to kill her by leaving the room, and both parents had been distracted from important conversation by rude behavior. Mr. and Mrs. Smith had since been coached not to let such comments throw an important conversation off track. I tried to bring the discussion back to the expected conversation.

MR. KEIM: You know, Beth will always be in the family, but you know, she's at the age where she's going to be making her own decisions and going on with her life and career.

MOM: Yeah, when Beth first came to us, she'd been with her mom for 10 years. Ten long years. And so her mom is, basically, that's her mom. You guys . . .

DAD: In her mind, that's her mom for life . . .

MOM: . . . even after she's come to us.

DAD: . . . no matter what.

MR. KEIM: Because at that age, especially, when you're 10, the person that you look at as—as your mom is the person you've considered your mom.

DAD: Um-hm.

SHERA: Well, I still consider her my mom, my old mom, but you guys just came and adopted us, and now you're treating us like nothing!

DAD: I hope not. You're very special.

SHERA: And you call people selfish!

Shera was trying once again to divert the discussion, and I coached the parents to stay on track. The attempts by the parents to discuss Beth continued. When attempts to discuss Beth's leaving failed, the parents and I resorted to soothing. If Shera would not allow direct soothing, we adults resorted to indirect soothing by talking to each other in a way that was complimentary to Shera.

DAD: Even without toe shoes, she can stand on the tips of her toes.

MR. KEIM: That's incredible.

MOM: Yeah.

DAD: Very well coordinated. And lately she's learning gymnastics routines. She can do a back walkover, very gracefully . . .

SHERA: Back walkover, front, front, back flip . . .

DAD: . . . front flip . . .

MR. KEIM: Um-hm.

SHERA: . . . splits. I can do anything I want to do.

DAD: . . . cartwheel . . .

SHERA: Right now, I don't want to do anything.

After more than 40 minutes of effort, a break occurred.

DAD: Yeah. I think when somebody has that ability that—even though it gets clouded by bad feelings, that they can always go back to the good feelings.

MR. KEIM: Um-hm.

MOM: Yeah. And it's, it's . . .

DAD: We're very lucky.

MOM: . . . she's very beautiful when she's like that. When she's—when she's very giving, her whole being is, like, really radiant, and it's really beautiful.

MR. KEIM: Um-hm.

MOM: And everybody wants to be with her.

MR. KEIM: Um-hm.

MOM: It's like . . .

DAD: Beth has that trait, too. She's just—she can be just a very, very good friend.

MR. KEIM: Um-hm. *(Pause)* What do you miss most about Beth? *(Pause)* Shera, what do you miss most about Beth?

MOM: Oh, let's see. I guess I miss those traits, those warm traits—you know, those traits where she's . . .

SHERA: I miss Beth because you take her away. No. You want to hear why I'm saddest? Because you take everything that's important to me away. Beth's important to me, and you just take her away from me.

DAD: And you feel great loss.

As Shera discussed her pain in the last few lines above, her voice changed from that of an angry pseudoadult to that of an age-appropriate young girl. She allowed herself to be vulnerable and was soothed by her parents. For the moment, she returned to the role of a 10-year-old girl. By the end of the interview, Shera was significantly less oppositional; she had taken the role of a child who accepted her parents' authority, and her tone and demeanor were once again age-appropriate. The expected conversation was starting to take place, and Shera was being soothed out of her oppositional behavior. Of course, it must be noted that one conversation of this sort doesn't by itself transform a severely oppositional child. Enduring change in the oppositional behavior requires repeated discussions of and soothing of the child's pain.

The therapy of Shera's oppositional behavior continued for several more months. As the oppositional behavior receded, concern turned to how the children were coping with the knowledge that their father had murdered their mother. The children had known that their mother had died, but hadn't known the details until Beth revealed the truth about the incident 6 months before the start of therapy. A new contract was then formed to work on the new issue, and therapy proceeded. Three years after the first interview, the family still returned from time to time for three or four sessions to deal with transitions (e.g., one of the children's starting at a new school), which tended to be accompanied by a short period of acting out, and also to deal with health problems that one of the children began to suffer from.

SUMMARY

The intervention described in this chapter doesn't focus on a global description of the etiology of oppositional behavior. For the purposes of facilitating change, the focus of therapy is on changing the sequence and hierarchy of interaction centering around the conflict. A clear contract is made, in which the therapist is hired to work on specific problems. Careful efforts are made to join with the clients and to avoid misperceptions (such as blaming of clients) that might interfere with a cooperative process. The therapist uses a combination of client-inspired and therapist-inspired directives, at times offering advice directly and at times coaching the clients to come up with ideas. One reason for the success of this intervention is that it facilitates cooperation among all those involved in the problem, including the identified patient, family, teachers, and others. Another reason for the success of this intervention is that it moves clients past the issue of who or what is to blame, and, in a cooperative and empathic manner, focuses the attention of the social system on solving the problem.

AUTHOR'S REPLY TO EDITOR'S COMMENTS

Therapists from different approaches often arrive at the same intervention, but have different explanations as to how and why they got there. For example, Dr. Dattilio's suggestions would absolutely be within the realm of good strategic therapy. I would take the actions he has suggested, but would explain them in a different way. For example, Dr. Dattilio suggests that a therapist might pursue the issue of self-blame with the parents of an oppositional child. I would accept this suggestion, although I would think of it in terms of removing a stumbling block to collaboration and in terms of preventing any perception of the therapist's "triangulating" with the child against the parents.

Scott Miller has suggested to me in personal conversations that comparisons focused on actions in different therapies tend to be fruitful, whereas comparisons focused on explanations for actions more often than not result in bad feelings between professionals. My personal experience has suggested that Scott is quite correct. The case comments by Dr. Dattilio are a nice example of this similarity on a level of action. His comments can best be appreciated if one is not threatened by the different language used to arrive at the interventions.

In a letter to the *Family Therapy Networker* just weeks before he died, John Weakland (1995) wrote of his concerns regarding conflict between schools of therapy. John wrote of a meeting of what has loosely been called "the Muddy Waters Group," a friendly gathering of therapists of different schools who strive to emphasize common ground. John wrote:

> Specifically, the meeting explored common premises and values shared at a general level despite specific differences, and avenues of cooperation and collaboration to present to colleagues and students.
>
> While not always easy, one of the strengths of the field from its earliest days has been constructive reflection and discussion of its diversity. The emphasis on having things "my way" and needing something new each year has distracted us from serious and useful dialogue about what aids people in distress and facilitates change. (Weakland, 1995, p. 16)

Dr. Dattilio's work stands in the tradition of such useful dialogue.

REFERENCES

American Psychiatric Association. (1994). *Diagnostic and statistical manual of mental disorders* (4th ed.). Washington, DC: Author.

Bateson, G. (1972). *Steps toward an ecology of mind.* New York: Ballantine Books.

Bateson, G. (1979). *Mind and nature.* New York: E. P. Dutton.

Fisch, R., Weakland, J., & Segal, L. (1982). *The tactics of change.* San Francisco: Jossey-Bass.

Gray, J. (1993). *Men are from Mars, women are from Venus: A practical guide for improving communication and getting what you want in your relationships.* New York: HarperCollins.

Grove, D., & Haley, J. (1993). *Conversations on therapy.* New York: Norton.

Haley, J. (1963). *Strategies of psychotherapy.* New York: Grune & Stratton.

Haley, J. (1973). *Uncommon therapy.* New York: Norton.

Haley, J. (1976). *Problem-solving therapy.* San Francisco: Jossey-Bass.

Haley, J. (1980). *Leaving home: The therapy of disturbed young people.* New York: McGraw-Hill.

Haley, J. (1981). *Reflections on therapy.* Chevy Chase, MD: Family Therapy Institute of Washington, DC.

Haley, J. (1984). *Ordeal therapy.* San Francisco: Jossey-Bass.

Haley, J. (1989). *Fifth profession ethics.* Unpublished manuscript.

Haley, J., & Weakland, J. (1987). *Remembering Bateson.* Chevy Chase, MD: Family Therapy Institute of Washington, DC.

Hoffman, L. (1981). *Foundations of family therapy.* New York: Basic Books.

Jackson, D. D. (1967). The myth of normality. *Medical Opinion and Review, 3,* 28–33.

Keim, I., Lentine, G., Keim, J., & Madanes, C. (1988). Strategies for changing the past. *Journal of Strategic and Systemic Therapies, 6*(3), 2–17.

Keim, I., Lentine, G., Keim, J., & Madanes, C. (1990). No more John Wayne strategies for changing the past. In C. Madanes (Ed.), *Sex, love and violence: Strategies for transformation.* New York: Norton.

Keim, J. (1993). *The Family Therapy Institute training handbook.* Unpublished manuscript.

Loeber, R., Lahey, B., & Thomas, C. (1991). Diagnostic conundrum of oppositional defiant disorder and conduct disorder. *Journal of Abnormal Psychology, 100*(3), 379–390.

Madanes, C. (1980). Protection, paradox and pretending. *Family Process, 19,* 73–85.

Madanes, C. (1981). *Strategic family therapy.* San Francisco: Jossey-Bass.

Madanes, C. (1984). *Behind the one-way mirror.* San Francisco: Jossey-Bass.

Madanes, C. (Ed.). (1990). *Sex, love, and violence: Strategies for transformation.* New York: Norton.

Minuchin, S. (1974). *Families and family therapy.* Cambridge, MA: Harvard University Press.

Minuchin, S. (1984). *Family kaleidoscope.* Cambridge, MA: Harvard University Press.

Minuchin, S. (1993). Keynote address presented at the Family Therapy Networker Symposium.

Price, J. A. (1996). *Power and compassion: Working with difficult adolescents and abused parents.* New York: Guilford Press.

Ruesch, J., & Bateson, G. (1951). *Communication.* New York: Norton.

Selvini Palazzoli, M. S., Boscolo, L., Cecchin, G., & Prata, G. (1978). *Paradox and counterparadox.* New York: Jason Aronson.

Stanton, D., Todd, T., & Associates. (1982). *The family therapy of drug abuse and addiction.* New York: Guilford Press.

Tannen, D. (1990). *You just don't understand: Women and men in conversation.* New York: Morrow.

Watzlawick, P. (Ed.). (1984). *The invented reality.* New York: Norton.

Watzlawick, P., Beavin, J., & Jackson, D. (1967). *The pragmatics of human communication.* New York: Norton.

Watzlawick, P., Weakland, J., & Fisch, R. (1974). *Change: Principles of problem formation and problem resolution.* New York: Norton.

Weakland, J. (1960). The double-bind hypothesis of schizophrenia and three-party interaction. In D. D. Jackson (Ed.), *The etiology of schizophrenia.* New York: Basic Books.

Weakland, J. (1995, September–October). Letter to the editor. *Family Therapy Networker,* p. 16.

Weakland, J., Fisch, R., Watzlawick, P., & Bodin, A. (1974). Brief therapy: Focused problem resolution. *Family Process, 13,* 141–168.

SUGGESTED READINGS

Haley, J. (1973). *Uncommon therapy.* New York: Norton.

Haley, J. (1976). *Problem-solving therapy.* San Francisco: Jossey-Bass.

Keim, I., Lentine, G., Keim, J., & Madanes, C. (1988). Strategies for changing the past. *Journal of Strategic and Systemic Therapies, 6*(3), 2–17.

Madanes, C. (1980). Protection, paradox and pretending. *Family Process, 19,* 73–85.

Madanes, C. (1981). *Strategic family therapy.* San Francisco: Jossey-Bass.

Chapter 7

Contextual Family Therapy

DAVID N. ULRICH

The contextual approach to counseling and psychotherapy is a school of therapy as well as a way of viewing the psychotherapeutic process. It maintains that the essence of what holds relationships together is reciprocal trust. Trust grows when a relationship is based on a fair balance of give and take, with each party responding to the interests of the other. Recognition of the other's interests is an ethical imperative (Boszormenyi-Nagy & Spark, 1973).

This isn't an easy concept to grasp. The sense of it suggests that human beings have evolved into a social matrix in which it is implicit that survival as a member is ultimately contingent upon one's awareness of and respect for the needs and interests of others, in a reciprocal fashion (Glanz & Pearce, 1989). Contextual therapists regard this as the "ethical dimension," and it cannot be reduced to a psychological or transactional dimension. It remains true whether it's recognized or not; hence it possesses an imperative quality. This imperative provides the best guarantee that any relationship will be satisfying and enduring.

The following may be considered different facets of the same phenomenon: deterioration of reciprocal trust, stagnation of a relationship, and the emergence of pathological symptoms. A major goal of contextual therapy is to help people reopen the question of who owes what to whom (in other words, how does the balance stand in the ledger of interpersonal accounts?) and to take "rejunctive" actions that will help to restore fairness and trust in a relationship (Ulrich, 1983). What's fair is determined not by the therapist or by one party, but by the willing negotiation of interests between parties. If one party holds more power (e.g., as a parent does over a child), he or she is under a heavier burden to protect the other's interests (Boszormenyi-Nagy & Spark, 1973).

Contextual therapy is based on certain premises about people. In any family, there is a deep synergism of interests. In exchange for their parents' creating and caring for them, children develop a profound sense of loyalty to their parents—a phenomenon that is often overlooked. Validation of the self as an individual and as a member of the family comes in substantial measure from what one can give; loyalty is one of the greatest gifts a child can offer (Boszormenyi-Nagy, Grunebaum, & Ulrich, 1991). This is the beginning of a lifetime paradigm of validating the self through acting on behalf of others. Such actions earn "entitlement"; that is, one may accumulate a legitimate claim upon those for whom one has acted. But if the parental couple is split by conflicting attitudes and values, then the child's loyalty may also be split, which will prove problematic for the child.

Far more devastating is the situation where one parent is split between caring and abusiveness. This poses a cruel dilemma for the child. If one of his or her caretakers abuses a child physically or sexually, the betrayal of trust, perhaps even more than the physical impact, is what traumatizes the child. As Denise Gelinas remarked to me (personal communication, 1996), "What happens when the person who is supposed to protect you from the boogey man turns out to be the boogey man?" The child may be able to preserve loyalty only by splitting off part of his or her own awareness. Thus, the attempt to maintain loyalty in the face of severe trauma may be a central factor in the formation of dissociative disorders. Any psychotherapeutic treatment that disregards this phenomenon of loyalty may eventually backfire.

Sometimes parents fail to recognize or acknowledge a child's best efforts at being a loyal participant in the family; for example, a daughter may relinquish a play date to take care of her sick little brother, only to get a scolding when he cries. If this kind of response occurs often enough, the child's loyalty may go underground or become "invisible" (Boszormenyi-Nagy & Spark, 1973). This may have long-lasting pernicious effects. For instance, a child may become a failure, in order to conform to the image imposed on him or her by the prior generation.

Even in cases of abuse, the assumption is never made that the deepest levels of family relatedness are adversary (Boszormenyi-Nagy & Spark, 1973). There may remain a residue of loyalty and caring that does not appear on the surface. This must not be destroyed by the therapist. It's hard to imagine a contextually oriented therapist encouraging a client to bring a lawsuit against abusive parents, or counseling a permanent break with the family.

Another significant aspect of contextual therapy has to do with "legacy." To a remarkable extent, our lives are guided by multigenerational directives concerning what we are to be and do. For example, five consecutive generations of males in a family may pass on to their sons, by betraying their trust, the lesson that the world isn't to be trusted. Stierlin (1976) refers to such directives as "mandates." My colleagues and I have found the term "designation" useful in discussing how people's careers are frequently shaped by multigenerational directives (Ulrich & Dunne, 1986). Loyalty, especially invisible loyalty, provides much of the incentive for acting according to one's legacy.

Of special concern is the issue of "destructive entitlement." The hurt and deprived child may seek to wrest from innocent parties what he or she did not receive from the parents, or to punish innocent parties in retaliation for his or her own wounds. The claims are legitimate, but the targets are not (Boszormenyi-Nagy et al., 1991). Establishing empathic "siding" with someone who is driven by a sense of destructive entitlement is one of the most difficult and challenging tasks a contextual therapist may face.

The contextual approach is also based on certain assumptions about therapy and the role of the therapist. First, the therapist is ethically bound to take into account the interests of all who will be affected by the therapy. This may involve making inquiries about people who don't attend the sessions, or in some cases pressing for those family members to participate. A therapist who finds against the father in a visitation dispute, without having even attempted to see the father, may be vulnerable to the charge of being a "hired gun." When conducting a session, the therapist doesn't have to strive for a sterile neutrality; instead, the aim is "multidirectional partiality," with the therapist serving as advocate in turn for everyone involved. This holds true regardless of whether the therapist is actually seeing one person or several.

Contextual therapists have developed a number of methods, all of which maintain the goals of (1) helping to clarify the often competing claims of family members concerning the "ledger," or the statement of who owes what to whom (some of these claims may have lain dormant for generations); (2) helping family members see why it's good to move toward resolution of these issues; and (3) assisting them in the task. This will obviously require the overcoming of resistance from intrapsychic factors working against change. These methods of contextual therapy include "loyalty framing," "balanced siding," and "holding accountable," among others.

Also, the therapist helps clients to "exonerate" members of previous generations. The therapist encourages clients to make room for the discovery of good things about parents, grandparents, and earlier ancestors (if facts are known about these). This will facilitate clients' finding something of value in their origins; thus, their loyalties may be to some degree validated. As one client observed, "It's nice to find that there was a good part of her. After all, everybody needs a mother."

The following two case reports serve to illustrate some of the concepts described above. I provide comments in notes throughout the text to explain the interventions. The first case demonstrates various facets of the dilemma faced by those who seek to retain ties of loyalty and attachment to their parents, and yet to break the bonds of abusive confinement that were imposed early by their parents.

CASE REPORT: LOYALTY FRAMING, EXONERATION

Contextual therapy is considered by its originators to be compatible with any other socially responsible school of therapy. However, the actual integration of contextual therapy with other therapies has been approached cautiously. In this first case, I was seeking as the therapist to coordinate such contextual strategies as rejunction, exoneration, and acknowledgment of merit with psychodynamic strategies. The underlying assumption was that contextual strategies for finding positive elements in the family mix would help the client to face and cope with the negative elements, including the sequelae of trauma.

The case revolved around the invisible loyalty of a son toward a father. As an adult, the son was still unable to contain the sense of outrage, loss, and despair resulting from the father's behavior toward him as a child. This fealty to the past prevented him from grasping emotionally what he perceived intellectually—that the occasion for outrage had passed, that he was by no means helpless, and that his gains outweighed his losses. Somewhat paradoxically, my support for various aspects of the son's family loyalty placed the son in a position to liberate himself from its pernicious aspects.

Donald was the youngest of three siblings in an intact upper-middle-class family. He portrayed his childhood as one of extensive isolation; although he didn't seem to lack social skills, he spent a great deal of his time either alone in his room or roaming the woods. He was aware of a growing conviction that if he did try to do anything, the results would be worthless. His parents pressured him to get out and find things to do, usually competitive things. This only caused him torment.

Reinforcing this torment was the fact that his father, an alcoholic, could be explosively critical. Although his father revealed virtually nothing to Donald about his own childhood, one or two clues slipped through indicating that he himself had been belittled as a child by an austere and condescending father. Donald's mother would be close with him at times, but for the most part she let her husband set the pace in the household.

By the time he reached high school, Donald was in the grip of intense, unremitting anxiety. He began looking for ways to induce oblivion; even a few moments' respite from the anxiety was a relief for him. His methods included using cigarettes, alcohol, and drugs; going on impulsive buying sprees; and reading pornographic magazines and masturbating. He felt a growing distaste for all of these, as well as a growing disgust with himself. Nevertheless, he proceeded through college in a pot-induced haze.

Several years out of college, with a wife and two children but with no essential change of ways of coping with anxiety, Donald found himself partially immobilized in performing life's tasks. He couldn't pick up a telephone to inquire about a job; he left household chores undone and bills unpaid. It was at this point that he first sought therapy. As treatment progressed, substantial shifts occurred, unquestionably aided by the use of antidepressive medications. He obtained a well-remunerated job, made a more substantial contribution to the household, became closer to his son and daughter, and became involved in Alcoholics Anonymous (AA), dedicating time and effort to his meetings. I assumed that these gains resulted from the continual reworking of Donald's basic fear of being unable to master the beginning steps of any enterprise. He was learning that his near-panic response to undertaking new ventures was derived from a family legacy laid down by endless repetitions of seemingly small traumas within the family. This dawning realization did not erase the sequelae of trauma, but it did open doors far enough for new, desirable functions to emerge.

In spite of all this, Donald's anxiety level remained unabated, and he still felt distant from everyone except his children. At the dinner table, for instance, his tension would become so acute that he felt almost irresistible pressure to get up and flee from the table. I assumed that the persistence of such symptoms as unremitting anxiety, a continuing sense of worthlessness, and an inability to be close to other adults, as well as a variety of physical signs that Donald described, could very well be indicators of underlying trauma. Although, despite many attempts at exploration, the deeper levels of trauma remained unidentified, it did appear that Donald's own futile attempts to preserve order in the family (e.g., trying to protect his older brother, Robert, from his father's onslaughts) had probably contributed both to his anxiety and to his constant sense of failure.

I relied heavily on the use of contextual strategies to bring Donald to the point where he would be more ready to investigate, face, and cope with whatever residue of trauma underlay his burden of anxiety. These strategies included helping to identify contributions Donald had made, or had at least wanted to make, to the welfare of the family; helping exonerate the father sufficiently that he wouldn't be so menacing; and helping Donald take rejunctive, reparative steps toward family members.

Excerpts from three sessions are provided. Here is the first:

DONALD: I've been feeling very raw, very vulnerable—all those feelings I was talking about last week. I feel very worried about my son, Charles. He seems to enjoy tormenting the dog, and gets very contentious, and it just makes me think, "What's his life going to be like? Is he OK?" I guess what it's about is, it makes me angry, and I feel like I have to exert some kind of control when that's not the way to deal with it—anger isn't the way to deal with it; control isn't the way to deal with it. . . . I'm at the stage in my life where I want the fear and anxiety removed from my life, but that's not the way to deal with it. You have to learn how to move through it.

ULRICH: Well, it's natural that you should want relief—

DONALD: Yeah, it's natural I should want relief, and that's fair enough. But relief comes from moving through it, not from trying to hide from it.

ULRICH: Well, whatever it is, it fuels your concern for Charles. On the one hand, you're feeling anger and resentment; on the other hand, you're feeling caring and concern.[1]†

> †In this statement, Dr. Ulrich used the term "feeling" with regard to Donald's reported anger and resentment. Although this was quite an appropriate response, particularly this early in the session, a cognitive-behavioral therapist might also have wanted to ask Donald what specific thoughts were accompanying his emotions. This would also have helped in setting the stage for gathering more information with regard to his internal schemas about himself and his present situation.

DONALD: Oh, yeah. I think in my heart of hearts that Charles is where he's supposed to be, given the kind of person he is. And he would be much better served if I helped him to move through things instead of trying to protect him, so he can have his life and be present in his life in a way that I was never really taught. What I learned growing up was to run hide, and I learned all kinds of ways to do this. I was thinking about that just this morning—it's incredible, the lengths I used to go to for relief. All of it was connected with relief.

ULRICH: We got to the point last week where you were describing when you were a kid, when you actually sat down to the table for a meal—which only occurred once a week anyway—the first person was through before the last person was even served.

DONALD: Yeah.

ULRICH: And during the week when you were having dinner with your brother and sister, and you saw your father coming, your impulse was to get out of there. And we could carry that over—to the dinner scene at your own house, where you've described repeatedly how it's all you can do to sit still with the kids. You want to get out of there. Well, it seemed to me last week that that was quite an important linkage. You wanted to run away from the table when you were a kid, and here you are an adult and you still do. But what's happening right now is that instead of pursuing that theme of fear and wanting to run, you start out with a lot of feelings—very uncomfortable ones, but then you're talking about Charles from the point of view of a concerned adult. Your concern for him gives you a kind of strength; here you are, functioning as an adult. So it's a remarkable changeover.

DONALD: Yeah, yeah, it's curious too—it's amazing, 'cause I identify with my father, even though I don't have any idea what his experience as a father was at the time when we were growing up. I imagine that he felt the same sort of fears and apprehension that I do. I don't know why. But I suspect that that was true.[2]

ULRICH: So you can look at it as an adult sympathetic to your father, and simultaneously you can look at it, not only with the memory of your being hurt, but the hurt's still there. And the anxiety and tension.†

> †*It was relayed to Donald here that he had a choice as to how he wished to view the situation, and that he could view it without being caught up in his current feelings about the situation. This is also a crucial aspect of cognitive-behavioral therapy, particularly as a prelude to the process of reframing.*

DONALD: In a very big way. The difference is, I'm able to think about it more clearly.

ULRICH: Well, one of the key liberating points you've just made is that your father must have had the same experience, because, you know, that observation which you made quite voluntarily—there's a world of empathy in it, to take the measure of it and to say that he suffered the way you're suffering.

DONALD: I think he suffered more, because he wouldn't have the benefit of self-reflection and guidance. And he still doesn't.

ULRICH: Let me go back to another piece of it. We spoke of your making a choice—in a sense, it's like a choice. You can either keep running the way your father ran, and the way he runs, looking for oblivion. Or you can say, in that respect, "I've been a loyal son to my father. I didn't do any better than he did, but now it's time for a change, and my children give me a reason for change. And I'm seeing that I'm free to make choices—the choice of how much of the past to bring with me, how much to leave behind. That can be under my control, rather than being controlled by some old destiny."[3]

DONALD: Yeah, I guess the confusing part for me is, it's hard to differentiate, I guess. . . . The past—when you talked about making the decision of what parts of the past to leave behind, I'm not exactly sure what that means. Maybe it's making the decision how to deal with the anxiety. It's really hard, though—it's really, really hard. This is the thing: It's a lot of hard work, it's distinctly uncomfortable, it takes a lot of awareness—and at the same time, it's OK. This is OK. I'm OK. I mean, sometimes I get—over the weekend I got this horrendous headache, oh, down my neck, and up to my head, and in the morning a little dizzy, sort of light-headed, and [this] persisted through the weekend. So there are some physical symptoms attached, and my stomach gets pretty uncomfortable too. There's some physical symptoms attached to it, but I think that those are transitory.

ULRICH: Well, in a sense it's like we're going through Mach 1, and feeling all the turbulence before you get on the other side. We also haven't yet uncovered all that we need to. We're right in the middle of it.

DONALD: Yeah, and there's a part of me that says, "How's this gonna ever end?" and a part of me that says, "That's not really relevant." And the point of it, too, is that I do get some relief from it. I'm happiest these days when I'm doing two or three projects at one time. That's what makes *me* happy. But that's not what makes my kids happy. So there are times when I just have to let that go. I feel like that's when it's really hard. It's difficult for me to be there for them in my present state of anxiety— hanging out with them, playing with them, being in their place and at their pace. It's really hard.

ULRICH: I suspect that's because it brings you back to a place that was really hard as a kid. I suspect it reminds you of when you were ready to jump and run—

DONALD: I hear what you're saying, but it's hard for me to understand it. I'm not sure of what you're saying here. Why would it be hard? Because I'm—

ULRICH: Simply a replay . . .

DONALD: But I'm the father now. I'm doing it differently. I guess that's where I—

ULRICH: Yes, but it's not either–or; it's two courses coexisting that aren't integrated yet. On the one hand, yes, you're the father, and that gives you a whole new leverage, for yourself as well as for your children. But yes, there is still the part of you that is the frightened child, that gets remembered and reactivated when you're with the children.†

> †*A cognitive-behavioral therapist would have regarded this as a childhood schema infiltrating the adult schema of Donald's role of the father.*

DONALD: It's like sitting at the dinner table.

ULRICH: Exactly. We haven't found out yet why your sister went through her meal so fast, or why you wanted to get out of there when you saw your father coming. So we have the two of you at the table, so to speak. We have "scared me" and then we have "father me," if I may phrase it this way. And as you get in touch with the caring part of yourself as father, that would make it easier for you to get in touch with the caring part of your actual father.

DONALD: I guess one of the goals I have—I'm very stuck on the whole concept of removal. I want to remove all this fear and remove this anxiety, but I guess what I really want to be able to do is manage it. And, to tell the truth, I think I am managing it OK right now, but it's this discomfort that is so difficult.†

> † *A cognitive-behavioral technique known as the "downward arrow" technique might have been useful at this point in the session in order to help Donald explore in more depth what his fear might be in expressing this disability of emotion. For example, a cognitive-behavioral therapist might have addressed Donald's feeling of being "stuck" by asking, "What would it mean to relinquish or remove this part of the 'scared you'?" This would then have been followed by the question "If so, then what?" in reaction to Donald's response, with adjoining arrows pointing downward (see Chapter 1). This might also have aided the therapist in uncovering Donald's core belief about himself, without negatively affecting the direction of the contextual approach.*

ULRICH: It sounds excessive. It shouldn't have to be that uncomfortable.

DONALD: I'm sitting here right now, and it's, like, I'm really uncomfortable. My stomach is knotted.

ULRICH: Well, we really are in the midst of Mach 1.

DONALD: I think so too. The good part of it is, I understand it. Before, it was "What's the matter with me?" And it occurred to me the other day, while I was driving, [that] I haven't been smoking at all. And that was a way of relieving some of the stress in the past, and I haven't had that. I really thought about it.

ULRICH: That's a real change.[4]

Here is an excerpt from the following session:

DONALD: I don't know what to call it any more. Sometime it's anxiety, sometimes it's a deep fatigue, sometimes it's an edginess—but it's pretty much always there.†

> † *Practitioners of many therapeutic modalities actually prefer to create a little bit of anxiety in clients, in order for it to serve as a motivator in treatment. If anxiety becomes too intense, however, it can also be a hindrance in treatment. Therefore, it may be helpful to*

> suggest the use of some behavioral relaxation exercises to help clients manage their symptoms. This could have been done in this case with Donald; he could have been taught a brief course of progressive muscle relaxation (Jacobson, 1938). This could have been incorporated nicely into this session. It might have allowed Donald to focus more closely on the important content of Dr. Ulrich's remarks, and it might also have set the stage for any imagery work in jogging some of Donald's uncovered memories about his family of origin.

ULRICH: Are there any physical signs?

DONALD: Yes, it's that weird feeling—a little bit jagged, a strong weariness to it—and that seems to be present a lot of the time. But there's more to it than just the physical part of it. In its more intense moments, there's this angry impatience where I'm quick to flare up.

ULRICH: With regard to?

DONALD: My job. There must be something I'm doing wrong; there must be something I can do to motivate these people.

ULRICH: You're driving yourself to make everything right.

DONALD: Yes, I'm trying to make the work exciting, and I just hit up against that brick wall, and I just say, "To hell with it." It makes me want to just get that oblivion.

ULRICH: You're really striving to make it come out the way you think it has to come out, and then you feel exhausted and discouraged, to a degree that—and it happens over and over. We're not clear why it's invested with that heavy, heavy sense of burden. The answer may come from some unexpected places. Would you reach into memory and throw a little more light on that scene at the dinner table? There's a part of you that wants to get through with the meal and get out of there.

DONALD: It's Dad, knowing he would be there. The way he talks about everything, the way he thinks, the words he uses—"fag," "nigger." I—I just don't like him. The awareness made it—made it very hard for me.

ULRICH: Can we hear what made that so hard?

DONALD: I don't like him. When I was 13, 14, 15, 16—you're supposed to like your dad. You're supposed to feel some sort of love and connection. But I didn't like the things he said. And I didn't like having to protect Mother against Dad. My brother would just sit and talk about himself, and my sister would just get up and leave the table.

ULRICH: So what does a child do, when you find that your dad is doing things you don't like to your mother?

DONALD: I feel real angry, and I feel really afraid to do any sort of confronting. I'd really want to say something.

ULRICH: What would you want to say?

DONALD: I'd want to say, "Why do you talk that way to her? Why do you talk that way to other people? Why are you so narrow-minded?" I feel so angry and disappointed—I guess I have this perception in my head [that] your dad is supposed to be like a paragon, but instead I feel so disappointed.†

> † *It might have been interesting to investigate where Donald developed this expectation for his father and how that impinged on his own role as a father.*

ULRICH: So what do you do with that?

DONALD: I withdraw, I hide out. I get afraid, too afraid to speak, and then I feel disappointed in myself.

ULRICH: Then you get to feeling bad about yourself. Like a child should be able to confront his father.

DONALD: That's reality crashing in again. Nothing is working out right. I wanted so much to have a relationship with my brother. But he's either not here, or when he is here he's just competing with Dad—and he was just an asshole. And Dad—he was an asshole too. I just wanted, I just wanted—

ULRICH: You wanted it to be right. What does your brother do when he's being an "asshole"?

DONALD: Well, there's either a dramatic problem, or else he's talking, talking—he doesn't shut up. He doesn't say anything, you know, he just goes on and on—

ULRICH: And if he's addressing someone in the family, how does he—?

DONALD: He doesn't address people; he just talks. I want to tell him to shut the hell up.

ULRICH: You want to straighten it out.

DONALD: This is home, where you're supposed to feel safe, and nobody feels safe. Mom doesn't feel safe because she has to deal with my brother and Dad. Dad doesn't feel safe unless he is the center of attention, and I'm just sitting there watching it.

ULRICH: You want to change it.

DONALD: Yeah, I want to scream out, "Will you calm down? Will you *stop!?*"

ULRICH: You want it to stop. What makes your brother keep talking? What would happen if he stopped talking?

DONALD: Well, people would probably just be silent.

ULRICH: What would happen in the silence?

DONALD: They wouldn't know what to talk about.[5]

In the following session, I sought to explore Donald's childhood relationship with his sister, Valerie. The possibility was raised that he might invite Valerie to join us, with the hope that she might prove to be a resource for information about the family. She might also be a significant resource if she could help Donald to mitigate his sense of isolation from his family. What I encountered was a virtually complete lack of memories of his childhood relationship to Valerie, and an almost panicky reluctance to consider asking her to participate in the therapy. The session proceeded as follows:

ULRICH: I'm curious that you raise the question about why it might be your sister that we ask to come in.

DONALD: So am I. I'm feeling really baffled. And threatened. I mean, I'm confounded by how inaccessible my relation with Valerie was. It really surprised me.

ULRICH: It threatened you. Like you got a tiger by the tail here or something.

DONALD: *(Long pause, then laugh)* It makes me think I did something absolutely horrendous to her when I was young, and now I've blocked it out. That's not true, of course.

ULRICH: Well, it's a possibility. We don't know.

DONALD: I'm only half facetious, saying that. A quarter facetious. I think I've invested a lot of energy in not knowing, my whole life. I think I've grown up believing that I would live a life of active denial, and that was going to be all right. That's the way Dad did it. That's the way the adults were. They seemed very untouched by the world at large—

ULRICH: Well, here we have a clear and present avoidance that is just so massive, it's like we're looking at the Rock of Gibraltar?

DONALD: It's very clear that we need to root around and see what's behind it. And I suspect in reality it might not be so steep and it might not be so rocky.

ULRICH: And eventually it might lead more into your father's own childhood.[6]

DONALD: *(Pause)* Boy, that makes me feel afraid.

ULRICH: When I mention your father?

DONALD: Yeah. It's sad, you know. I'm afraid of my own empathy, because it's so strong sometimes.

ULRICH: That could really turn your head around.

DONALD: Yeah.

ULRICH: How could you have any really warm empathy for this "asshole"?

DONALD: Ha ha ha. Ha ha ha ha ha. You know what my first thought was when you said that? "Wait a minute, he's not so bad!" *(Pause)* It's so complex.

ULRICH: Maybe not.

DONALD: How can I say of my father that he's an asshole?

ULRICH: That's part of your pleading. There was a real pleading there. Would he please listen? Would he stop being an asshole and listen and see what's going on? And act accordingly? Why can't he see what's going on here, and do something about it? Why does this have to fall in your lap, to be the only one who's aware and reacting? *(Pause)* I don't know. Maybe I'm missing your part in this.

DONALD: Well, no, I don't think you are. That's the emotional part, the intellectual part of me saying he was hamstrung from the get-go. So how can you hold that against him?

ULRICH: Well, it doesn't mean that you have to go into another kind of denial. You don't have to deny that he hurt you. But you can sure see why he hurt you.†

> †*This was a good move. Helping Donald separate the affect from the cognitive component might also have helped him to see that he had a choice and could modify his thinking toward a more salubrious disposition.*

DONALD: The program [AA] talks about forgiveness.

ULRICH: This is quite different.

DONALD: How so?

ULRICH: Because forgiveness means "I'm going to erase my memory of what you did," which leaves us vulnerable to a repetition of it—whereas this means we're going to look at what you did, and we're going to acknowledge the pain it caused, and then we are going to redeem you by recognizing that there was a time when you were the victim, in exchange for which we expect you to be more accountable.†

> †*This was an excellent example of reframing what was a difficult situation for the client.*

DONALD: That's the first time it's ever made sense to me. *(Pause)* So where do we go from here?

ULRICH: Valerie?

DONALD: Imagine my surprise. Imagine my surprise. That—that—that our connection goes deeper with each other than I ever imagined. That she's more than just another person in my life.

ULRICH: You had accepted the belief that this was just superficial.

DONALD: I mean, I don't even see myself having a relationship with her. You know, we were well into adolescence. It's strange, you know, I can't remember having a conversation with her, doing anything with her, or—until she was probably 12—

ULRICH: And you have no idea how she felt about that.

DONALD: I have no idea. I can't—I have no idea. I have no idea, I have no idea what went on in her life. What life was like for her, growing up. I haven't got a clue.

ULRICH: This is really blank city.

DONALD: It's a total blank. I mean, I thought that life for her was just water rolling off a duck's back. You know, and I know, that can't possibly be true. I mean, if my experience was any indication, she really would have had to be a piece of wood not to be affected by the things I was affected by.

ULRICH: Consideration for your sister's life is something new and unfamiliar. Will you forget about Valerie?

DONALD: No, I won't forget. This has got to be done. I would really like to find a little—psychic peace.

ULRICH: You might find you have a sister in there somewhere, and one can always use a sister.[7]

In spite of my attempts encourage him, Donald did not take hold in subsequent sessions of the idea of actually bringing in his sister. Nevertheless, it seemed as if by now some rejunctive work had been accomplished— that is, restoration of some sense of positive connection with his family, or at least the demonstration of some positive concern for his family. In this respect, I felt that Donald might be less resistant to the idea of attempting to uncover the trauma presumed to be underlying his stated symptoms.

Toward this end, he and I first established that our goal was to pursue a better understanding of his sense of failure and worthlessness. Next, we employed a hypnotic induction technique (with which Donald was already familiar), and then I introduced the theater technique, in which the client is invited to imagine that he or she is observing events unfolding on a movie screen. This led to a recollection vastly different in quality and quantity from anything Donald had ever produced. It was the story of a family event, and as it emerged, I could see that virtually all of Donald's symptomatic behavior could be viewed as recapitulations of the core behavioral and affective ingredients of this event.

In his recollection, Donald was starting out with his family for his first time on skis, at the age of 10. His mood shifted from elation to despair as he realized on his first trip down the slope that he would have to grapple with a tow rope at the foot of the slope. Except for his father, the family seemed to have disappeared. He made three attempts to grasp the rope; each time, he found himself being jerked off his feet. As he recalled it, his father flew into a rage, turned his back, and went up the tow rope by himself, leaving Donald sprawled at the bottom. Even before he fell, Donald was sure that everyone was looking at him; that they could see that he was a beginner; and that, as such, they considered him worthless. Obviously, this wasn't the first such experience that Donald had had. Reviewing the entire scene, Donald summed it up: "In our family, there was no room to be a beginner."

At this writing, Donald is now addressing a career situation in which he is struggling through the "Mach 1" of being a beginner in a strange place and reexperiencing some of the original attitudes and affects generated by trauma. This time, of course, he possesses more of a sense of awareness and control. When Donald speaks of work he still focuses on the tensions he feels toward his employees, yet he did mention to me that he had been asked to present at a state-wide conference, describing a new method he had developed to help his employees achieve more effective results. He had also mentioned in passing that his supervisor had said to him, "I have learned a lot from you."

What makes it possible for Donald to forge ahead, I believe, is the recurring emergence of his empathy for his father, who had shown that he too had been allowed no room for beginnings. The fact that Donald can now exonerate, instead of simply exercising hatred, has relieved his fear of rediscovery. Thus this case illustrates the performance of trauma recovery work in a family-oriented, contextual framework.

To recapitulate, the foundation of the contextual framework is in the basic premise that the deepest levels of family attachment are not adversary; each person retains some claim on the others and owes something of value to the others, no matter how bad the real-life situation of the family has become. There is still a bond of loyalty, even when this bond is most vehemently unwanted.

It is not uncommon for therapists to encourage clients to demonize significant others, as if the clients were victims entitled only to counterattack or to cut themselves off from the demons. This approach goes against the grain of contextual therapy. There are many reasons why this is so. We are, of course, compelled to recognize that parents are capable of acting persistently like monsters. But contextual therapy expands the frame to include the enduring acknowledgment of a residue of parent–child connection.

If there is no hope left for any good in a parent or for developing an understanding of what in the parent's life turned him or her into a demon, then by the unconscious dictates of legacy, which sometimes prescribe very powerfully that the child can be no better than the parent, there is no hope left for the child either. Contextual therapists work from the conviction that although the child's self-esteem will be much enhanced if the child can learn to hold his or her own vis-à-vis an abusive parent, that self-esteem will nevertheless be impaired if the child sees himself or herself as compelled to go through life being nothing more than the immediate descendant of a monster. This is a sentence that no therapist should allow a client to impose on himself or herself.

In contextual terms, possibly the strongest incentive for a therapist to demonize a parent is the operation of invisible loyalties that compel the therapist to displace his or her unresolved hostility toward his or her own parent onto the client's. To put it another way, the therapist may be compelled endlessly to reenact a rescue fantasy, with the therapist as the parentified child saving others from the family demon.

Sometimes clients are all too reluctant to relinquish the victim role. They often seem to be awaiting their "day in court," when they can get recognition for what has been inflicted upon them. A victim may claim a negative entitlement: "The world has hurt me; I deserve reparations wherever I can find them." But there may exist in many people a deeply embedded part whose emerging, even more compelling litany is this: "I am the part that carried the pain. I have carried it in isolation and in silence. Now, by God, I want the rest of you to know what it feels like before I will even begin to relinquish my rage." Paradoxically, this can be heard as a cry to begin the reintegration of this with the other facets of the personality. An effective therapist, whether designated "contextual" or not, will seek to empathize with this aspect of a client and of the client's forebears. If some measure of hope for the parent can be preserved, then (as noted above) the parent need not seem so terrifying, and the client's sense of entrapment may not be so nearly complete.

For the contextually oriented therapist, all of this remains true even if for therapeutic purposes it becomes necessary at least temporarily for the client to separate from other family members.

CASE REPORT: MULTIDIRECTIONAL PARTIALITY

The second case illustrates how a therapist engages in "multidirectional partiality"—serving as advocate first for one member of a couple or family and then for the other, in order to bring both individuals into the rejunctive effort.

Jon and Sally presented themselves as a husband and wife who had never known how to communicate or solve problems. Instead, Sally said tearfully, it was no time at all before Jon would raise his voice to a shout, deliver a brief rebuttal, and then walk out. Jon and Sally had met while each was dating someone else; they began a covert relationship, which led to their engagement. Their respective families were old friends. It seemed as though everything simply fell into place. In fact, they were so enamored of each other they hadn't even realized that they might have differences to work out.

When Sally was a child, everything fell into place for her as long as she managed to play the part of "little golden girl." But if she incurred her father's displeasure, his reaction was swift and severe. For her to negotiate with him was unthinkable; she could only pretend to succumb to his wishes and then try to find ways to act behind his back. In a family system built upon superior power, the only way Sally knew how to respond was to exploit the position of helplessness. Jon, in contrast, dealt with a severe mother by taking severe countermeasures. The mother came to believe that once Jon embarked on one of his outbursts, there was no way she could keep the upper hand. With such a potential for interlocking patterns of response, it isn't surprising that the members of this couple found each other!

The following is an excerpt from one of their early therapy sessions:

ULRICH: If neither one of you has an item for the agenda, I would like to pick up on something that emerged during our last session. There seemed to be an impasse: Sally reports feeling abused by what Jon says, but Jon doesn't think she even listens. Can we work from an example here?

SALLY: We were rushing to get ready for a party, and I put some stuff in the upstairs hallway. Then Jon threw it onto my side of the bed. And he said, in that tone of his, "Next time you leave stuff there, I'm going to throw it out." And he does throw my things around. The reason I left it in the hallway [was that] I do have time restrictions. So the hallway is a good place to leave things. His reaction was extreme.

ULRICH: How did you feel when he spoke to you in that tone?†

> † When clients are asked, "How does that make you feel?", they will commonly respond by also revealing their automatic thoughts. From a cognitive-behavioral perspective, it's believed that this is due to the close connection between cognition and affect. This might have been something to point out with Sally, particularly in later attempts to introduce change in her emotions and behavior.

SALLY: I was upset. It was "Here he goes again." I can't converse with him. I can't say, "I'll do it later," because he'll just say, "No, you promised you weren't going to do it any more." We can't talk about it. I feel he doesn't want to hear from me. If I try to talk, he'll just be angry and shut down.

JON: This has been going on for 10 years. We've talked many times, and she always says, "I won't do it again." There's a long history of this.

SALLY: It's you saying, "Don't you do this again," and me saying, "No, I won't." But there's no effort to really look at it to see what's going on . . . and I'm just appeasing your anger.

JON: Well, it's my house, too. It's not that she has to conform. She can go make a mess where I can't see it. But she can't force me to accept chaos. She can't mess things up when it infringes on me. I have to have order in my life.†

> † *I would have been very curious about this statement, which seemed to suggest that Jon felt he had little control over his ability to be flexible. It might have been worthwhile to explore his automatic thoughts and to reveal his schema regarding rigidity versus flexibility.*

ULRICH: Why can't Sally call it just like you're calling it?

JON: *(Making a big gesture)* Because I'm *right*.

ULRICH: You are a courageous, man, sir. *(To Sally)* You don't often hear a man talking like that any more. It's kind of refreshing.[8]

SALLY: *(To Jon)* There have been times when you could be a little bit flexible about it.

JON: I wish I could be more flexible.

ULRICH: Again, let me ask, does Sally get equal time here?

JON: There are times when she has freedom to say she's right, even if I say she's wrong. Like when she's planting. She digs one hole, puts in the plant, then digs the next hole. The right way would be to dig all of the holes first. But I let it go. But there are times when she does not have the right to make the call, because what's right is right; it's universal. It's not up to her. And I'm not just having my way.

ULRICH: And you are the custodian of the universal?

SALLY: I want him to know that there are different ways of looking at things.

JON: I know—who died and left me in charge?

ULRICH: That could be an important consideration. There could indeed be a legacy here.[9]

JON: It's when it's so damn obvious.

ULRICH: Is it obvious to the other?

JON: Sometimes. But there's no argument for leaving stuff in the hall, other than "I'm just too lazy to take the six steps needed to put the stuff away." I just don't want the mess in my face. So there's no use having a discussion about when it's going to be put away.

ULRICH: Jon, in the field of family therapy, there are some people who seriously believe that in order for a marital relationship to work and be healthy, there has to be observance of a kind of universal order of things, whereby each spouse has equality with the other. Looking at it from this perspective, you are an advocate for disorder. How do you reconcile that?

JON: There are certain things I can't give up—things I can't live with and be happy. I can't be happy surrounded by chaos. I am going in 27 ways at once. I have such a tenuous grip on holding myself together. Why am I so busy? I'm innately a lazy person. If I let myself stop, I'd stop for good. I don't do well with shades of grey. Whether it's unfair or not, I have to live with some degree of order.

ULRICH: Now you are pleading a very human kind of equity. You're asking for your needs to be seen and considered.[10]

In the following session, Jon made an explicit reference to the "personal issues" that were having an impact on his life. When I asked him whether he was interested in working on these issues, he seemed to ponder for a while and then came back with a "No!" that left no room for discussion. Following this session, Jon sent word via Sally that he did not think we were getting anywhere and he wasn't coming back.

Under certain conditions— an open acknowledgment that problems exist, and a commitment to finding another way of dealing with them— such a refusal could be considered valid from an ethical perspective. But in this case, Jon's abrupt withdrawal from therapy, without even coming face to face with me, might perhaps be better understood as a flight from the realization that he was indeed having a hard time holding himself together. After he made this revelation, I did side with him, but evidently this didn't go far enough in addressing his fears.

AUTHOR'S REPLY TO EDITOR'S COMMENTS

My initial response to Dr. Dattilio's commentary is that much of what he suggests is already familiar to me. Virtually all of it would prove useful in contextual practice. In my opinion, there is very little sense of dissonance. I would, however, like to respond to a few specific points.

The "downward arrow" technique described on page 166 should lend itself very well not only to exploration of core beliefs, but also to the therapeutic task of getting the client to consider rejunctive alternatives (e.g., "If so, then what might you do that would help repair this situation? Do you think that might work or not?").

Dr. Dattilio's later comment on Jon's rigidity–flexibility schema is especially interesting in view of how the work with Jon turned out. As I have speculated at the end of the case report, Jon's withdrawal from treatment might have resulted from his being thrown into a panic at the suggestion that we might upset his rigid defenses; to him, the only possible outcome of that course of action might have seemed to be ego dissolution and chaos. It's certainly conceivable that had the therapy dealt more actively with his fear of letting go (i.e., his "schema regarding rigidity versus flexibility"), his panic might have been alleviated enough that he could have managed to stay in treatment.

Despite the fact that in the present exercise, the cognitive-behavioral approach appears to work well with the contextual approach, I would like to express concern about a possible divergence of underlying goals. To cite an example, I recently saw a cognitive-behavioral training videotape in which the therapist seemed to be leading the client through a series of real-life moves designed to make him less dependent on his spouse. The result, at least for the moment, was as desired, but the client's moves included no dialogue with the spouse. A contextual therapist would encourage at least an attempt at dialogue in which the needs and concerns of each spouse would be reviewed together, so that external change would result from reciprocal efforts at enhanced understanding and acceptance. This may also facilitate the restoration of this reciprocity, rather than a shift in the behavioral interaction pattern of the couple. This would clearly be the goal of treatment. I merely wonder whether the goals of contextual and cognitive-behavioral therapy might sometimes be divergent in this respect. Certainly I do not find any such divergence in Dr. Dattilio's commentary.

NOTES

1. This was a contextual move. I acknowledged the socially and ethically responsible part of what Donald was saying. I recognized that Donald had, in his concern for his son, performed an "act of merit." Thus the client engaged in a kind of giving, and through giving he validated himself. Eventually, this could help him to stabilize.

2. Contextual therapy regards any positive statement about a parent, unless it is coerced, as an asset to be acknowledged, remembered, and built upon. There is nothing to be gained by undoing whatever good remains of the parent–child connection.

3. "Destiny" has meanings at many levels. At one level, it could mean the narrowed view of self and world imposed by trauma. At another level, it could mean the "legacy" laid down by generations of family members designating what an offspring is to become. These two levels interact.

4. This may have been a significant change. Although the cessation of smoking added to Donald's current sense of discomfort, I suspected that the continual effort being made in therapy to integrate the client's positive perceptions with his negative ones was beginning to reduce the inner tension.

5. In this sequence of exchanges, I repeatedly acknowledged the impossible burden carried by the parentified child; the futility of his efforts to make things right became in itself a source of trauma. Although this acknowledgment alone would not restore fairness, at least the child-become-adult might finally be able to sense that the failures were not his fault.

6. Here, because I was concerned that the references to Valerie might become

too threatening, I got back to a more familiar track. This was in line with the contextual principle that it's necessary to hold people accountable, but it should not be done harshly.

7. Thus it was demonstrated that relief for the self and consideration of the welfare of the other were actually parts of a single rejunctive process.

8. Here I sided with Sally ("You don't often hear a man . . . ") but bracketed this with remarks offered in a fraternal voice that I hoped would sound supportive to Jon. Jon's response seemed positive.

9. This was not being pursued simply as a feminist issue; it was pursued as an ethical issue of equal consideration for the rights of all concerned.

10. Here I switched abruptly from confronting Jon on Sally's behalf to supporting Jon's open expression of his own difficulties. Thus a therapist's partiality is expressed in whatever direction it is needed, with the eventual aim of helping the members of a couple find their way to a balanced reciprocity of interests.

REFERENCES

Boszormenyi-Nagy, I., Grunebaum, J., & Ulrich, D. (1991). Contextual therapy. In A. Gurman & D. Kniskern (Eds.), *Handbook of family therapy* (Vol. 2). New York: Brunner/Mazel.

Boszormenyi-Nagy, I., & Spark, G. (1973). *Invisible loyalties: Reciprocity in multigenerational family therapy*. New York: Brunner/Mazel.

Glantz, K., & Pearce, J. (1989). *Exiles from Eden*. New York: Norton.

Jacobson, E. (1938). *You must relax*. New York: McGraw-Hill.

Stierlin, H. (1976). The dynamics of owning and disowning: Psychoanalytic and family perspectives. *Family Process, 15*, 277–288.

Ulrich, D. (1983). Contextual family and marital therapy. In B. Wolman & G. Stricker (Eds.), *Handbook of marital and family therapy*. New York: Plenum Press.

Ulrich, D., & Dunne, H. (1986). *To love and work*. New York: Brunner/Mazel.

SUGGESTED READINGS

Boszormenyi-Nagy, I., & Krasner, B. (1986). *Between give and take: A clinical guide to contextual therapy*. New York: Brunner/Mazel.

Goldenthal, P. (1996). *Doing contextual therapy: An integrative model for working with individuals, couples, and families*. New York: Norton.

Krasner, B., & Joyce, A. (1995). *Truth, trust, and relationships: Healing interventions in contextual therapy*. New York: Brunner/Mazel.

Chapter 8

Symbolic-Experiential Family Therapy for Chemical Imbalance

DAVID V. KEITH

Symbolic-experiential family therapy is a relatively atheoretical, or at least unsystematic (or not formulaic), approach to psychotherapy. The conceptual basis includes fragments of psychoanalytic theory, systems theory, existential therapy, dialectical ideas, Zen, hypnotherapy, and play therapy. The therapy is organized around the dialectics of individuation and belonging, creativity and adaptation. Health is rooted in the group spirit of the family. We believe that experience produces change (growing and maturing), and that experience is nonrational. A symbolic experience is a response to a biopsychosocial context, to a metaphorical event, often psychosomatic in nature and perturbs the pattern of everyday life. Symbolic-experiential family therapy has a poetic relationship to language and experience, which takes the therapeutic process beneath the surface of the family's lived experience into the realm of myth. Not the overdeveloped myths of the culture's literature, but the myths that murmur in our blood, and are tangled in our relationships.

The relationship between the family group and the cotherapy team is important to therapeutic experience. Our metaphorical model for therapy is the foster home: The family members come in to be cared for while they get through a difficult period in their lives. The foster home's effectiveness depends on the maturity of the foster parents and the desperation of the family about their problems. The dynamics of therapy are in the person-hood of the therapist(s), in interaction with the emotional currents of the family (Betz & Whitehorn, 1975).

Some of the goals of symbolic-experiential family therapy are as follows:

1. To increase anxiety in the family ("It's really much worse than you think"). Increased anxiety forces the family members to take more respon-sibility for their living.

2. To increase ambiguity. Increasing ambiguity forces more of each person's self to be present as a stimulus to growth, and pushes the existential dialectics (independence–dependence, love–hate, creativity–adaptation) toward synthesis—that is, to a new experiential level.

3. To complete each person's symbiotic dance with parents, spouse, and siblings, so that more affect is available for investment in the self.

4. To increase each person's investment in the self, which is a symptom of individuation/differentiation and allows for healthier affective investment in spouse, marriage, parents, and children.

5. Similarly, to make more affect available for investment in the therapist(s) and therapeutic project by each person in the family.

Being a patient is a laboratory experience in forming a relationship in the interest of growth. The transferential relationship to a therapist (fantasies and identifications) becomes a model for how to use transfer-ence in the interest of growing, so that the patient can later have a therapeutic relationship with any person and that person does not have to know about it. The goal of psychotherapy, the definition of growth, is for the patient to have as much access to the self as possible. Access to the self is greatest in the context of a deeply intimate relationship (e.g., marriage). Marriage is one of the best ways of getting a PhD in being a person. Being grown up means accepting my endless ambivalence about myself.

All this is by way of introduction, and obviously too condensed. Let me proceed to the case.

INITIAL TELEPHONE CONTACT AND FIRST INTERVIEW

I make all of my own appointments. The psychotherapy project begins on the phone. It is a blind date, and it is important to establish some parameters for what our first meeting will be like.

My work with this family began when I returned Helen Vanderpoehl's phone call.

HELEN: We would like an appointment.

D. V. K.: Why don't you tell me a little about the situation so as to be sure I am the right man?

HELEN: We were referred to you because you're a psychiatrist and you do marital counseling. Our marriage is kind of a mess right now. I mean, we're separated—I think my husband needs medication.

D. V. K.: You may not have the right man. I don't use medication.

HELEN: But I thought you were a psychiatrist.

D. V. K.: I am, but I use a different kind of system. It involves including the whole family. Who referred you?

HELEN: The Bread of Life Counseling and Growth Center. We went there for counseling, but they don't know what to do about his chemical imbalance.

She indicated that they had been involved with five different mental health practitioners, and they had learned that her husband had a bipolar disorder or manic–depressive illness, based on a "chemical imbalance." They also learned that although manic–depressive illness affects relationships, relationships do not affect manic–depressive illness. Those who treated chemical imbalances did not work with marriages and families, and those who worked with marriages did not work with chemical imbalances. The culture of mental health taught them to think dichotomously and linearly.

D. V. K.: My way of dealing with chemical imbalance is to add people.

HELEN: I don't think I understand. Does it work?

D. V. K.: Not always.

HELEN: But what if someone *needs* medication?

D. V. K.: I get someone to see them who believes in medication.

HELEN: So you are saying he might not need medication?

D. V. K.: That's right.

HELEN: Should he come alone first?

D. V. K.: No, you should all come.

HELEN: You mean the kids, too?

D. V. K.: Sure.

HELEN: But I don't think he'll want them to come.

D. V. K.: So tell him you talked to me, and I said that's how I work. If you don't bring the kids, you'll be starting into the same setup that led to him being on medication, so you will probably be better off seeing someone else. If he has any questions, he should call me.

They all came. They surprised me; I was expecting cautious, conventional people who formatted all experience in conservative Christian theology. Instead, they were an attractive, energetic group. Helen Vanderpoehl, 39, was blond and athlete-slender. Her skin had a Dutch ivory tint. William Clark, 42, was a husky African-American man, whose skin tended toward the red brown of mahogany. Their children, Sarah, 7, and Saniqua, 3, were lightly tanned, with almost blond, kinky hair. I, the therapist, was aging; I had dark hair with flecks of silver, and a white, trimmed beard. My skin was tan with mauve and olive undertones.

D. V. K.: How can I help?

WILLIAM: *(With a tone of incredulity)* Help? Help? You think you can help a ship that hit a goddamn rock and sank? She's still on the ship and it's on the bottom. Me—I may not have a PhD, like her, but I'm smart enough to know when a ship isn't going anywhere. But she and her therapists and her psychiatrists say I'm crazy—and I need medicine. If they load me up with their drugs, then I can have the privilege of getting back on a ship that's going nowhere. *(He smiled suddenly at his own outburst, and at what I assumed was the absurdity of saying this after showing up in my office.)* If you can help this mess, Doc, you're some kind of a miracle man.

HELEN: We need help—but I'm not sure you are the right one. William has this bipolar disorder, mixed type. He has moved out and I am still working. I *do* have a PhD in political science. I am a policy adviser on cultural affairs to the Mayor. I want this marriage to go somewhere, but to tell you the truth, Dr. Keith *(she began to choke back tears)*, I am just about out of energy. I have an interesting but demanding job; I am taking care of the kids because he's living in a room downtown. And I just can't count on William. His mood swings make it totally impossible.

WILLIAM: Sure. My mood swings. What about your damn righteousness swings? Anybody'd be crazy living with you.

Despite the angry intensity of their parents, the children quietly explored my office and my toys. They glanced at their parents, or moved close to them, but did not seem anxious about the emotional conversation. Helen continued, "When I hear him say the marriage is sunk, I sometimes think it is just this awful illness talking, and sometimes I think he may be right. I am just too dumb, too Lutheran to see that this is no longer a marriage." Tears appeared in her eyes, and Sarah moved to her side. William looked away; he appeared to be reading the book titles in my bookcase.

The interview continued with bilateral complaints and definitions of differences. I eventually turned to Sarah, the older daughter, and said, "Do you know anything about how I can help?" She slid shyly behind her mother's chair. Both parents responded warmly and reassuringly to their daughter, and said, almost in chorus, "Sarah, you can tell him what you think. You can say whatever you want."

SARAH: I wish Daddy wouldn't make my mommy cry.

WILLIAM: See, Doc! She's got them brainwashed.

SARAH: Be quiet, Daddy. You told me to talk.

The girl's manner was self-assured, unafraid; she sounded like a mother talking to her son. Both parents were responsive and kind with the children, in contrast to their bitter, adversarial attitude toward each other. Helen's account suggested that William was abusive and dangerous, but his natural warmth with the girls, and Sarah's self-assurance in addressing him, contradicted Helen's picture of him. I said to Sarah, "I think you are right. It's time for you to say what you think."

I interviewed the children while holding a medium-sized teddy bear. Our discussion was a playful digression, but listening to their children created a new thoughtfulness in the parents, and gave me a relationship with Sarah and Saniqua.

When I had finished talking with the girls, William described part of his background. "Doc, I was in show business for 20 years. On the road. It's a very different world—and if I say it's crazy, you still won't get what I'm talking about. I never really had my own band; I was a backup singer." He mentioned some of the people he'd traveled with and sung behind. They were familiar names. "Sometimes it was fun. Sometimes it was just weird, too weird to talk about or even remember. But the thing you ought to know, Doc, is that I was the guy who sort of took care of people. I talked them down when they were too high. I stayed with them when they were depressed. It was really crazy sometimes, Doc. I mean, there were bad trips and there were people being suicidal. And if we could take care of it ourselves, we took care of it ourselves. I mean, if some of those people would have showed up in a psychiatrist's office, they would have left in chains." (He said this playfully, with considerable nonverbal embellishment.)

Helen and William had met when Helen was teaching at a college in a different city, and William took one of her courses. They had started living together a month after the course ended. She had been married before and divorced after 1½ years. He had never previously married. They lived together for 4 years. Sarah was born after 2 years, and they married when Sarah was 2. They had been married nearly 6 years.

Helen described the early years of their relationship. William had bouts of depression and despair, in which he would plead with her to help him, to take him to a hospital; these episodes would subside. They had separated about four times before now (though she'd never felt as estranged as she did this time). Six years into the relationship, she managed to get an appointment at a large medical center so that William could be treated. She ended up taking him to the hospital emergency room. She was interviewed by a psychiatrist, and then William was interviewed. The psychiatrist determined that William had a bipolar disorder, and started him on lithium and Prozac.

WILLIAM: *(Interrupting)* So after I got my prescriptions, Helen asked the psychiatrist, "What am I supposed to do while the medications are taking effect?" And the doctor said something I felt real good about. She said, "Get a new man."

HELEN: *(Interrupting)* We have always disagreed about this. I thought she said, "Get a support group."

WILLIAM: What I was depressed about was that my family was coming apart. I did not want to lose this family. And the "helpers" were saying, "Get a new man."

Since then, William had been on and off medication. Sometimes it seemed to help; sometimes it did not. He said he did not feel like himself on the medication, and the part of him that was missing was too important to him. He lost his creative side on medication.

HELEN: But if you have a sickness, and the medicine helps, I just don't understand why you wouldn't take it. I like his fun, creative side, but I hate the mood swings that go with it.

WILLIAM: Doc, I am not sick! What you see here isn't any bipolar, manic–depressive freak. Doc, what you got here is an angry black man. And you know and I know—and this you can think of as crazy—but you know and I know that black men end up on drugs, whether they get them in some doctor's office or if they get them on the street. You must be smart because of those diplomas I see over there, but no doctor, no therapist yet, smart or not, has been able to do anything about me being a black man. I love this woman. You probably can't see it very well today. But we come out of different worlds, and right now, I don't see any way those worlds are going to fit together.

As the end of the hour came near, I asked, "Do you have any questions?"

Helen asked, "Can you help us?"

I leaned back in my chair and talked toward the ceiling—as if to myself.

D. V. K.: I really don't know. The way I hear it, William is after a divorce, and Helen is trying to hold the marriage together. It sounds to me like the marriage might be dead, beyond resuscitating.

WILLIAM: *(Interrupting, excited)* Then I'm coming back. If he's honest enough to say he doesn't know, if he's honest enough to face the fact that we're probably going to get divorced, then he's good enough for me.

HELEN: What about the medication? *(William looked at her. They both looked at me.)*

D. V. K.: This really isn't a medication problem. I believe what he says; he's an angry black man. And I'm used to working with people as upset as you two seem to be.

HELEN: Do you have any advice?

D. V. K.: Sure. My standard advice is that you do not continue this discussion after you leave. Do not discuss any of this for at least 24 hours. And do not fight. If you catch yourself heating up to one, stop it. And continue it when you come back here.†

> † *At this point it might have helped Helen and William if they had been provided with a more specific technique for circumventing their expressions of anger, as Dr. Keith suggested appropriately. (This might have been particularly important since there was a history of violence between them, if only one incident years ago. See the second interview, below.)*
>
> *One cognitive-behavioral strategy that might have been helpful here would simply be to suggest that if they "catch themselves heating up," they actually separate themselves physically in designated areas and consider utilizing some form of cognitive self-talk in order to defuse the situation more effectively. For example, William might have tried doing some deep breathing and simultaneously examining his inner thoughts by weighing their veracity and considering alternative modes of expression. At least this might have provided more of a game plan to insure the partners' mutual safety.*

SECOND INTERVIEW

I asked Anne Marie Patti Higgins, a family therapist who started out as a nurse practitioner, to be my cotherapist. She had very dark hair and a skin color not unlike mine, except that her darker hair caused the olive tones in her skin to attract blue tones. So from the standpoint of skin tones, we were an interesting, multihued group.

William and Helen were very welcoming to her. However, they were still cool toward each other. Their friendly reaction to Anne Marie demonstrated their social skillfulness. They seemed somewhat uneasy with me and my professional distance. I was wary of them, and of the fact of the previous failures in psychotherapy. I also found much to like in both of them as persons, and in what they did. I am captivated by pragmatic intellectuals like Helen. And among my current hobbies is a deep enjoyment of the blues, the kind of music William performed. I had recognized and admired the names he mentioned when he recounted his professional history.

I reviewed the case for Anne Marie while they listened, telling her what I had learned in the first interview. Helen and William seemed to like the experience, both paying careful attention. I concluded by saying that they were seriously divided, and that I needed a partner. I was concerned I could fail with them, and I didn't want to fail alone.

Anne Marie questioned them about how they'd experienced the first interview. "Did Dr. Keith leave anything out?"

Helen said, "No. He got the facts right. But I felt very lonely afterwards. I felt blamed. I feel Dr. Keith was blaming me or accusing me of being naive."

That did not sound like me. In fact, I thought I had been fairly supportive of her, though not of her clinical opinion of William. I was inviting her out of the position of "assistant psychiatrist," to which she probably had been appointed by earlier practitioners. Afraid of excluding William, I must have overcompensated. This is another reason why a cotherapist is important: The family is not put in the position of needing to take care of the therapist. Here, in fact, they were invited to comment on their new therapist.

HELEN: *(Continuing)* Also, I don't think he understands what it's like to live with blame. William doesn't understand what he's like when he is angry.

A. M. P. H.: Are you afraid of him?

HELEN: Yes. I don't know what he's going to do when he is angry.

A. M. P. H.: Has he hit you?

HELEN: Yes. Well, not really. I mean, I blocked the door last month and he pushed me out of the way. He did push me once about a year after we started living together, but only once.

WILLIAM: Yes, I did push her once, but for some reason she is leaving out what happened before and after. And keep in mind, this was 9 years ago—not last month, not last week. We were having a really heated argument, and she got mad. Madder than I had ever seen her. She was real clear about what was wrong with *me*. I mean *real* clear. She was making these points and started pushing me. She said something like, "You're the one who gets to be upset, and I always have to be so nice and so organized." Then she pushed me. Like some kind of a punctuation mark. That went on for about six pushes, and then I blew up and pushed her. Then I think I got more scared than she was. I couldn't believe I had done that. I swore that I would never do that again. And I haven't. Why do you leave that stuff out, Helen?

HELEN: I don't know why. Maybe it's because I'm afraid they won't understand what it is like to live with you. I want some attention here too, you know. Don't you get it? I want some attention.

WILLIAM: You want attention! But what her friends think is that I'm a barely controlled mass murderer. I admit I get pretty angry, and my voice gets loud and forceful and I say things that hurt, but I am *not* a violent *person.* I've seen a lot of violence, but I'm always the one who settles other people down. I bet if I was a white man, like her dad, she wouldn't be afraid of me when I got angry. Part of what she sees when this black face gets angry is the danger of the slums—a world she doesn't understand. So far, we haven't seen anybody who gets that. I think from what the Doc said to you, Anne Marie, that he gets it. I think we both see something we want in the world the other one comes from, but in her case, she feels scared of parts of my world, and I feel like I . . . I don't know, I feel like sometimes in her world I can't be *me.* I mean, it's like that Prozac and your lithium. It makes me whiter or something.

D. V. K.: *(To A. M. P. H.)* This sounds to me like on the one hand, he is trying to fit into her world. But on the other, when he is in, he has to be someone he isn't. It sounds deeply painful—on both sides.

Helen and William had been so angry and wary of each other in the first interview that it had been hard to get a full history. They were less anxious at this second interview. Anne Marie asked each of them how they got together: "What attracted you to William [or Helen] in the first place?" We usually do this with couples in the first interview. It is especially important when there is anger and polarization, because it recalls a sense of togetherness and recalls the partners' being in love.

William had been in Helen's political science class—a night class at a university in a large city. As Helen recalled, they went out for coffee one night and ended up walking by a river for 2 hours. "He was so much fun to be around . . . although sometimes I felt afraid of him . . . but I had confidence in myself." William commented, "She was such a gentle soul. I felt like she needed protection. But then I admired how smart she was. And I liked the fact that she liked me, even though I—and I think I was kind of showing off so she'd know I was smart—even though I hadn't been to college."

Helen said that she experienced a lovingness she had never known. She had been married for 1½ years to "someone with whom I had much in common, but it was desperately boring, and we divorced. . . . But with William, there was such wonder in our talking. Until we met we were like two halves. Incomplete. And we joined together to make a whole." She wished they could go back to the joy and romance of that time. William shared in this nostalgic sense of their beginning

The interview then led into the question of what kind of families they came from. Helen came from a loving family in the Midwest—politically liberal, and morally Protestant conservative. She had one sister younger than herself, and she believed herself to be loved, admired, and supported by her family. On the other hand, William came from the underside of the Bronx, where his mother still lived but his father was seldom seen. He grew up tough; he made his way in the world of show business.

THIRD INTERVIEW

William, Helen, and the children returned a week later. Helen said things weren't any worse. In fact, she seemed refreshed and elated. They'd had some suppers at home that were "great." I was surprised. I hadn't expected the therapy to go in this direction; I thought Helen and William were going to get divorced. The children were very much at home in my office. This was a good sign—a measure of a reduction in anxiety. The children moved the doll house, the dolls, and the animals out of the toy corner and into the center of the room.

William said, "You know, Doc, that rule about not talking about the therapy for 24 hours has been a real help. We have been taking this thing apart for years. I can see, it's part of our problem. I think half the time we aren't even speaking the same language. I can hear her a lot better now." I sensed in him an undertone of desire to reunite—a sense of loneliness and appreciation of Helen that I hadn't noticed in the first two interviews. But I was concerned that they had just put the brakes on; they had not really shifted gears. I said, "I think you're both being too careful. I can understand the reason for it, but usually it's a mistake."

The rest of the third interview likewise had an air of calmness to it, as if they had decided it might be safe to get back together again. They talked more about of their early life together. Helen said she had liked herself better then. She said she was not sure she liked the person she had become.

FOURTH INTERVIEW

The fourth interview was uneventful. There was no change. They had all done something together as a family, and there had been some sexual interaction between Helen and William. But he held back. He was concerned about being seduced back into too much togetherness before he was ready. He did not want to return to the status quo.

HELEN: *(To D. V. K. and A. M. P. H.)* I do not really understand what you are up to. Where are we going? What are you doing? William and I were talking, and we don't know what it is you are doing.

A. M. P. H.: I think we are still waiting for you two to decide what you're going to do. And until you do, we provide a neutral zone—a time and a place for you to talk about it. My guess is that you both need to do a little growing up, but you are so preoccupied with the other, you don't know it yet.

WILLIAM: I don't exactly get it either. It seems like you just sit there. Isn't there something we could be working on? We haven't found much to agree about recently, but we do agree that you aren't doing anything.

They were teasing us. It represented a healthy way of securing our relationship.

HELEN: Could you recommend something for me to read? Maybe I could understand you better if I had something to read.

D. V. K.: I don't think reading is a good idea when you are in therapy. It interferes with your own processing. It runs the risk of turning this into another intellectual exercise. As I see it, I think the project right now is focused on each of you trying to locate yourself in the marriage relationship. According to our philosophy, there are at least three patients here. There's William, there's Helen, and there's the marriage, the relationship itself. It is interesting to me that you both feel cheated and deprived of something you had. How can *both* be cheated? Why doesn't one of you feel gratified? The reason is [that] the marriage, the relationship, is in charge. The people have disappeared in the relationship. So I assume that what you are up to is refinding yourselves, so that then you can bring the marriage contract up to date.†

> † *Dr. Keith made a cogent point when he said that each partner was focused on trying to locate himself or herself in the relationship. An interesting question might also have involved asking them what they each imagined their relationship would look like if it were where they would each want it to be. In this respect, the therapist might also have gained some insight into the partners' respective expectations about where they wanted the relationship to be.*

HELEN: Don't you think we could do a better job if the kids weren't here?

D. V. K.: No, I don't. I think the kids force you to be more honest.

WILLIAM: I know that's true for me.

HELEN: *(In a pseudosarcastic tone)* Thank you for telling us something.

But, really, I would like something I could read. That's how my mind works.

A. M. P. H.: So we are trying to screw up how your mind works—to get you past thinking and talking about living into just living. I think that's what was going on during that time when you were first together. You were describing a time of being more fully alive. I bet you weren't reading much back then—you were too full of life.

D. V. K.: Besides, you should never read a book or go to a movie your therapist recommends, anyway.

HELEN: Are you serious? Why not?

D. V. K.: Because my recommendation would come out of my fantasy about you. And when you read it you probably would not see in it what I see that pertains to you.

FIFTH INTERVIEW

The fifth appointment was at 10 A.M. William said he awoke at 4:00 in the morning. He had a dream but could not remember it. He woke up feeling very sad, then began to cry.

WILLIAM: I couldn't stop crying. I cried until 7:00. I don't know what it was. I didn't understand it, but for some reason, I didn't want to stop. There was something purifying in it. When Helen and the kids came to pick me up, I was glad to see them. But I felt sort of defensive, I suppose, like I wanted to be alone. But I do love them. When they came, my crying stopped. But before that it was just overwhelming. This has never happened to me before.

D. V. K.: Were you talking to yourself when you were crying?

WILLIAM: I suppose. But, Doc, I have no words for it. This has never happened to me before. You haven't known me for long, but can you imagine me speechless?

Helen started to say she was glad to hear of it. I gently told her to be quiet; he wasn't crying to make her feel glad. This was an important experience for him. She should let it be. He did not know what to do next.

Disrupting the marital symbiosis can seem rude. When a marriage is in therapy, there is a tendency for all events to be linked to the marital dynamics. This impulse is related to the marital symbiosis, and it is important to allow that condition to be disrupted. Then each partner can have experiences (self-to-self, or self-to-therapist), and the other does not need to do anything about them.

I was impressed by William's experience. It gave me the feeling that he had entered therapy, despite his early reservations. He had become a patient, our symbolic child (Whitaker & Malone, 1953). He was questioning himself in a deep way. My impression was that Anne Marie's presence made it safer for him to form a connection to us. This is one of the hidden benefits of cotherapy. A mature cotherapy partnership (such as I have with Anne Marie) has a powerful therapeutic component; it both induces and allows a therapeutic regression such as this. William was into therapy, and that was a surprise. We had gone from the zone of "Let's define our problems; you give us advice, and we will go on from here" to that of "We are on a journey together."

HELEN: I'm jealous. I wish I could cry like William.

D. V. K.: I think you may be too preoccupied with him.

HELEN: How do I get over it?

D. V. K.: What comes to mind is [that] you need to go crazy.

HELEN: What? *I* need to go crazy? I thought we came here so *he* would *stop* being crazy, but now you are telling me *I* need to be crazy? I thought I was the sane one—"the good lady" who would lead him into the heaven of Protestant mental health. Now you tell me I'm supposed to be crazy.

She was outraged and a little surprised, but she was also mocking herself. This capacity for self-mocking and their pleasure in double entendre were signs of health—hints that they could tolerate the pain of getting lost in this process we call experiential psychotherapy.

Helen continued, "William's always had this kind of emotion or passion about him. I know that's why I fell in love with him, and I know, despite the hard times we've had, this is why our relationship has continued. Sometimes I have to say that I *am* jealous of how open he can be emotionally, but me, I always feel, 'I don't know how to do this,' like I got—like I can only get it wrong. I don't even know how to be *crazy* the right way."

There was a switch here. Both of them had now entered into the therapy, had become what I refer to as "patients." They had detached from each other ever so slightly. They were allowing the process to take them over. Some families never leave the first-interview stage of therapy, which I am suggesting can go on for five interviews. They stay safe, sane, controlled. We call it "in-sanity"—being trapped inside of sanity.

To some, William might have seemed symptomatic; his uncontrolled crying episode following anger could have been taken as evidence of bipolar "rapid cycling." But we would think of his episode of crying as an episode of a therapeutic regression induced by the therapeutic process. In this context, "regression" refers to a nonrational, out-of-the-head experience.

An openness to change is the usual implication, but pain, loneliness, and confusion are common concomitants (Keith, 1989).

Helen and William were detached from each other as the symbiosis was disrupted; he was in pain that she did not cause, nor could she repair it. The structure of her fantasy world, with him at the center, crumbled a bit. As we came to the end of the interview, both partners said in their own ways that they were feeling better—unburdened, but confused. I told them, "If you are confused, then we must be getting somewhere. . . . But don't worry, the feeling better won't last. Enjoy it while you can."

SIXTH INTERVIEW

Helen had been thinking. My suggestion that she needed to "go crazy" became an existential *koan* for her. What would "crazy" be like? She and her two daughters were all dressed alike. She said this was her version of "keeping it crazy." We were impressed and touched by this sophisticated woman and her two daughters, all dressed in matching red outfits, their hair done up in ponytails. And for William, their entertainer father, they sang "The Barney Song": "I love you, you love me, we're a happy family." Three-year-old Saniqua was their proud director. Helen and the girls had driven separately from William to the interview, so it was a surprise to William. It was innocent, touching, sweet, and corny. He was appreciative and proud of his wife and daughters.

"That's what I love about her," he said. "And when that spontaneous part of her goes away, I start to feel like I am not here any more. That may be weird, Dr. Keith, but that's how it is. I think that's how it is."

The interview continued with Helen's taking the lead and interviewing us about what I meant by being "crazy." Craziness is linked to creativity and spontaneity. It is linked to health. Being crazy is a part of the dynamics of intimacy. Like any experience, it is not easily definable. Being crazy is being joyful and expansive. Or it is being lost inside oneself, feeling the pain of depression, confusion, or insignificance. Preoccupation with the other is escape from craziness.

HELEN: But isn't crazy something you *don't* want to be?

D. V. K.: Yeah, in our culture I think the fear of craziness is a powerful, however covert, determinant for behavior. A phobia of craziness in the parents puts a lot of pressure on the children. What makes craziness pathological is when it occurs in too much isolation. If you get extruded from a group and locked out, that's when it turns pathological, especially if you get taken to some doctor who places the right cultural diagnostic stamp: "Bipolar," thump, "Next!" "Manic–depressive," thump, "Next!" "Clinical depression," thump, "Next!" Craziness can feel free and exhilarating, or it can feel deeply painful and lonely, or even both.

HELEN: You're clever. If your motto is "keep it crazy," then you can't lose.

D. V. K.: Hmmm! I hadn't thought of that. I still think I lose. I am aware I still fail.

I mention failing a fair amount in therapy. I suspect my unconscious motive is to keep patients from sitting there waiting for Dr. All-Knowing to work his magic on their problems. It keeps them thinking, "How are we going to get out of this?", instead of "How will they get us out of this?" If they hear me being concerned about my failing, they stay more alert and responsible for the outcome—for the success of the therapy.

SEVENTH INTERVIEW

The seventh interview was uneventful. It began with more discussion of what therapy was about.

HELEN: Do you remember last week when I was asking you for something to read? Well, I have a friend who teaches [educational psychology] at the university. She told me she had heard of you from some place, and she told me you might do something unexpected. She gave me that book by your friends Napier and Whitaker [*The Family Crucible*, 1978].

D. V. K.: I better reread it so I don't disappoint you.

A. M. P. H.: You're talking about intellectual preoccupations. I wonder if you thought of not coming today?

HELEN: Actually, I was looking forward to coming.

WILLIAM: Yeah. She wanted the Doc here to know that she had disobeyed him.

D. V. K.: Naughty, naughty. No dessert for you, little mayor, and early to bed. (*They laughed. It was quiet for a few moments.*) By the way, I ran across a weird novel about families and craziness. I think you both should read it: *Let the Dog Drive.*

HELEN: Oh, God! You *are* crazy.

D. V. K.: You don't have to call me "God." "Doctor" is good enough.

HELEN: Why would I want to read something like that?

D. V. K.: It is about craziness and the pain of searching for self.

EIGHTH INTERVIEW

When the family came back, things were not going well. It sounded as though Helen had become overly optimistic and tried to induce William into her optimism, and he had backed up. She called the day before the next interview to say she was upset, worried that he was symptomatic again. I was worried that she was pathologizing again, diagnosing him. I talked with her on the phone for about 20 minutes. I suggested that if the situation was getting worse, we should increase the size of the group; they could bring one of their friends, or include their parents by telephone. She didn't want to bring a friend because the friend would side with her and William wouldn't come. She said she would talk with her parents and his mother, to see if they would be willing to participate by speaker phone.

When they arrived, Helen had talked to William's mother and her parents, and all of them were available by phone. I called William's mother's number, but there was no answer. I did not try her parents. I was uneasy about them; I worried that they would be too conventional and too supportive, and that including them would further exclude William. Not calling them may have been a mistake, however.

The tension between Helen and William was high, as if they were turning the responsibility for the marriage over to us so they could have more freedom. She was angry at him for letting her down, for "playing like this poor black man that no one can understand." He was angry at something going on in their church. It had to do with her friends, who had invited him to sing, but wanted to see the arrangement first; it sounded as if they wanted to tone him down. He said it was like he was their token black. They would all get into heaven sooner if they helped him out, especially in light of the fact that he was mentally ill at that, and if they rehabilitated him it would make it even more likely they would get into heaven. He was irritated and upset. She said that he had it wrong; her friends loved him and were trying to be helpful. She went on to say that part of the problem was that he thought he was "too good" for them, because he was this "famous show-business professional." William retorted, "This really gets under my skin. You don't know what you're talking about."

William was very angry. I had two ways of looking at it. On the one hand, it sounded as if he might have gone into some sort of paranoid thing. On the other hand, it sounded as if he was being marginalized and Helen did not see it.

The tension continued. Almost 30 minutes into the interview, Sarah said, "I think I'm going to throw up." She moved closer to her mother. Casually, I reached over, grabbed my large wastebasket by the rim, and put it in the center of the room. "Here's the wastebasket," I said.

It was quiet for a few moments. There was then further definition of resentments, with the sense from both that "I've had enough of this." Time ran out. As we were closing, it felt as though something painful was happening and I wasn't getting it. It was like surgery, where the abdominal cavity is open and there is bleeding, but its source is not clear. I commented, "I worry I might not be black enough to be helpful." I said this for two reasons: First, I thought it was true; and, second, I felt it was important to keep the race issue on the table. No one responded. All were tight-jawed as they got up and left.

NINTH INTERVIEW

The girls went to a picnic with some friends. And Helen felt she needed some time away from them. Helen and William had been squabbling all week.

Helen said they'd received a letter from William's mother in which she urged him to stay with Helen. William said that he thought his mom had been at her phone when we'd tried to call her earlier, but that she just didn't want to get involved because she was worried he would come back to her, and she wanted him to count the blessings he had with Helen and the kids.

In the letter William's mother said, "I am no longer your mother." I had never heard anything like this before. It suggested that there was too much pain in her life—the life he came out of—and that she did not want him to be reinvolved in it. This was a painful, unfamiliar idea to me. It recalled William's earlier remark about a "different world."

WILLIAM: Doc, what will I do? I don't have a mother, I'll never go back to show business, and this life has become too stifling.

D. V. K.: My impression is that there is something about this white world that attracts you—some vindication in it. But on the other hand, it may be costing you too much to join into it.

HELEN: *(Changing the subject)* You know last week when Sarah was nauseated, and you said, "Here's the wastebasket," I was *so* angry with you. Your response seemed so cold, so indifferent. But then I thought, "Yeah. A wastebasket. If you are going to throw up, that's what you need." This may not quite make sense, but then I thought that if William was feeling upset, I did not need to fix it. I just say, "OK, there's the wastebasket. OK, go be crazy. But we are going to the Smiths' for dinner at 6, so be back to normal by then." I think it works better. Whenever I try to help him, I think whatever is happening happens worse.

TENTH INTERVIEW

Helen and William returned without the girls. They had tried to recover their togetherness during the interim, but with no luck. He seemed to have clarified something for himself, and she seemed desperate. He was keeping his distance and was unwilling to reunite with his wife. His distance and calm seemed to make her more anxious; it was a role reversal.

WILLIAM: I'm not the crazy one here, and she can't get over the [idea] that just because that psychiatrist said I have a mental illness that I need to be on medication, and I refuse. I'm not going to do medication again. They just don't see how this is a problem between us; it's not just me. See, Doc, we like you and Anne Marie, but I'm not sure that's enough. And Helen doesn't really trust you and the stuff you talk about. I think you had it right, Doc, when you said she's got to learn to be crazier. It's just so easy for her to turn into the great Protestant standard for normal when I get excited. I don't pretend I'm an easy man to be married to, but this is not about me being *sick*.

HELEN: He's right; I am worried that your ideas are too simple. And he's right; I don't know if you *are* doing anything.†

> † Would it have detracted from the basic spirit of experiential therapy to inquire into Helen's schema about William's "craziness" and what it would mean to her if she were to be "more crazy" herself? It would also have been interesting to operationally define the term "crazy" and what it meant to each of them.

WILLIAM: *(Chuckling)* That's one thing we agree on: Anne Marie and the Doc aren't doing anything.

HELEN: *(Suddenly)* William, you keep accusing me of being no fun, of being too serious and too self-righteous. But I think it's because I have to take too much responsibility for the details of our life. You want to be the only one who can be crazy in this family. Why can't we be crazy together for once? I do know how to be playful. *(She rose up wide-eyed and vibrant.)* You want crazy, you can have crazy! *(She danced slowly across the office then straddled him face to face on the sofa, with her arms extended out to the side. She sang to him:)* I'm crazy for you. I'm crazy for you, William. *(She said to us:)* And it's easy for me to be like this. *(She caressed his face with her hands. He was nonresponsive. He sat calmly, like a patient father with a silly daughter. She stood up and turned toward us.)* See? I *am* being crazy. I love being crazy! But I don't know if he can stand it when I'm crazy. Maybe I should start taking lithium.

WILLIAM: *(Grinning)* I don't know where this is going. It just seems crazy to me.

But there was some rapprochement. The hour ended with him rubbing her back.

When they left, I said to Anne Marie, "They are lively, unpredictable characters. I enjoy working with them. I think I am still worried about the marriage."

Anne Marie answered, "I am so impressed by the way they change roles. You have talked about the idea before, but I have never seen it happen so clearly. He gets so straight when she is being playful, it's almost laughable."

ELEVENTH INTERVIEW

Again, William and Helen returned without the girls. They were uneasy with each other. They had had an argument about who was going to watch the children. He had an appointment about the possibility of a new job. She had a temper tantrum; he asked her to stop. She refused, insisting that she had every right to be as upset as he was. "And he doesn't like it when the shoe is on the other foot," she said. William looked annoyed. There was a deeper anger simmering in him today—deep in the same way his earlier sadness had been deep.

WILLIAM: This therapy isn't helping. You are nice people. But I'm not sure you know what you are doing. Half the time you just sit there. And when you do say something, it seems like a joke. *(He paused. We did not respond, but gazed back at him.)* I don't know where this is going.

HELEN: *(Uneasy with our continuing silence)* I know where I want it to go. I want it to go towards us being back together again, but I hate it when you act like Mad Face. [She had told us before that she had two names for him, Mad Face and Chocolate Face.] *(To us)* Now you are seeing the angry William who frightens me. I hate to see this William, but I'm glad you are seeing him. Maybe it will change your mind about medication.†

> † *At this point it is my impression that Helen was more calculated with her statements than she appeared to be. She actually pushed William into angry modes, consciously or unconsciously, even though she claimed that she feared his anger. I wonder whether making her consciously aware of her behaviors would have been helpful to both of them. Perhaps several behavioral strategies could have been employed that might have helped her to elicit less animosity from William.*

I wished she had not said that. It was like sticking him with a stiletto.

WILLIAM: This is too dumb. This is not me you are talking about. Just cut it out. If you don't stop this shit, then I'm done. I'm just plain done.

HELEN: I don't want our marriage to end, but you can't keep putting this load on me. *(He looked at her and shook his head. He then got up and started for the door.)*

WILLIAM: I'm leaving!

D. V. K.: *(Firmly)* If you're leaving, you better take her with you.

WILLIAM: I don't want her. You can have her. *(The door slammed. He was gone. She sat in the chair, saying nothing.)*

D. V. K.: We need to quit. I don't want to go on without him.

HELEN: I can understand that, but what will I do now? I'm afraid to go home. I don't know what he will do. Don't you think he needs medication?

D. V. K.: No. This is not about medication. Like he said, he's an angry black man. He wants to be in your world, but he can't stand to be in your world.

Anne Marie questioned Helen further to get a better sense of her fear. Anne Marie suggested that if she had problems, she should contact the shelter for abused women in our city. I was troubled by the hint of violence that Helen feared, but that had never been present thus far. Anne Marie was even more anxious about the possibility of violence. More than anything, Anne Marie's discomfort made me uneasy, but Helen had to take care of herself.

When I'm working with a family, I don't want to get cornered with one fragment of the family, so I made sure Helen left early so as not to exclude William. I also made sure she knew that I was not indifferent to her plight.

When she was gone, Anne Marie seemed uneasy and wondered what I thought. I reiterated what I had said before—that I thought William knew how to be angry, but that I didn't view him as abusive. However, the next day I was aware of my continuing apprehension about the situation. Anne Marie called me in the morning to see if I had heard anything, and again asked what I thought. Because I was still apprehensive, I called Helen. Nothing upsetting had happened. William had called in the evening and then come over to take care of the girls while she went to a meeting of the city council—but they were not speaking.

They did not return. Two weeks later, Helen sent a check for the copayment. She thanked us for trying and for caring; she said that she had been hopeful, but no longer. I was unhappy about the outcome. I have been doing this for over 20 years, but divorces still hurt and cause me to feel like a failure. But I believe firmly that people must take care of their own lives, and that when we mental health practitioners try too hard to rescue people, we are undermining their capacity for surviving emotionally, physically, and spiritually.

About 6 months later, I ran across an article in the morning paper about a church in our city whose congregation was largely made up of racially mixed couples. I cut out the article and sent it to Helen and

William, with a note saying that I hoped things were working out for them, one way or another. My assumption was that they were probably in the process of divorce. Two days later, I had a call from William. His tone was warm when he thanked me for the note and told me how receiving it had been "kind of an ESP experience." He had seen the article in a coffee shop the day before and meant to take the paper with him; he forgot it, but was very heartened by it. He was glad to know we had been thinking about them. He said, "Doc, I'd been meaning to call you and thank you, because you probably don't know how some of these cases turn out. Especially with nuts like us. We got back together 3 weeks after that last appointment, and things have never been better between us. I want to thank you for caring about us the way you did."

CONCLUSION

This case provides a good example of couple therapy in the context of symbolic-experiential family therapy. The marital subgroup went through what I call a "therapeutic psychosis" (Keith & Whitaker, 1986) as a result of our disrupting the rhythms and patterns of their living. This perturbation, combined with our caring and their desperation, produced confusion. We were prepared to deal with any change that resulted from this temporary disorganization. The children were present for most of the interviews; although I have not highlighted much of their participation, it was very important. The children's presence forced the parents to see their individual and marital struggles as part of a greater whole; it demanded more honesty from them.

Eighteen months after our last interview, Helen and William agreed to participate in a seminar, in which some physicians interviewed them and us about the therapy and their previous experiences in seeking mental health services. The seminar was great fun. It seemed that the shifts in the couple's living were stable. And although William and Helen were appreciative and grateful, they took great pleasure in teasing Anne Marie and me for "doing nothing."

AUTHOR'S REPLY TO EDITOR'S COMMENTS

There is considerable continuity between cognitive-behavioral methods and symbolic-experiential methods. It looks as though we are trying to get to the same place. I have selected a case in which the family had a good response to our pattern of working. At the end of the therapy, I thought we had failed; I felt discouraged about it. My interaction with Helen and William later, however, demonstrates something I believe to be true about therapy—that it is an experience that *establishes the conditions* for growth or healing, and that its benefits are often not immediately apparent. There are other cases in which my methods may more closely resemble those of a cognitive-behavioral therapist (or, at least, a playful cognitive-behavioral therapist). I sense in Dr. Dattilio's comments a gentleness and awareness that lead me to believe we are headed in the same direction. I can imagine us working together. I would be amused by his carefulness, earnestness, and attention to thinking things through. He would be amused by my nonrational, intuitive style. I have discovered that in these struggles out in the ocean of human pain, there can be no competition for ignorance.

   1. (p. 185) The advice given here is standard for me at the end of the first interview with a couple. Most couples have been conducting at-home seminars on what's wrong and how to fix it. The effort to fix it becomes part of the problem. My instruction not to talk is not paradoxical; I get grumpy when couples misbehave. The instruction has at least two purposes beyond interrupting the amateur therapy they are doing with each other. First, it induces individuated meditation on "I" and "we." The conversation in the therapy room is different from social conversation. Social conversation tends to neutralize any change in thinking or perception that may have occurred as a result of the therapeutic interaction. Second, it disrupts the impasse that results from trying to fix what's wrong. At this point, I did not know of any history of violence; what was involved here is fear of violence. The "heating up" I was referring to was verbal arguing. However, Helen and William had already built in a cool-off zone: They had decided on their own to live separately. *(He had a room downtown.)* My sense here was that they were already into being too intellectual about their problems. She had evolved into an assistant psychiatrist, with him as her full-time, live-in patient. I am not quick to offer solutions to a couple like this one, because it sets up a situation where I take over the problem and suggests that I know how to live the partners' lives. It has the same quality that giving medication at the first interview does. It says, "You shouldn't feel this way, and I have the magic to make it better." I think a better ending is "It sounds painful. It looks to me like you are going to have to learn how to suffer." I am making the partners responsible for what happens in therapy by letting anxiety and ambiguity increase. In this case, I had no anxiety that anything dangerous might happen. I was most concerned about the marriage coming apart, about both William's and Helen's feeling in need, and about my being pulled between them. Dr. Dattilio's advice might feel useful to some therapists, but for me, it seems too careful and concrete. It would be awkward for me to use it, akin to making me pitch left-handed.
   2. (p. 189) This is a good point, and in some situations a useful point. I have used variations of that question at times. It would not have fit well with William and Helen, however. They had seen other therapists who guided them and asked good questions, and they had not gotten anywhere. My intuition

told me to stay covert, more Zen-ish with these two. They were verbal, and accomplishment came easily to them. The fact that they were experiencing change even though we were "doing nothing" was engaging them, and I preferred to keep this therapeutic double bind in place. In the follow-up interview about 18 months after the last interview, they talked about how this pattern pressured them into looking out for their own welfare instead of trying to live up to our expectations.

3. (p. 196) I think it would have detracted from the therapeutic process if we had become too concrete about "craziness." Essentially, "craziness" is the mystery, the unknown—the shadows and the darkness at the edges of our experience. I have, on several occasions, started a paper with the title "Craziness as a Clinical Concept." The paper has never been concluded, but I have a lot of ideas. My belief is that in our culture, the fear of craziness is widely prevalent, and many decisions about life are organized around avoiding the "feeling" of being crazy. But "resisting madness may be the maddest way of being mad," says Norman O. Brown (1991, p. 2). Curiously, Helen and William not only embraced the idea, but feasted upon it. They easily translated it into their experiences, into their roles in the relationship. The suggestion to "keep it crazy" was a counterbalance for the pathologizing of behavior they had experienced in their interactions with psychiatrists. However, many families are challenged or spooked by the word, so it may lead to more discussion and need for desensitization. Craziness is health; it is a whole person living in the present. Craziness is creativity. Craziness is the reluctance to adapt. Health is a balance between craziness (dedication to "I") and social adaptation (dedication to "we"). The overtly identified patient in any family is usually the one who is dedicated to "I," but he or she is a counterbalance to the covert, unidentified patient, who is the one dedicated to the "we."

4. (p. 197) There is some truth in this observation. It is not unusual for me to ask patients like Helen whether they have any idea what they contribute to their problems. However, it did not come to mind at the time. I was surprised by William's anger. It seemed to me to be like his deep crying earlier. It was coming from a place where there were no words. I also believe that the depth of his feeling was augmented by his relationship to us. I do have a concern that sometimes an interpretation, an attempt at education, or a push for a solution can trivialize emotional experience. Such interventions are often driven more by a therapist's anxiety than by a patient's need. I am not suggesting that I knew this in this situation. But it felt important to let the situation heat up in order for it to produce change. This issue raises a question about the teaching of experiential therapy. How can it be learned? Learning this kind of therapy is like learning to do surgery. Therapists must face the fact that there is some danger. The pattern is best learned in an apprenticeship pattern. I suggest that less experienced experiential therapists do nothing that makes them anxious. However, sometimes I suspect it may be that what

therapists learn is a certain facility for explaining their behavior, even when they do not understand it themselves.

ACKNOWLEDGMENTS

I wish to thank Noel Rahn Keith, MA, and Anne Marie Patti Higgins, MA, BSN, FNP, for their helpful suggestions in preparing the manuscript.

REFERENCES

Betz, B., & Whitehorn, J. C. (1975). *Effective psychotherapy with the schizophrenic patient*. New York: Jason Aronson.

Brown, N. O.(1991). *Apocalypse and/or metamorphosis*. Berkeley: University of California Press.

Keith, D. V. (1989). The family's own system: The symbolic context of health. In L. Combrinck-Graham (Ed.), *Children in family contexts*. New York: Guilford Press.

Keith, D. V., & Whitaker, C. A. (1988). The presence of the past: Continuity and change in the symbolic understructure of the family. In C. Falicov (Ed.), *Family transitions*. New York: Guilford Press.

Napier, A. Y., with Whitaker, C. A. (1978). *The family crucible*. New York: Harper & Row.

Whitaker, C. A., & Malone, T. (1953). *The roots of psychotherapy*. New York: Blakiston.

SUGGESTED READINGS

Keith, D. V. (1993, Winter). Alternative psychiatry: Replacing medication with family members. *AFTA Newsletter*, pp. 10–14.

Keith, D. V., & Whitaker, C. A. (1980). Play therapy: A paradigm for work with families. *Journal of Marital and Family Therapy, 7*, 243–254.

Neill, J. R., & Kniskern, D. P. (Eds.). (1982). *From psyche to system: The evolving therapy of Carl Whitaker*. New York: Guilford Press.

Whitaker, C. A., & Bumberry, W. (1988). *Dancing with the family: A symbolic experiential approach*. New York: Brunner/Mazel.

Whitaker, C. A., & Ryan, M. C. (1989). *Midnight musings of a family therapist*. New York: Norton.

Chapter 9

Solution-Focused Couple Therapy
Helping Clients Construct Self-Fulfilling Realities

MICHAEL F. HOYT
INSOO KIM BERG

> What we talk about and how we talk about it makes a
> difference (to the client). Thus reframing a "marital problem"
> into an "individual problem" or an "individual problem"
> into a "marital problem" makes a difference both in how
> we talk about things and where we look for solutions.
> —Steve de Shazer (1994b, p. 10)

Solution-focused therapy is an intervention approach that has been described and applied in a wide variety of situations by Steve de Shazer (1982, 1985, 1988, 1991, 1994b), Insoo Kim Berg (1994a; Berg & Miller, 1992; DeJong & Berg, 1997; Miller & Berg, 1995), and others (Dolan, 1991; Duncan, Hubble & Miller, 1997; Kowalski & Kral, 1989; Kral, 1987; Quick, 1996; Miller, 1994; Miller, Hubble, & Duncan, 1996; Miller, Duncan, & Hubble, 1997; Walter & Peller, 1992; see Miller & Hopwood, 1994). Initially, the approach emerged in a deductive manner—that is, from studying what clients and therapists did that preceded their declaring problems "solved." It was noticed that problems were described as solved (or resolved, dissolved, or no longer problems) when clients began to engage in new and different perceptions and behaviors vis-à-vis the presenting difficulties. This recognition led to the "basic rules" (de Shazer, in Hoyt, 1996a, p. 68) of solution-focused therapy:

1. If it ain't broke, don't fix it.
2. Once you know what works, do more of it.
3. If it doesn't work, don't do it again; do something different.

Following from these rules, some basic heuristic questions can be derived: What is the client doing that works? What does the client want? What can the client do toward what is wanted? What can help keep the client going in the desired direction? When should therapy end?

FOCUS ON SOLUTIONS, NOT PROBLEMS

Solution-focused therapy can be understood as a constructivist, postmodern, poststructural approach (de Shazer & Berg, 1992)—one that conceives therapy as a process of clients and therapists co-constructing more desirable "realities." The basic guiding principle is that as therapists we are actively involved—whether we realize it or not—in helping clients construe different ways of looking at themselves, their partners, their situations and interactions. How we look influences what we see, and what we see influences what we do; and around and around the process goes, recursively (Hoyt, 1994a, 1996b). All questions are leading questions, directing attention and consciousness here rather than there, there rather than here. Solution-focused therapy is just that: intervention that purposely directs attention and energy toward the expansion of desired outcomes. "Building solutions" is not simply the reciprocal or inverse of "having problems"; indeed, development of a solution often involves a reformulation or different construction, such that the former "position" loses its relevance or simply "dis-solves."

A "problem" arises and a couple seeks "therapy" (intervention) when the partners view their situation in such a way that they do not have access to what is needed to achieve what they consider reasonable satisfaction. Although support can be given and skills taught, solution-focused therapy's primary emphasis is on assisting clients to make better use of their own strengths and competence; it is recognized that how clients conceive their situation will either empower them or cut them off from existing resources. The solution-focused therapist thus interviews purposefully (Lipchik & de Shazer, 1986; Lipchik, 1987) in order to "influence the clients' view of the problem in a manner that leads to solution" (Berg & Miller, 1992, p. 70). As de Shazer (1991, p. 74) writes:

> The therapeutic relationship is a negotiated, consensual, and cooperative endeavor in which the solution-focused therapist and client jointly produce various language games focused on (a) exceptions, (b) goals, and (c) solutions (de Shazer, 1985, 1988). All of these are negotiated and

produced as therapists and clients misunderstand together, make sense of, and give meaning to otherwise ambiguous events, feelings, and relationships. In doing so, therapists and clients jointly assign meaning to aspects of clients' lives and justify actions intended to develop a solution.

ORIENTATION

A few general points about solution-focused therapy may be highlighted in preparation for the case to be described below.

1. There is usually a "future focus," with the therapist drawing attention to what the clients will be doing differently when they have achieved a desired outcome or solution. The language presumes or presupposes change ("After the miracle . . . "). Questions are designed to evoke a self-fulfilling map of the future (Penn, 1985; Tomm, 1987). The purpose is therapy, not archeology; blame talk and escalation of negative affect are avoided in favor of eliciting movement in helpful directions.

2. The therapist assumes a posture of "not knowing" (Anderson & Goolishian, 1992), allowing the clients to be "experts" rather than having the therapist tell the clients what is "really" wrong and how to fix it. This is not to say that the therapist abdicates his or her role as skillful facilitator, but it does imply that the clients' language and ideas—their ways of "storying" their lives—will be given full respect and seen as valid and real.

3. Focusing on strengths, exceptions, solutions, and a more favorable future inspires clients (and therapists) and promotes "empowerment." The therapist–client relationship is evolving and dynamic. Flexibly renegotiating goals, and appreciating and working *with* clients' sense of their situations maintain therapist–client cooperation and vitiate the concept of "resistance" (Berg, 1989; de Shazer, 1984).

4. Well-formed goals have the following general characteristics: They are (a) small rather than large; (b) salient to clients; (c) articulated in specific, concrete behavioral terms; (d) achievable within the practical contexts of clients' lives; (e) perceived by clients as involving their own hard work; (f) seen as the "start of something" and not as the "end of something"; and (g) treated as involving new behaviors rather than the absence or cessation of existing behaviors (de Shazer, 1991, p. 112).

5. Questions are asked and responses are carefully punctuated to build or highlight a positive reality facilitative of clients' goals. All questions are, in effect, leading questions, inviting clients to organize and focus their attention and understanding in one way rather than another (Tomm, 1988; Freedman & Combs, 1993). As Hoyt (1996c) has written elsewhere, the therapist functions like a special kind of mirror that can become convex or

concave and swivel this way or that. Rather than providing a "flat mirror" that simply "reflects and clarifies," the solution-focused therapist purposely and differentially expands and contracts the reflected image, so to speak— opening parts of the story and closing others, making "space" for (or "giving privilege" to) discourses that support the realization of clients' goals. The therapist endeavors to help the couple build a solution. As the story about the three baseball umpires disputing their acumen (Hoyt, 1996d, p. 315) has it:

> The first umpire, who prides himself on ethics, says, "I call them as I see 'em." The second ump, who believes in objective accuracy, says, "Not bad, but I call 'em the way they are." Finally, the third ump speaks: "They ain't nothing until I call 'em!"

In the following transcript, we want to show the details of how a solution-focused therapist selects what to highlight, how the therapist and clients co-create how they will "call 'em," and what results.

CASE EXAMPLE[1, 2]

Leslie and Bill had been married for approximately 7 years and had two children, aged 5 and 3. Bill also had another child from a previous marriage, but he rarely saw this child, even though he made child support payments. Bill was an attorney working for a large law firm, and Leslie was a consumer services director for a large telephone company. Leslie initiated therapy; when she told Bill she was "unhappy" and wanted "marriage counseling," he agreed to attend. This was their first session, held at the Brief Family Therapy Center (BFTC) in Milwaukee. Insoo Kim Berg (I. K. B.) was the therapist.

Redirection from Problem Talk to Solution Talk

The session began with socializing and joining, in which the therapist and clients introduced themselves and started connecting. The partners then quickly began to present their conflict, both in words and in action. Leslie complained that Bill worked a great deal entertaining women clients, while Leslie did her full-time job outside the home and also maintained the children and household; Bill countered that he was working 70 hours a week to make partnership in his law firm and thus to provide better for his wife and family. Tensions mounted. The storyline Bill and Leslie were enacting did not seem to be taking them where they wanted to go, so at this juncture the therapist interrupted the escalating cycle of complaints and "problem talk" to elicit the clients' view of a desirable outcome of therapy.

This redirected their attention to progressive narrative by refocusing the interaction on constructing "solution talk."†

> †This is very similar to what cognitive-behavioral therapists try to do with couples in conflict: To zero in on what the specific conflict is, and to operationally define terms so that they may be clearly framed in a manner that everyone involved with the case can understand.

I. K. B.: What do you suppose needs to happen as a result of your being here today, so you can look back—oh, let's say a few months from now, when you look back at this period in your life—so you can say to yourselves, "That was a good idea that we went and talked to Insoo; that was helpful"? What needs to happen?

LESLIE: I would hope that Bill could come up with some kind of understanding of what are his responsibilities, and that in these sessions he could really hear what I am saying—because at home he really doesn't listen—and, therefore, he could change his behavior so that we could be as we were earlier in the marriage.

I. K. B.: Really? [The therapist was responding to indications of a more satisfying life in the past. Leslie laid out her complaints: When Bill understood his responsibility, he would change his behaviors, and they would return to how they had been earlier in the marriage. Notice how the therapist built consensus between the partners.]

LESLIE: You know. Listening to one another and communicating.

I. K. B.: Right.

LESLIE: But he seems to have strayed from that.

BILL: That's what, that's what we need.

I. K. B.: What? [She was trying to refocus the conversation.]

BILL: Communication.

I. K. B.: OK.

BILL: If we can come out of this with some ground-level communication, I will think that it has been successful.

I. K. B.: OK.

LESLIE: You know, I appreciate him as a husband. I do love him.

I. K. B.: You do? [The question laid emphasis on this positive aspect of their relationship.]

LESLIE: And I know he does work hard.

I. K. B.: You do love him. [This further highlighted the positive.]

LESLIE: Yes, I do. I do.

I. K. B.: OK. When he is more responsible, what will he be doing that he's not doing right now that will let you know he's being more responsible? [Notes presupposition of change with "when" rather than "if."]

LESLIE: He will take more responsibility for our children. He will take more responsibility for his own son, whom I love very much, too.

I. K. B.: OK.

LESLIE: He will take responsibility to include me—have respect for me. Include me in his activities and have respect for me.†

> †*Already in this case, the therapist identified a very common issue in couple therapy—"expectations." Among the most common areas of violation in a relationship are the partners' expectations of each other and of the relationship as a whole. A common area of focus in cognitive-behavioral therapy is to identify each partner's expectation of the spouse and the relationship, and to attempt to make some early determination as to whether or not the partners' expectations are realistic. Here, the therapist was already identifying this as a "positive goal in general terms" and attempting to support her understanding with a behavioral description.*

Having identified a positive goal in general terms, the therapist now asked for a specific behavioral description:

I. K. B.: What will Bill be doing exactly that will let you know that he is being responsible around the house, with his children, with his son? [Answers to this question would establish behavioral indicators of how Bill would be more "responsible."]

LESLIE: Well, right now I'm always reading the bedtime stories because he's out doing whatever.

I. K. B.: OK. So he will be doing some of those? [She refocused on positive behavioral criteria.]

LESLIE: Yes. Especially on weekends, when you don't have to carry the load that you carry during the week.

I. K. B.: OK.

LESLIE: I would like some help around the house. He thinks that I'm the built-in maid, it feels like.

I. K. B.: What would he be doing?

Leslie responded by complaining that she did all the washing, ironing, and cooking. Bill suggested hiring someone to do housework; Leslie replied that they couldn't afford it; and Bill rejoined the argument with a comment about Leslie's not wanting anybody else taking care of the kids. At this point, the therapist refocused on the thread of Leslie's small but specific behavioral goal that Bill help at bedtime. She tried to amplify the positive possibility, rather than the complaint, in order to build a shared vision of their life; however, the couple began to bicker about "responsibility." The therapist persisted in attempting to refocus the conversation toward the desired outcome. It is common for members of a couple to become distracted and embroiled in "problem talk" when their "trigger words" are used. Therefore, it is particularly helpful for a therapist to focus on what the clients want and not on what may interest the therapist.

I. K. B.: I need to know from both of you what needs to happen, so that I am helpful to both of you. So let me come back to this. What would he be doing different, let's say 6 months down the road?

LESLIE: I think even though it's important that he is building a partnership, and I realize it takes time and I try to be supportive . . .

I. K. B.: Right. OK.

LESLIE: He also has to build a relationship at home. *(To Bill)* We have little ones that don't even know you.

I. K. B.: So what would he be doing to build a relationship at home?

LESLIE: He would be communicating more with me.

I. K. B.: OK.

LESLIE: He would be taking an active role with our children. Our children. He is just someone who comes in during the morning and leaves. I mean, they don't even have a concept of who you are. And I think that's a shame.

I. K. B.: OK. Now . . .

BILL: Uh, you, uh . . . [He was starting to argue back.]

I. K. B.: Let me come back to you, Bill, on this. I'm assuming you want to have this relationship with Leslie also? [The therapist returned to the shared vision and refocused toward the goal.]

BILL: Yes, of course. I love her as well.

I. K. B.: You do.

BILL: Yeah.

I. K. B.: Does she know how much you love her?

LESLIE: Do I know?

BILL: She should. I mean, you know.

I. K. B.: Yeah? What do you think? Does she know?

BILL: You know. We've been together for 7 years. I love her and I haven't left her. I wouldn't leave her. This is my wife. I love her. I love my children as well.

LESLIE: Do you see this? *(She held up Bill's left hand, which was ringless.)* He has a wedding ring. I wear mine. He doesn't wear his. He doesn't wear his.

I. K. B.: Uh-huh.

BILL: I figure that they're [the children] 3 and 5 years old; that if I put in these hours now, when they are older they'll be able to appreciate me more; [and] that I will then have more time to spend with them.

I. K. B.: I see.

BILL: That's the principle that I'm operating on. Either I can stay at home and wash dishes, or I can spend 70 hours a week trying to build up this practice, so that as an eventuality you won't even have to work, and you don't seem to have any patience or understanding or cooperation.

LESLIE: I don't have to work?

I. K. B.: Oh, wow. So you really are working for the future. [She was building the shared vision once more.]

BILL: Yes. Absolutely. I'm trying to secure a future not just for myself, but for all of us.

As the interview proceeded, the therapist then introduced the "miracle question" (de Shazer, 1988). Notice how as common goals began to emerge, the affect changed. Also notice how detailed and specific were the elicited behavioral descriptions of what would indicate the beginnings of a desired outcome.

I. K. B.: OK. I'm going to ask both of you some very strange questions that will take some imagination on both of your parts. Let's say as a result of a miracle, the problem that brought you here today is gone *(snapping her fingers)*. Just like that.

LESLIE: That would be a miracle! *(She and Bill laughed.)*

I. K. B.: That would be nice. But this miracle happens in the middle of the night when both of you are sleeping. Like tonight, for example. So you don't know that this has happened. *(Both Leslie and Bill chuckled.)* So when you wake up tomorrow morning, what will be the first small clue to you that, "Wow! Something must have happened during the night! The problem is gone!" How will you discover this?

BILL: I'll smile first thing in the morning, instead of avoidance.

I. K. B.: You will smile at Leslie.

LESLIE: He would put his arm around me.

I. K. B.: He'll put his arm around you. OK.

LESLIE: That would be a real sign of a miracle at this point.

I. K. B.: OK. All right, so suppose he does. What will you do in response to that?

LESLIE: I won't turn my back to him *(laughing)*.

I. K. B.: All right. OK. Is that right? Is that what she would do? Would that be a miracle for you?

BILL: Yeah. That definitely would.

I. K. B.: That would be a miracle for you.

BILL: It would be very different.

I. K. B.: It would be different. OK.

BILL: Yeah. It would be a miracle.

LESLIE: Mmm-hmm.

I. K. B.: OK. So when she turns her back towards you—I mean, so she's facing you—when you smile at her, she'll face you instead of turning her back towards you. What will you do when you see her do that?

BILL: I don't know. I suppose I'll embrace her, probably.

I. K. B.: Uh-huh. So you will give her a hug.

BILL: Yeah.

I. K. B.: What about you, Leslie? What will you do when he gives you a hug?

LESLIE: Well, if he hugs me, I'll hug him back.

I. K. B.: Uh-huh. OK. OK. What will come after that?

LESLIE: Tomorrow's Saturday, you never can tell! *(Said sexily; Bill and Leslie laughed.)*

I. K. B.: *(Laughing)* OK.

BILL: A miracle!†

> †*A cognitive-behavioral therapist might have considered focusing here on what specifically was occurring cognitively with both Leslie and Bill. For example, when the therapist asked Leslie, "What will you do when he gives you a hug?", it might also have been interesting to inquire, "As you imagine him doing that right now, what thought goes through your mind, and how does that thought affect how you feel?" Not only would this have exposed Leslie's schemas, but it would also have given Bill firsthand insight into the mechanisms of Leslie's thoughts and feelings and how they were processed. This would also have set the stage for them to begin to learn each other's "cognitive dance" for the future.*

The therapist then posed an "exception question," to find recent problem-free times that the partners might may have already achieved on their own. Once identified, such exceptions often can be built upon.

I. K. B.: When was the most recent time when you had a morning like that? Maybe not all of it, but just pieces of that—part of that miracle picture?

BILL: It's been a while.

LESLIE: Probably right after Evelyn was born.

I. K. B.: Is that right?

LESLIE: That's almost 2 years—almost 3 years ago.

I. K. B.: Wow. That was a long time ago.

LESLIE: Yeah. I think so. Am I right? Can I be right sometimes?†

> †This was another trigger statement for what cognitive therapists refer to as a "hot cognition." A cognitive strategy might have been to address this statement right up front as it accompanied the emotional tone; it implied that there was an issue in Leslie's mind as to whether she was ever right. This could have opened a door to her self-esteem issues or any oppression existing in her mind regarding her role in the relationship.

BILL: Well, I don't know if it's quite that long—somewhere in that framework, but I wouldn't say it's been that long.

I. K. B.: Well, not all of it, but just pieces of it? [The therapist sought a small positive exception, rather than buying into the bickering.]

LESLIE: It's been a couple of years.

BILL: It's been a while.

LESLIE: But we've been avoiding. He's out a lot. I take care of the kids. I bury myself in my job. But I don't—I'm not married to my job.

I. K. B.: Right.

LESLIE: You know. I'm married to him. And my job is important. My children are precious to me. But I want the whole thing, and I want to . . .

I. K. B.: You want this relationship back.

LESLIE: Right. I know it won't always be, you know, peaches and cream, but it's not supposed to be, you know . . .

Not getting a more recent exception to build upon, the therapist returned to their positive response to the miracle question by using "relationship questions"—that is, each client's perception of others' perceptions of him or her.

I. K. B.: So let me come back to this tomorrow morning. When the children see the two of you tomorrow morning, what would they see different about the two of you that would tell them, "Wow! Something happened to Mom and Dad"?

BILL: Wow.

I. K. B.: I mean, if they could talk. I realize they're very young and they may not be able to have the right words for it, but if they could talk.

LESLIE: Well, Carl knows something is going on, because he always asks me, "Why are you and Daddy always yelling at each other?" You know, I tell him not to yell at his little sister and—see, I haven't told you this—and then he says to me, "Well, you and Daddy are always yelling."

I. K. B.: Yeah. So what would he notice different about the two of you tomorrow morning? [The therapist persisted in returning to the image of the desired positive outcome.]

BILL: Some warmth.

LESLIE: Yeah. I don't think our kids have seen us embrace lately. They probably won't even remember it.

I. K. B.: So he may see the two of you embracing. What else? What else would he see?

LESLIE: We would go somewhere together. That would really be a miracle. You know, instead of me . . .

I. K. B.: You mean the family of four. [The therapist interrupted to maintain the solution-building set.]

LESLIE: All four of us.

I. K. B.: All four of you will go somewhere. Someplace fun? [This kept the focus on the solution, not the problem.]

LESLIE: Yeah. Someplace fun where we're not just dropping them off on the way to work, you know.

I. K. B.: OK.

BILL: Just all of us being in the same space would be a miracle.

LESLIE: Not getting ready to go to the babysitter's or day care, and not getting ready to go to bed. It would really be different.

I. K. B.: That would be different.

The therapeutic task now was to bridge the emerging images of changes and possible solutions by highlighting the interactional aspect of this new and different vision. The partners' shared vision for how they wanted their lives to be—in concrete, behavioral, measurable detail—was examined from several points of view, including that of the children ("if they could talk").

I. K. B.: I'm not sure if this is realistic or not, but suppose you do [move toward the desired outcome], how would Leslie be different with you? What would she do different?

BILL: Well, I suppose she'd be warmer.

I. K. B.: She'll be warmer with you?

BILL: We'd get along better. We would communicate.

I. K. B.: OK. Say some more about this "getting along." What would go on? What would go on between the two of you?

BILL: If we just try to get along, we could get along. But if we have to get along at the cost of me suddenly, you know, not giving the time that I need to give to my job, as an eventuality it's going to affect us financially. I'm trying to look out for our future, and I think that we have to invest some time in that in order to make the whole thing work.

I. K. B.: Got you.

LESLIE: There are some ways that we could be investing and doing our money differently . . .

BILL: I love our children and I love you, you know, but I'm trying to build something.

LESLIE: There's some ways we could be saving money and doing better financially that doesn't require you to be out of the house 70 hours a week and meeting with these female clients. "Clients" in quotes, OK?

BILL: Well, then, you tell me what it is then (said angrily).

LESLIE: Because if you were home every night . . .

BILL: You tell me what it is, then (again angrily).

I. K. B.: Hang on a minute. What has to come first? In order to do whatever you'd like to see happen between the two of you, what might be the first small step to help you move toward that?

The therapist actively intervened to stop the negative escalation. She did not ignore the angry affect, but attended to Leslie's insistence that Bill become an active partner in raising the children and responding to her wishes. This was pursued by refocusing the discussion on what small steps would move them toward their vision of greater closeness and cooperation, rather than on another round of accusations and rebuttals.†

> † This refocusing was an excellent strategy—to stay on track. She could come back and address Leslie's automatic thoughts later on. Addressing her automatic thoughts would have been important, since it had already been intimated several times and almost surely had something to do with Leslie's individual schemas regarding her insecurity.

LESLIE: He could be honest.

I. K. B.: What would it take, do you think—knowing Leslie as well as you do—what would it take for her to believe you that you are being honest? [The therapist tracked Leslie's comment while highlighting progressive interaction and constructively using Bill's position as the expert on Leslie.]

BILL: I don't know. What would it take? I'm willing to try.

I. K. B.: Oh, you are? [Bill's positive motivation was highlighted with this question.]

LESLIE: It would help if you would call. If you would let me know about what time you're going to come home. I don't need to know every client that you're going to meet, but I would like to be included in your life in a way that I think is respectful.

I. K. B.: Ahh. That's what you really want, isn't it?

This was a good example of how partners often do not know initially what are the first small steps toward better communication. The jump between the issue of "honesty" and Bill's calling to let Leslie know what time he will come home was not obvious.

I. K. B.: You want to be part of Bill's life.

BILL: I'll call. I can do that. That's not unreasonable. And sometimes I get caught up in business and I don't call.

I. K. B.: I see.

BILL: OK. But I can call. That I can do.

I. K. B.: *(To Leslie)* What do you need so that you feel that Bill understands how hard you are working to make this marriage work? What do you need from Bill?

LESLIE: I need some support from Bill. I work more than 8 hours a day also, and I come home. I mentioned that I need him to take more responsibility with the child care arrangements, everything. Doctor appointments, shoes, clothes. I do all that. He doesn't even ask me any questions about how was the day with the kids. You come in and say, "How are the kids?" And, you know, sometimes you're not even listening. You walk right by.

I. K. B.: So his asking?

LESLIE: I could say they had both been in a train wreck and you wouldn't even hear it.

I. K. B.: So his asking and being concerned—sounds like that's what you want.

BILL: Well, I mean she's made an assumption that I don't hear. I mean, if I didn't want to know, I wouldn't ask.

LESLIE: I don't think so. When you come in the house it's common courtesy, you're going to ask how your kids are, but one day I think I'll try that. You know, "The kids have been in a train wreck." I'm going to see if you hear me.

BILL: That's not common courtesy. These are my children.

LESLIE: See, I'm female. I wouldn't come in the house without asking how are the kids. I mean, I guess you just expect that to happen, you know. [This was a possible invitation for the female therapist to join in a discussion against the husband. Instead, the therapist attempted to refocus on what would be helpful.]

I. K. B.: So what . . .

LESLIE: OK. I know he loves the kids. I'm not accusing you of that.

I. K. B.: Oh, you do! Does Bill know how much you love him?

LESLIE: Well, earlier in the marriage . . .

BILL: No, not earlier. Let's talk about right now.

Leslie went on to complain that she felt her husband no longer found her attractive; that she wondered whether he had other "romantic or sexual interests"; and that he might be staying because, "like the saying goes, 'It's cheaper to keep her.' " When the therapist said, "You really want to change that," Leslie responded, "It's going to have to change, or else I'm going to be someplace else." The therapist then posed a series of "scaling questions," each designed to "make numbers talk" (Berg & de Shazer, 1993)—that is, to help the partners articulate their conceptions of their relationship and what would be needed to help it progress in the directions they desired.

I. K. B.: Let's say on a scale of 1 to 10, as things are right now—and you know what you've been through, the two of you know what you've been through, and you know what the issues have been and you know what the issues are better than I do right now—let's say 10 stands for that you will do just about anything humanly possible to make this marriage work. That stands for 10. OK? And the 1 stands for you're ready to throw in the towel and you're ready to walk away from this. Where would each of you say you're at on this scale of 1 to 10?

BILL: *(Pausing and thinking)* Hmm.

LESLIE: Honestly?

BILL: Seven.

I. K. B.: Seven. How about for you, Leslie?

LESLIE: Well, the past year or so I think I've been at a 10, quite frankly, but the way I'm feeling now I'm probably—well, let's put it this way—I've talked to a lawyer. I've talked to a lawyer, just to inquire about what my rights would be. I'm probably about a 5.

I. K. B.: About a 5.

LESLIE: I'm in the middle somewhere.

I. K. B.: Yeah.

LESLIE: I don't want it to go to the 1, but . . .

I. K. B.: You don't want to be at 1.

LESLIE: No, but I can't . . . I feel like I'm pulling it alone.

I. K. B.: Right. Uh-huh.

LESLIE: *(To Bill)* I'm surprised you're at a 7.

I. K. B.: Now I have another set of numbers questions here. Knowing how things are right now between the two of you, let's say 10 stands for you have every confidence that this marriage is going to survive. OK? Ten stands for this marriage has every chance of making it. And 1 stands for the opposite—there's no chance this marriage is going to make it. Where would you say things are right now?

LESLIE: Well, if we worked at it, I could say it would be more than a 5.

I. K. B.: Really? So you see a lot of potential in this?

LESLIE: Well, we do love each other. I know it doesn't sound like it, but I think we do.

I. K. B.: You do.

LESLIE: I know I love him.

I. K. B.: Does he know? Does Bill know how much you love him?

LESLIE: He ought to.

I. K. B.: Bill, what would you say the chances are of this marriage making it?

BILL: Umm . . . I would really say an 8.

I. K. B.: Eight.

BILL: You know, I mean, I want this to work. I'm willing to try to make it. We have to find some kind of way to compromise, though. I mean, I didn't go through undergrad and law school, working in the mailroom— all that bullshit—just to now, suddenly, chuck it all away. I mean, we can't . . .

LESLIE: I don't want you to chuck it all away.

I. K. B.: What would it take, do you think, from your point of view, Leslie—what would it take for you to go from 5 to 6, so you can say it's just a little bit better? It's not perfect yet, it's not all the way up to 10, but it's just a little bit better. What has to happen between the two of you so that you can say that to yourself?

LESLIE: Well, he could call like he said he would, and . . .

I. K. B.: That would help?

LESLIE: Yeah, if he could just make some effort with trying to share some of the responsibilities. I would recognize it. I know he has to work.

I. K. B.: So calling would help you a little bit.

LESLIE: I mean, I don't know. Maybe if he could hug me sometimes.

I. K. B.: He could what?

LESLIE: He could hug me sometimes. To make me feel like a wife.

I. K. B.: OK. That would help also. Now what would that mean? What does that mean? How would that help? His hugging you and calling you and . . . I don't understand that. How would that be helpful for you? [The therapist was trying to understand Leslie's personal construction of what hugging and calling meant in the context of their relationship.]†

> † This was exactly the type of question that a cognitive-behavioral therapist would ask in attempting to understand Leslie's schema or "construction" of her world and her needs in the relationship. Once again, it is very important—as the therapist demonstrated so nicely in this case—that this be done in the presence of the other partner, so that the other can become attuned to the first partner's needs and eventually assimilate it into his or her own thinking.

LESLIE: Because for me, first of all, he doesn't believe it, but I do worry about him. It can be dangerous out there. And, two, I could—we could talk just about what his day has been like. I would know what time he was going to come home. Maybe I would sit up and we could have, you know, a late dinner together.

I. K. B.: Uh-huh.

LESLIE: Sometimes I sit up and I don't know what time . . . I just fall asleep and then he comes in and the next thing I know he's in the bed, but then he's asleep and . . .

I. K. B.: . . . so some more personal and private time together.

LESLIE: Right. The kids still go to bed relatively early, and I'm just, you know, doing some paperwork or I end up watching TV alone. I don't know what time he's coming in.

I. K. B.: OK. What about it will be helpful for you? Having those kind of private times between the two of you?

LESLIE: We used to have those private times.

I. K. B.: You used to have those.

LESLIE: Before the kids were born, and it was something I looked forward to. You know, I mean, we—he was working long hours. But that was our special time and we talked. I mean, I knew people at his office before—not always personally—but because we talked about those things, and I talked about problems on my job.

I. K. B.: So when you have this private time talking about what his day's been like, what his work is like, and he also asks you about what your day has been like and having this time without children . . . how would that be helpful?

LESLIE: It was close. Your husband is your main confidant. We would have the relationship, and then I remember the times we would even go to bed and make love, and it would be nice. And it was beautiful.

I. K. B.: Uh-huh.

LESLIE: And that doesn't happen any more, either.

I. K. B.: Right. So that's what you're looking for. Some special moments with Bill that you feel close to him and you feel like he's your confidant.

LESLIE: *(To Bill)* Didn't you like those? I mean, I thought it was fun. I looked forward to it. I mean, no matter how bad the day was, I could look forward to it at some point, you know, over salad or whatever. Maybe even a glass of wine. We would talk. We would have good times.

I. K. B.: *(To Bill)* Is there something that Leslie can do to make it easy for that to happen?

BILL: Yeah!

I. K. B.: What? What can she do to make it easier for that to happen?

LESLIE: I'm listening. I'm all ears. What can I do? I'll do it . . . within reason.

BILL: Just be understanding.

I. K. B.: What does that mean, "be understanding"?

BILL: I mean, don't pressure me.

I. K. B.: OK.

BILL: And know that I love you and I love our children. You know, I'm really and truly trying, and it's difficult, and a lot of times I just don't have the time, you know, but that . . .

LESLIE: You're going to be able to make time? Is that what I'm hearing?

BILL: I'm going to try the best I can, you know? But I have a vision, and you need to help me with this vision, and if the vision calls for you maybe to do a little more now, I guarantee you'll do a little less later.†

> † *Goals are extremely important in a couple's relationship, particularly since it sets a direction in the relationship. Often when these goals are not clear, or the partners do not have similar or at least*

> complementary goals, conflict develops. One question that I fre-
> quently ask a couple is this: "Do you have some type of concrete
> plan both of you agree to?" The therapist addressed this issue quite
> nicely in the dialogue presented below; in my opinion, it is a very
> important issue, regardless of the therapeutic modality that one
> espouses.

Feedback and Suggestions

At this point the therapist took a 5- or 10-minute break, asking the clients
to sit in the waiting room. This pause can be used to reflect upon what has
occurred and to plan a message or feedback to present to the couple when
the session is resumed. This time can also be used to consult with
colleagues, including any team that may have observed the session.

The session presented here was difficult, and not atypical. Both
partners brought up important issues. For Bill, his way of caring about his
family was to be a good provider and to be successful financially. He
referred to his vision of the future, which was to be a good provider so
that Leslie could even stay at home and not have to go to work—a view
that in some ways was very traditional. At the same time, he recognized
that there needed to be some balance. On the other hand, Leslie's issues
had to do more with the here and now: the family relationship, time with
the children, helping her out, doing things together, more of the sort of
intimate moments they used to share earlier in their life together. What she
wanted and what he wanted both had to do with the relationship; they
were coming from very different angles, but were moving toward the same
vision of their life. The therapist's task was to help them somehow figure
out how they could see themselves working cooperatively together, incorporating both the vision of the future as well as what needed to happen in
their current life. They would then be in a position to bring their skills and
resources to bear in a more mutually satisfying way.

When a therapist invites a couple back into the room, there are
typically three components to what is said (de Shazer, 1985, 1988): (1) an
acknowledgment and validation of the clients' point of view; (2) a bridging
statement that leads to the suggestion or directive to be offered; and (3)
the suggestion or directive, a message designed to guide the couple toward
perceptions and behaviors that are more consistent with their goals. The
dialogue that follows shows how the therapist complimented and positively
framed Leslie and Bill's coming to therapy and their expressed concerns as
the beginning step. She then offered suggestions for each person to notice
what the other was doing to make the relationship better, but not to tell
the other what had been noticed. This task was carefully constructed to
shift attention from what was *wrong* to what was *right*—to help the
partners watch each other from a different point of view, each noticing
positives about the other. The suggestion not to tell the other what had

been noticed was given for two reasons: (1) to make the task interesting and capture the partners' attention and cooperation; and (2) to permit each partner even to give favorable credit to the other for something that was inadvertent. Consistent with the social constructionist ideas that we all make meaning and build "reality" out of ambiguous circumstances, that how we look determines what we see and what we see determines how we act, and that this feeds back self-recursively, this observational task purposefully directed the partners' attention toward constructing a more mutually fulfilling relationship.[3]†

> † *What the authors state here about "what we see determines how we act" is one of the main tenets of the cognitive-behavioral model. This notion of working with a couple's "construction" is essential and is very similar to the notion of the "cognitive triad" introduced by Aaron Beck in the early 1960s (see Beck, 1967, 1976, 1988) which is essential in understanding how clients view the world and their future.*

I. K. B.: I really have to tell you that I think that your calling to set up this appointment was really good timing. It sounds like you both are very concerned about what's not happening between the two of you, and you want to do something about that. And I am very impressed, Bill, that you responded to Leslie's initiating this meeting and your willingness to take time from your very busy schedule, and obviously this relationship is very important to you.

BILL: Yes . . .

I. K. B.: And that's why you are here, to do something about this. Both of you really care about this relationship a great deal. But both in a very different way. Let me explain to you about this. Bill, your way of caring about this relationship is to have this vision of the future—how you want things to be. That is, you're accustomed to sacrificing a lot for the future, and that's how you still see it—in order to have a better future, even to the point of maybe Leslie staying home one of these days.

BILL: Yeah.

I. K. B.: That finally you could earn enough money so that she could stay home. And so you have this vision of the future, how you want things to be. And that's how you care about this relationship. On the other hand, Leslie, your way of caring about this relationship is to be paying attention to now, when the children are young.

LESLIE: Mmm-hmm.

I. K. B.: You want the two of you to do more things with the children. You want to share this experience of raising children together. You want to stay close and have more intimate moments and somehow try to make it—sort of like have it all, right? And that's how you care about this relationship. So there's no question in my mind that both of you care about each other in a very different way. And that gets misunderstood. And I think that both of you need both ways. Any relationship needs both—that is, to pay attention to here and now as well as the future. You need to do both. You need to—like Bill said, it's a matter of a balance. How to balance here and now, and also worrying about the future.

BILL: Mmm-hmm.

I. K. B.: And so I think that you two have a very good start, because you're already thinking about right now as well as the future. So the next task for the two of you is to figure out how to fit your concerns together. [This was the bridging statement.] I don't think it's either your way or your way. It's the blending of the two. In order to do that, both of you have to work together to strike this balance. And I really like the way that you want to get started on this. You have lots of ideas of how to get started on that—like sort of stealing those few moments here and there without the children; that certainly would help. So what I would like to suggest to you between now and the next time we get together is for each of you to keep track of what the other person is doing. For you *(to Leslie)* to keep track of what Bill does, and for you *(to Bill)* to keep track of what Leslie does, to make things a little bit better for the marriage. And it's important for you not to discuss it, but just keep track of them. And when we come back together, we will discuss this more—the details of them. But I want you to sort of observe, file it away, and then when we get together we'll talk about it. OK?

The couple agreed to perform the task; a subsequent appointment was scheduled; and the session was adjourned.

Follow-Up

When Bill and Leslie returned for their appointment 2 weeks later, they were smiling and looked relaxed. Bill announced that he had taken time off from his busy schedule to go with Leslie and the kids to the zoo on Saturday morning. The therapist complimented them on this and explored with them how they had managed to accomplish it. Consistent with the thrust of the first session, and in keeping with the second basic rule of solution-focused therapy ("Once you know what works, do more of it"), throughout the session efforts were made to elicit, reinforce, amplify, and extend favorable changes (see Adams, Piercy, & Jurich, 1991; Weiner-Davis, de Shazer, & Gingrich, 1987). This included getting details of positive movement and exploring the meanings each partner assigned to favorable developments; complimenting each partner's efforts and accomplishments; asking scaling questions about their hopefulness and what would strengthen it; refocusing on goals and finding out what each person did do and could do to further solutions; and developing future goals to help them stay on track.†

> † This strategy parallels the "quid pro quo" and "positive replace-ment" strategies introduced by the early behaviorist movement and social learning theorists in working with couples (Stuart, 1969; Liberman, 1970; Patterson, 1971).

Throughout this session—and the therapy—the therapist worked to help the couple avoid escalating past complaints (which usually triggers a cycle of blaming/accusing/defending/blaming the other/etc.). Instead, the therapist asked questions and otherwise directed the clients forward—"es-calating the future" by helping them create a view consistent with how they would like to be. Their communication style was reframed as "passionate" rather than "conflictual," to help them remain engaged and move in a positive direction rather than falling into the stalemating perceptions of "right and wrong," "black and white," and "husband versus wife." As a task to keep them on track, Bill was asked to notice what Leslie did, in her own way, to stay in communication with him, and Leslie was asked to notice what Bill did, in his own way, to keep her included; this shifted their noticing from "noncommunication and exclusion" to "communication and inclusion."†

> † Once again, this is very similar to cognitive-behavioral techniques for helping couples restructure their thinking and behaviors. In fact, the technique of reframing is used in a number of modalities and is quite effective, along with identifying cognitive distortions such as "black and white" thinking.

THINKING ABOUT PRACTICE:
SOME QUESTIONS AND POSSIBLE ANSWERS

1. There did not seem to be a lot of attention given to exploring underlying issues, including anger. Is this typical? Throughout the thera-peutic interaction, the emphasis was on doing what works. The therapist repeatedly focused on those aspects of the clients' presentation that sug-gested movement in the direction (outcome) they wanted to go. It may sometimes be useful to facilitate the expression of anger and other so-called negative affects, especially if this is part of what the clients require to feel that therapy can be useful, although experience suggests that an "abreac-tive" approach often simply leads to more animosity and further alienation. Reinforcing Leslie's "victim" position in the case presented here would not have been likely to move things forward. The therapist, by word and demeanor, acknowledged the couple's frustration and unhappiness. Patients

need to know that their experience has been heard and appreciated as valid. It may be more therapeutically helpful in the long run, however, to look for positive intentions that have not yet worked out and to highlight them.[4] Each case is unique, so guidelines have to be general.

2. *Was Bill having an affair? Why wasn't this important issue focused on?* It is important to be reminded of the "big picture" of what these partners wanted and how they imagined their lives could be different. Leslie—in her frustration and anger at being treated as if "it's cheaper to keep her," and feeling unappreciated for her own long hours of work—said many negative things, such as that Bill was indifferent and unconcerned about his children. It is interesting to note that when viewing the videotape of this session (Berg, 1994b), many therapists immediately become focused on the issue of whether Bill was having an affair and not on other issues, such as why Bill thought he was too busy to wash dishes or help with the shopping or child care as Leslie wanted him to do. We believe that therapists tend to hear selectively, according to their own constructions of what leads to marital conflict (and resolution). What proved to be therapeutic in this case was to address what would help the couple move in the direction of greater trust in the here and now. Once the present reality improves, it is easier for persons to let go of what may (or may not) have happened—to let it be "past." We once heard John Weakland say to a client who was focused on a particular idea, "Would it be OK with you if we solve the problem and then come back to that if you're still interested?" This helped move the client into a present-to-future orientation and allowed therapy to occur. We also have to be careful, of course, that a client does not feel discounted. However, when we say that an issue is "important," we need to ask, "Important to whom?" Sometimes it is the therapist more than the client who feels something has to be "addressed" or "dealt with directly," and this may lead to the kind of "either–or" thinking that can produce a therapeutic impasse.†

> †*I concur completely with this statement. Even though cognitive-behavioral therapists are concerned with elements of the past, such issues can also serve to sidetrack or in some cases even to derail a course of treatment. Consequently, a here-and-now focus is important, since a therapist can always return to a prior issue if it is still deemed important or continues to resurface repeatedly.*

3. *How does solution-focused therapy address issues of ethnicity and cultural diversity?* By working within the goals, ideas, values, and world views that clients present, solution-focused therapy is sensitive to the cultures that clients bring to the consulting room. It should be *their* therapy, not the therapist's. The solution must fit their frame of reference, not that of the therapist. Moreover, the therapeutic alliance is foremost, and this is based on a high regard and respect for what makes sense to a client, not to a therapist. This means that as therapists we have to have skills to join

and work with folks of varying ethnicities, and we also have to be clear about what our values (tacit as well as explicit) may be, so that we do not impose them. In the case presented here, the couple was African-American; the therapist was Korean-American.

4. *What are some similarities between solution-focused therapy and other therapeutic approaches?* Although a thoroughgoing review is beyond the scope of the present discussion, we are glad to acknowledge a few connections and related perspectives.[5] As Shoham, Rohrbaugh, and Patterson (1995) have noted, solution-focused therapy especially shares certain important commonalities with the strategic therapy (Watzlawick, Weakland, & Fisch, 1974; Fisch, Weakland, & Segal, 1982) practiced at the Mental Research Institute (MRI) of Palo Alto; these include a Batesonian interactional constructivist orientation that eschews "normative–pathological" theorizing, a preference for "minimalist" interventions, and an Ericksonian interest in utilizing whatever the client brings. However, the approaches are distinct in that MRI attends more directly to changing behaviors that maintain a problem, whereas the BFTC solution-focused model assumes that behavior change will follow naturally after clients see things differently. Summarizing the two approaches, Weakland and Fisch (1992, p. 317) wrote: "We focus primarily on attempted solutions that do not work and maintain the problem; de Shazer and his followers, in our view, have the inverse emphasis. The two are complementary."[6] There are also connections between solution-focused therapy and narrative therapy (White & Epston, 1990; White, 1995; Freedman & Combs, 1996), including a postmodern, nonpathological perspective and an emphasis on client–therapist collaboration. Although both approaches are interested in "exceptions" (solution-focused) or "unique outcomes" (narrative) as keys to "solutions" (solution-focused) or "alternative life stories" (narrative), there are major differences between the approaches in terms of perspectives, intentions, and procedures as outlined by Chang and Phillips (1993) as well as by the prime enunciators of the respective approaches themselves (de Shazer, 1993b; de Shazer & White, 1994; White, 1993; White & de Shazer, 1996). Finally, there are similarities between solution-focused therapy and cognitive-behavioral couple therapy (Beck, 1988; Dattilio & Padesky, 1990; Baucom & Epstein, 1990; Jacobson & Margolin, 1979), since these latter approaches are also directly concerned with how clients may be construing their psychological realities. The solution-focused approach, because of its strong constructivist and antipathologizing slant, may place more emphasis on assisting clients to develop a new perspective that allows them to draw more effectively upon existing resources and areas of competency (e.g., finding exceptions to help build solutions); whereas cognitive-behavioral therapists may spend more time assessing deficits in thinking and acting, as well as teaching specific skills.

Examination of various effective brief therapies suggests that they all share certain basic characteristics (Budman, Hoyt, & Friedman, 1992; Hoyt, 1995):

a. Rapid and positive alliance.
b. Focus on specific, achievable goals.
c. Clear definition of clients' and therapists' responsibilities and activities.
d. Emphasis on clients' strengths and competency with an expectation of change.
e. Assisting the clients toward new perceptions and behaviors.
f. Here-and-now (and next) orientation.
g. Time sensitivity.

Whatever our particular theoretical orientations, it is incumbent upon us as therapists to join with our clients to notice and amplify what works for them in achieving their goals.

Authors' Reply to Editor's Comments

The editor's interspersed comments highlight differences in assumptions about therapy and the therapist's role in the process. We have elsewhere described this paradigm shift as one of "problem solving" compared to "solution building" (DeJong & Berg, 1997). Although, as noted above, there are similarities between solution-focused therapy and cognitive-behavioral therapy—such as an emphasis on the importance of the social construction of meanings and the specification of clear behavioral descriptions—the differences seem much more fundamental. In order to "problem solve" it is generally believed that one must understand the nature of the problem and then find the solution that will fit the problem—in the case described here, identifying Leslie's "insecurity" and addressing it, and then finding strategies to "solve" and "replace" it with appropriate behavior. In contrast to this way of thinking, solution-focused therapy eschews the imposition of concepts of deficit or pathology (see Hoyt & Friedman, in press), and may even say that there may not be any relationship between the problem and solutions. This is a rather radical departure from the prevalent scientific view of cause-and-effect relationships.

Consider the editor's recommendations to "zero in on what the specific conflict is, and to operationally define terms." We believe that this is a "problem-solving" way to conceptualize the therapeutic task. Taking a solution-focused approach, the therapist in the present case bypassed the "problem talk" and "zeroed in" on the details of solution-generating behaviors and meanings. Especially early in a session, when the partners may be likely to conceive themselves, each other, and their situation in terms of "problems" to be attacked and addressed, it is important to sidestep conflicting views and meanings that result in blame talk by shifting attention toward more hope-engendering and cooperative new behaviors, such as Bill's calling to let Leslie know that he would be home late. The therapeutic task is to construct a detailed description of what solutions might be like and to build consensus around these solutions, not to tear down barriers.

When clients articulate their vision of a favorable outcome (goals), the therapist does not assume the "expert" position to "make some early determination as to whether or not the partners' expectations are realistic," but rather purposefully steers the conversation to help the couple negotiate mutually agreeable and achievable expectations. In the case presented here, the therapist nicely sidestepped conflict in favor of pursuing "the first small step to help you move toward [your goal]." In our view, thinking about Leslie's "automatic thoughts" and her "insecurity" (which is a clinician's interpretation, not her description) would not have been a useful way to conceptualize the therapeutic task, since Leslie's request for service did not center on her "insecurity" but on getting Bill to be more attentive and helpful to her and the children. Solution-focused therapy is client-driven, whereas we read in the editor's comments a more therapist-driven approach.

As we note in discussing the case follow-up, behavioral exchanges, homework tasks, and *quid pro quo* strategies help structure a positive feedback loop for the couple to move into and expand their self-fulfilling realities. Helping clients become aware that they have a choice in how to construe their reality (as cognitive-behavioral therapists know—see Lyddon, 1990; Mahoney, 1991; Meichenbaum, in Hoyt, 1996e), and that they already have some successes in that direction (focusing on exceptions to the problem), is the most helpful task we can perform as therapists.

We appreciate the opportunity to clarify these issues, and we favor "diversity" ("both–and" heterogeneity), rather than obscuring or reducing important distinctions in the "melting pot" of "integration." Consistent with the solution-focused model, we are interested in what works and recognize that there are multiple perspectives and paths toward that goal.

ACKNOWLEDGMENTS

The case dialogue in this chapter is drawn from the first session of a reconstructed case presented on a professional training videotape by Berg (1994b). Copyright 1994 by I. K. Berg. Used by permission. A fuller case report is also available in Hoyt (1998).

NOTES

1. Particularly in the spirit of the postmodern perspective informing the work to be reported, it is important to realize that what follows is a construction about a construction, not "what happened." Therapy, as John Weakland (quoted in Hoyt, 1994b, p. 25) said about life, is made up of "one damn thing after another." Any report can only be a gloss, a few brushstrokes that can suggest (or obscure). Still, some useful approximations (or "misunderstandings" or "misreadings," since each person takes his or her own meaning—see de Shazer, 1991, 1993a, 1994a, and de Shazer & Berg, 1992) may be receivable.

2. For additional applications of solution-focused principles to couple therapy, see de Shazer and Berg (1985), Friedman (1996), Hudson and O'Hanlon (1991;

O'Hanlon & Hudson, 1994), Johnson and Goldman (1996), Lipchik and Kubicki (1996), Nunnally (1993), Quick (1996), and Weiner-Davis (1992).

3. A related example is provided by Furman and Ahola (1992, p. xix) in their book *Solution Talk: Hosting Therapeutic Conversations*. They tell of a woman who complained about the rudeness of a man she knew. A friend offered to intercede, and a few weeks later the woman reported that the man was completely changed. When she asked her friend whether the man had been confronted, the friend replied, "Well, not really. I told him that you think he is a charming man." If we see someone in a positive light, we are more likely to respond in kind; this may help produce a "virtuous," not "vicious," cycle.

4. After watching portions of the videotape (Berg, 1994b) depicting the case presented here, then-7-year-old Alexander Hoyt (personal communication) remarked, "Dad, that's good. Instead of letting them fight, she's getting them to talk about ways they could be happier."

5. At a conference held in Saratoga, California, in March 1995 (see Efron, 1995; Hoyt, 1997), a number of leading brief therapists of varying theoretical persuasions discussed the importance of acknowledging connections and collaboration, rather than promoting a divisive pitting of one approach against another. We applaud the "both–and" idea that everything is not "revolutionary" and "completely different."

6. Recall the observation task that the therapist gave at the end of the first session in the case example presented here: for each member of the couple to notice what the other person was doing to improve the relationship (but not to reveal what had been noticed). This task is somewhat similar to the "jamming" tactic an MRI strategic therapist (Fisch et al., 1982, pp. 156–158; Shoham et al., 1995, p. 149) might employ—that is, having one partner randomly perform a negative behavior and having the other try to guess (without telling) when the behavior is "real" or "fake." The intention of the MRI strategy is to disrupt a problematic interactional pattern by reducing the informational value of interpersonal communication, whereas the BFTC observation task (noticing the positive) is designed more to shape viewing to support a more favorable interaction.

REFERENCES

Adams, J. F., Piercy, F. P., & Jurich, J. A. (1991). Effects of solution focused therapy's "formula first session task" on compliance and outcome in family therapy. *Journal of Marital and Family Therapy, 17,* 277–290.

Anderson, H., & Goolishian, H. (1992). The client is the expert: A not-knowing approach to therapy. In S. McNamee & K. J. Gergen (Eds.), *Therapy as social construction* (pp. 25–39). Newbury Park, CA: Sage.

Baucom, D. H., & Epstein, N. (1990). *Cognitive behavioral marital therapy.* New York: Brunner/Mazel.

Beck, A. T. (1967). *Depression: Causes and treatment.* Philadelphia: University of Pennsylvania Press.

Beck, A. T. (1976). *Cognitive therapy and the emotional disorders.* New York: Signet.

Beck, A. T. (1988). *Love is never enough.* New York: Harper & Row.

Berg, I. K. (1989). Of visitors, complainants and customers. *Family Therapy Networker,* 13(1), 27.

Berg, I. K. (1994a). *Family-based services: A solution-focused approach.* New York: Norton.

Berg, I. K. (1994b). *Irreconcilable differences: A solution-focused approach to marital therapy* [Videotape]. New York: Norton.

Berg, I. K., & de Shazer, S. (1993). Making numbers talk: Language in therapy. In S. Friedman (Ed.), *The new language of change: Constructive collaboration in psychotherapy* (pp. 5–24). New York: Guilford Press.

Berg, I. K., & Miller, S. D. (1992). *Working with the problem drinker.* New York: Norton.

Budman, S. H., Hoyt, M. F., & Friedman, S. (Eds.). (1992). *The first session in brief therapy.* New York: Guilford Press.

Chang, J., & Phillips, M. (1993). Michael White and Steve de Shazer: New directions in family therapy. In S. Gilligan & R. Price (Eds.), *Therapeutic conversations* (pp. 95–111). New York: Norton.

Dattilio, F. M., & Padesky, C. A. (1990). *Cognitive therapy with couples.* Sarasota, FL: Professional Resource Exchange.

DeJong, P., & Berg, I. K. (1997). *Interviewing for solutions.* Pacific Grove, CA: Brooks/Cole.

de Shazer, S. (1982). *Patterns of brief family therapy.* New York: Guilford Press.

de Shazer, S. (1984). The death of resistance. *Family Process, 23,* 79–93.

de Shazer, S. (1985). *Keys to solution in brief therapy.* New York: Norton.

de Shazer, S. (1988). *Clues: Investigating solutions in brief therapy.* New York: Norton.

de Shazer, S. (1991). *Putting difference to work.* New York: Norton.

de Shazer, S. (1993a). Creative misunderstanding: There is no escape from language. In S. Gilligan & R. Price (Eds.), *Therapeutic conversations* (pp. 81–90). New York: Norton.

de Shazer, S. (1993b). Commentary: de Shazer and White: Vive la difference. In S. Gilligan & R. Price (Eds.), *Therapeutic conversations* (pp. 112–120). New York: Norton.

de Shazer, S. (1994a). Freud and Erickson said it all. *Journal of Systemic Therapies,* 13(1), 15.

de Shazer, S. (1994b). *Words were originally magic.* New York: Norton.

de Shazer, S., & Berg, I. K. (1985). A part is not apart: Working with only one of the partners present. In A. S. Gurman (Ed.), *Casebook of marital therapy* (pp. 97–110). New York: Guilford Press.

de Shazer, S., & Berg, I. K. (1992). Doing therapy: A post-structural re-vision. *Journal of Marital and Family Therapy,* 18(1), 71–81.

de Shazer, S., & White, M. (1994, July). Dialogue held at Therapeutic Conversations 2 Conference, Washington, DC.

Dolan, Y. D. (1991). *Resolving sexual abuse.* New York: Norton.

Duncan, B. L., Hubble, M. A., & Miller, S. D. (1997). *Psychotherapy with "impossible" cases: The efficient treatment of therapy veterans.* New York: Norton.

Efron, D. (1995). Conference review. *Journal of Systemic Therapies,* 14(3), 1–3.

Fisch, R., Weakland, J. H., & Segal, L. (1982). *The tactics of change: Doing therapy briefly.* San Francisco: Jossey-Bass.

Freedman, J., & Combs, G. (1993). Invitations to new stories: Using questions to explore alternative possibilities. In S. Gilligan & R. Price (Eds.), *Therapeutic conversations* (pp. 291–303). New York: Norton.

Freedman, J., & Combs, G. (1996). *Narrative therapy: The social construction of preferred realities.* New York: Norton.

Friedman, S. (1996). Couples therapy: Changing conversations. In H. Rosen & K. T. Kuehlwein (Eds.), *Constructing realities: Meaning-making perspectives for psychotherapists* (pp. 413–453). San Francisco: Jossey-Bass.

Furman, B., & Ahola, T. (1992). *Solution talk: Hosting therapeutic conversations.* New York: Norton.

Hoyt, M. F. (Ed.). (1994a). *Constructive therapies* (Vol. 1). New York: Guilford Press.

Hoyt, M. F. (1994b). On the importance of keeping it simple and taking the patient seriously: A conversation with Steve de Shazer and John Weakland. In M. F. Hoyt (Ed.), *Constructive therapies* (Vol. 1, pp. 11–40). New York: Guilford Press.

Hoyt, M. F. (1995). *Brief therapy and managed care: Readings for contemporary practice.* San Francisco: Jossey-Bass.

Hoyt, M. F. (1996a). Solution building and language games: A conversation with Steve de Shazer. In M. F. Hoyt (Ed.), *Constructive therapies* (Vol. 2, pp. 60–86). New York: Guilford Press.

Hoyt, M. F. (Ed.). (1996b). *Constructive therapies* (Vol. 2). New York: Guilford Press.

Hoyt, M. F. (1996c). Some stories are better than others. In M. F. Hoyt (Ed.), *Constructive therapies* (Vol. 2, pp. 1–32). New York: Guilford Press.

Hoyt, M. F. (1996d). A golfer's guide to brief therapy (with footnotes for baseball fans). In M. F. Hoyt (Ed.), *Constructive therapies* (Vol. 2, pp. 306–318). New York: Guilford Press.

Hoyt, M. F. (1996e). Cognitive-behavioral treatment of posttraumatic stress disorder from a narrative constructivist perspective: A conversation with Donald Meichenbaum. In M. F. Hoyt (Ed.), *Constructive therapies* (Vol. 2, pp. 124–147). New York: Guilford Press.

Hoyt, M. F. (1997). Unmuddying the waters: A "common ground" conference. *Journal of Systemic Therapies, 16*(3), 195–200.

Hoyt, M. F. (Ed.). (1998). *The handbook of constructive therapies.* San Francisco: Jossey-Bass.

Hoyt, M. F., & Friedman, S. (in press). Dilemmas of postmodern practice under managed care and some pragmatics for increasing the likelihood of treatment authorization. *Journal of Systemic Therapies.*

Hudson, P. O., & O'Hanlon, W. H. (1991). *Rewriting love stories: Brief marital therapy.* New York: Norton.

Jacobson, N. S., & Margolin, G. (1979). *Marital therapy: Strategies based on social learning and behavior exchange principles.* New York: Brunner/Mazel.

Johnson, C. E., & Goldman, J. (1996). Taking safety home: A solution-focused approach with domestic violence. In M. F. Hoyt (Ed.), *Constructive therapies* (Vol. 2, pp. 184–196). New York: Guilford Press.

Kowalski, K., & Kral, R. (1989). The geometry of solution: Using the scaling technique. *Family Therapy Case Studies, 4,* 59–66.

Kral, R. (1987). *Strategies that work: Techniques for solution in the schools.* Milwaukee, WI: Brief Family Therapy Center Press.

Liberman, R. P. (1970). Behavioral approaches to couple and family therapy. *American Journal of Orthopsychiatry, 40,* 106–118.

Lipchik, E., & Kubicki, A. D. (1996). Solution-focused domestic violence views: Bridges toward a new reality in couples therapy. In S. D. Miller, M. A. Hubble, & B. L. Duncan (Eds.), *Handbook of solution-focused brief therapy* (pp. 65–98). San Francisco: Jossey-Bass.

Lipchik, E. (Ed.). (1987). *Interviewing.* Rockville, MD: Aspen.

Lipchik, E., & de Shazer, S. (1986). The purposeful interview. *Journal of Strategic and Systemic Therapies, 5,* 88–89.

Lyddon, W. J. (1990). First- and second-order change: Implications for rationalist and constructivist cognitive therapies. *Journal of Counseling and Develeopment, 69,* 122–127.

Mahoney, M. J. (1991). *Human change processes.* New York: Basic Books.

Miller, S. D. (1994). Some questions (not answers) for the brief treatment of people with drug and alcohol problems. In M. F. Hoyt (Ed.), *Constructive therapies* (Vol. 1, pp. 92–110). New York: Guilford Press.

Miller, S. D., & Berg, I. K. (1995). *The miracle method: A radically new approach to problem drinking.* New York: Norton.

Miller, S. D., Duncan, B., & Hubble, M. (1997). *Escape from Babel: Toward a unifying language in psychotherapy.* New York: Norton.

Miller, S. D., & Hopwood, L. (1994). The solution papers: A comprehensive guide to the publications of the Brief Family Therapy Center. *Journal of Systemic Therapies, 13*(1), 42–47.

Miller, S. D., Hubble, M. A., & Duncan, B. L. (Eds.). (1996). *Handbook of solution-focused brief therapy.* San Francisco: Jossey-Bass.

Nunnally, E. (1993). Solution focused therapy. In R. A. Wells & V. J. Giannetti (Eds.), *Casebook of the brief psychotherapies* (pp. 271–286). New York: Plenum Press.

O'Hanlon, W. H., & Hudson, P. O. (1994). Coauthoring a love story: Solution-oriented marital therapy. In M. F. Hoyt (Ed.), *Constructive therapies* (Vol. 1, pp. 160–188). New York: Guilford Press.

Patterson, G. R. (1971). *Families: Applications of social learning to life.* Champaign, IL: Research Press.

Penn, P. (1985). Feed-forward: Future questions, future maps. *Family Process, 24,* 289–310.

Quick, E. K. (1996). *Doing what works in brief therapy: A strategic solution focused approach.* San Diego, CA: Academic Press.

Shoham, V., Rohrbaugh, M., & Patterson, J. (1995). Problem- and solution-focused couple therapies: The MRI and Milwaukee models. In N. S. Jacobson & A. S. Gurman (Eds.), *Clinical handbook of couple therapy* (pp. 142–163). New York: Guilford Press.

Stuart, R. B. (1969). Operant–interpersonal treatment of marital discord. *Journal of Consulting and Clinical Psychology, 33,* 675–682.

Tomm, K. (1987). Interventive interviewing: Part I. Strategizing as a fourth guideline for the therapist. *Family Process, 26,* 3–13.

Tomm, K. (1988). Interventive interviewing: Part III. Intending to ask lineal, circular, strategic and reflexive questions. *Family Process, 27,* 1–16.

Walter, J., & Peller, J. (1992). *Becoming solution-focused in brief therapy.* New York: Brunner/Mazel.

Watzlawick, P., Weakland, J. H., & Fisch, R. (1974). *Change: Principles of problem formation and problem resolution.* New York: Norton.

Weakland, J. H., & Fisch, R. (1992). Brief therapy—MRI style. In S. H. Budman, M. F. Hoyt, & S. Friedman (Eds.), *The first session in brief therapy* (pp. 306–323). New York: Guilford Press.

Weiner-Davis, M. (1992). *Divorce busting.* New York: Simon & Schuster.

Weiner-Davis, M., de Shazer, S., & Gingrich, W. J. (1987). Using pretreatment change to construct a therapeutic solution: An exploratory study. *Journal of Marital and Family Therapy, 13,* 359–363.

White, M. (1993). Commentary: Histories of the present. In S. Gilligan & R. Price (Eds.), *Therapeutic conversations* (pp. 121–135). New York: Norton.

White, M. (1995). *Re-authoring lives: Interviews and essays.* Adelaide, Australia: Dulwich Centre Publications.

White, M., & de Shazer, S. (1996, October). Narrative Solutions/Solution Narratives Conference, sponsored by Brief Family Therapy Center, Milwaukee, WI.

White, M., & Epston, D. (1990). *Narrative means to therapeutic ends.* New York: Norton.

SUGGESTED READINGS

Berg, I. K. (1994). *Family-based services: A solution-focused approach.* New York: Norton.

De Jong, P., & Berg, I. K. (1997). *Interviewing for solutions.* Pacific Grove, CA: Brooks/Cole.

de Shazer, S. (1985). *Keys to solution in brief therapy.* New York: Norton.

Hoyt, M. F. (Ed.). (1994). *Constructive therapies* (Vol. 1). New York: Guilford Press.

Hoyt, M. F. (1995). *Brief therapy and managed care: Readings for contemporary practice.* San Francisco: Jossey-Bass.

Hoyt, M. F. (1996). *Constructive therapies* (Vol. 2). New York: Guilford Press.

Chapter 10

Integrative Marital Therapy

WILLIAM C. NICHOLS

Integrative marital therapy is concerned with the treatment of the individual in context. It is unlike pure individual-oriented therapies, which focus strictly on an individual's intrapsychic processes or behaviors. It is also different from purely systemic therapies, which are concerned solely with systemic interaction. Integrative marital therapy deals with both the major systems and subsystems in which one functions and with the individual's feelings, thoughts, and dynamics. Viewed from a broader perspective, marital therapy with a lasting relationship has both process and product aspects; it is a process of problem discernment and intervention/solution, combined with incremental and systemic enhancement aimed at producing a more effective marital relationship. In some instances, depending on the wishes and decisions of the clients, it may shift over to focusing on divorce and ending the marriage in the most benign and responsible ways possible.

Marital therapy, in my judgment, is the most complex and most difficult form of outpatient psychotherapy. Dealing as it does with a relationship that may or may not continue, and combining the individual personalities and problems of both spouses as well as their interaction in their subsystem, it requires that the therapist "juggle" individual dynamics and marital dynamics in an ongoing struggle to achieve some semblance of balanced understanding. What I look for in a marriage is the "complementarity"—that is, how two individuals are fitted together, what attracted them originally (as best I can determine), and what holds them together currently. What kinds of needs do they meet for each other? In addition, what kind of commitment do they have to each other, to the relationship, and to the process of change? What kind of commitment do they have to working in therapy? Also, what is their individual condition? That is, do they have any kind of psychopathology that is affecting the marital and therapeutic interaction? What kind of diagnostic description fits them, if any? As I am attempting to understand these factors during the juggling, I am also attempting to understand the presenting complaints and the problems the clients wish to solve. The context in which I work with these people essentially consists of the major systems into which they fit and the kind of processes that go on with the clients. There is a fairly straightforward segue from the larger contextual perspective into that of interpersonal relations in the marital subsystem and into how these dig down into the individual psyche and behavior of each person—and, conversely, into how the individual processes engage in feedback processes.

Integrative therapy attempts to combine major theoretical approaches. It is different from eclectic therapy, which seeks to meld various techniques of treatment and intervention. The integrative approach presented in this chapter combines theory from family systems, psychodynamic, and social learning approaches. Attempts to synthesize selected emphasis of these three therapeutic models have been presented elsewhere (e.g., Nichols, 1996, pp. 52–56). The selected features of psychodynamic psychotherapy include an emphasis on the individual, intrapsychic dimension; an emphasis on unconscious processes; and an interpersonal emphasis derived from the work of Harry Stack Sullivan (1953a, 1953b, 1954). They also include an object relations focus (dyadic and choice factors) derived from the work of W. R. D. Fairbairn (1952, 1954, 1963) and Henry V. Dicks (1963, 1967), including specific attention to projective identification, introjection, projection, and collusion. Emphases from the behavioral model include attention to individual, observable behavior; attention to teaching/learning processes (cognitive processes and techniques for change); and a stress on change. The family systems emphases include the contextual (interactive, systemic) dimension mentioned earlier; a new epistemology; a broad systems perspective (stress on organization, subsystems, wholeness, boundaries, hierarchy, open systems, closed systems, equifinality, feedback, nonsummativity, communication, stability and change, structure, and process); and an emphasis on change.

Integrative marital therapy is not particularly concerned with technique. Treatment is tailored to the needs of the client system, to the personality and mentality of the clients, and to the personality and mentality of the therapist. (See the description in Nichols, 1985, of adapting language and descriptions to fit the perspective of an engineer). This tailoring aspect makes integrative marital therapy much more difficult to illustrate and demonstrate in workshops than approaches that are based on specific techniques for intervention.

This chapter is concerned with marital therapy, not couple therapy per se. Both long-term study of marital and family research findings, and my own clinical observation and experience, lead me to the conclusion that there are some significant differences between marital relationships and couple relationships in which marriage is not part of the picture. There has been some recognition that differences prevail between group therapy with previously unrelated persons and family therapy with persons who have a long and deeply shared history. Interestingly, there has been less awareness that marriage carries with it specific sets of expectations ("models of relationship"; see Nichols & Everett, 1986, p. 275) derived from one's experiences in growing up in a family of origin. Such shaping models of relationships are typically not found in couple relationships that do not involve the commitment to marital roles and relationships.

Integrative approaches to family and marital therapy have included Feldman's work (Feldman, 1979, 1992; Feldman & Pinsof, 1982) as well as my own (Nichols, 1988, 1996; Nichols & Everett, 1986). For more comprehensive discussions of the approach represented in this chapter, see Nichols (1988, 1996).

ASSUMPTIONS AND VALUES

The assumptions and values underlying the integrative approach of this chapter deserve at least a brief summary (Nichols, 1996, pp. 75–83). They are as follows:

1. *The client system.* "Client," rather than the more passive term "patient," is used because the expectation is that therapy will be an interactive, cooperative process. Marriage is both a subsystem of a family and a system in its own right in which what affects one partner affects the other. Therapy can influence each marital partner by working with the system, and on the other hand can affect the system by working with one partner.

2. *Respectful treatment of clients.* The therapist respects each client's right to self-determination, while striving to support an appropriate balance between group rights and needs and those of the individual partners, and maintaining what Boszormenyi-Nagy (1966) and Boszormenyi-Nagy and Krasner (1986) have labeled "multidirectional partiality." As I use this term, it does not mean remaining morally or ethically neutral, as in the instance of abuse of one spouse by another (in which ethical and perhaps legal imperatives require taking a stance); it refers to being equitably committed to the clients and the treatment process.

3. *The relationship and alliance with clients.* The assumption here is that forming a relationship of trust with the client system, leading to the establishment of a therapeutic alliance, is a crucial—perhaps the *most* crucial—element in therapy. "What one is" significantly affects the effectiveness of "what one does" in the therapy.

4. *Direct and indirect intervention with clients.* Stated briefly, the point of view here is in agreement with Williamson (1991), who states that "paradox is always the second choice. It is always preferable to deal with clients in a straightforward way" (p. 81). Straightforward and direct interventions include giving clients logical explanations, suggestions, and tasks, and dealing with them in similar ways. One can deal playfully with clients, as Williamson (1991), Everett (Nichols & Everett, 1986), and others do, and accomplish many of the results sometimes regarded as possible only through the use of paradox.

5. *The responsibility for change.* Clients, not therapists, are responsible for their own change. Rather than a director who is totally responsible for change, the therapist is a facilitator who creates conditions of relationship and reasonable hope and brings appropriate knowledge and interventions to the client system. Use of what therapy offers and use of their own resources to effect change in themselves is the responsibility of clients. They should, whenever possible, leave therapy with an improved knowledge of how they function and how they can continue to improve.

6. *The assumption of least pathology.* Two questions guide this approach: (a) whether the client's problems arise from major pathology or whether a more parsimonious explanation is available; and (b) whether long-term, in-depth treatment or briefer intervention is required. One implication is that therapy often deals first with simpler issues, and that it proceeds to deeper exploration and intervention only when working with the more apparent issues does not suffice.

7. *The education of clients.* Helping clients learn what they need to do and to know is one of the most significant things a therapist can do. This includes learning new skills, such as more effective communication. It may involve working with one or both families of origin (Framo, 1992; Williamson, 1991), in conjunction with beginning to free a client or the client system from acute and/or chronic anxiety.

8. *The motivation of clients.* Therapists can influence, encourage, persuade, and support clients, but they do not motivate the clients. They can try to create conditions in which clients can develop essential motivation to make needed changes.

9. *Gender considerations.* Recognizing the possibilities and effects of gender inequities, and working to change them in a marriage whenever possible, are fairly recent but significant considerations in marital therapy.

10. *Ethnicity considerations.* Being knowledgeable about and respectful of customs, characteristics, common history, and language effects among the various divisions of humankind as they are reflected in marital assessment and therapy is an ongoing challenge for therapists. Therapists need not only to do formal study, but also to "read" the messages clients put before them and to ask clients sincerely, "Teach me" and "Help me understand."

CASE EXAMPLE

Names and other details have been changed to protect identities in the case used to illustrate some of the principles described above. The case also contains some composite features representing fairly simple and straight-forward clinical situations and a minimum of individual psychological difficulties.

Initial Conjoint Sessions

Background Information

The Bensons could have been the model for a "distinguished couple" advertisement. Tanned, tall, and slender, Ben and Nancy carried themselves with the ease and confidence of people who are usually successful and know how to be comfortable in almost any social situation. Except for their steely gray hair, they could have been taken for several years younger than Ben's 63 and Nancy's 55 years. Only their hesitation and their body postures when I asked, "What brings you in? What are you looking for?" betrayed their underlying tension and anxiety.

Glancing at the background information forms that Ben and Nancy had completed in the reception room prior to the appointment provided me with some helpful information. A few questions quickly filled in some of the blanks. They had been married for approximately 3 years. For Nancy, it was a third marriage. She had married first at age 24, had a child 2 years later, and lost her husband in an automobile accident 5 years after that. Her second marriage had come 2 years after she was widowed and had ended in divorce after 7 years (a "rebound" situation). Ben had been married once previously and had two married sons in their 30s. His first wife had died of congenital heart problems after 35 years of marriage. Two years after her lingering illness had ended in her demise, Ben married Nancy, whom he indicated he had known slightly and viewed with respect and admiration for several years.

Additional data on the background information form permitted a quick sketching of the structure of both spouses' families of origin. Both came from lower-middle-class Protestant families in the Midwest. He was the youngest of five children, having two brothers and two sisters; she had two younger brothers. These items of information and others provided not only some immediate clues for questions, but also a framework for exploration of patterns in the spouses' respective families of origin. Genograms were completed subsequently in individual sessions with each of them.†

> † *Similar to this modality, the cognitive-behavioral approach explores the background of each partner in order to understand the impact*

> *on each of his or her family of origin, particularly the family's effects on his or her self-perceptions, relationships, and styles of thinking. Cognitive-behavioral therapists usually do not go as far as to construct genograms; they place more emphasis on the individual and conjoint schemas about the marriage.*

Things had "worked out very well" for Nancy and Ben to get married. Nancy had retired 3 years previously from her position as executive director of an endowed foundation, which provided her with a nice medium-income pension for her 30 years of service. Ben, an entrepreneur who had "struck it rich" with a computer business that he had developed, sold the company, established trust funds for his children and grandchildren, and retired at the same time as Nancy. All three children—Nancy's son and Ben's two sons—had approved of the match, as had the extended families and friends of both partners. There seemed to be general agreement that they were well matched and would be "good for each other," since they were both "honest, decent people, who are caring and kind." Each spouse regarded the other in similar terms, pointing out that there were no problems with alcohol, drugs, extramarital affairs, or gambling, and that they held similar values.

What, then, were the complaints that brought them to my office? Ben said that coming in to see a therapist had been Nancy's idea. He admitted that he had wanted to "handle things ourselves, but we haven't been making any progress," and that "things are at an impasse." He described his own need to have somebody to rely and depend on him (i.e., to have somebody to take care of). As we probed a bit into a deeper emotional level, it appeared that Ben's need was to make certain that he secured love and affection from a dependable source. He would establish an unspoken *quid pro quo* ("something for something") agreement in which, in exchange for taking care of a needy spouse, he would receive the undivided loyalty and affection of a companion who would remain available. Privately, I was reminded of a widowed client in his early 40s who dated and pursued relationships with much younger women because, as he eventually realized, they were not likely to die and leave him.

The spouses described their problems in terms of differences in relating to each other and in dealing with those differences. Ben wanted to take life at a slower pace, to sleep late, and to spend most of their time together. Nancy, although retired, wished to spend her days essentially as if she were still employed—getting up early, working seriously at some volunteer activities, and getting together with Ben at the end of the day. "We have quite different energy levels," she declared. "I'm up and running, I tackle things head on, and I want to spend a lot of time by myself. I had a lot of years in which that's what I had to do in order to support myself and my son."

The Relationship of Assessment and Intervention

Assessment and intervention are interrelated, ongoing processes in therapy. Feedback continually informs assessment and shapes the interventions used. An integrative approach involves being able to hold some ideas about the clients and their interaction both firmly and loosely at the same time. As feedback is available, perceptions tend to be either confirmed or changed.†

> † *One of the advantages of using questionnaires and inventories in the cognitive-behavioral approach is that the results serve as supplementary information to the assessment, which, much as in the integrative approach, can be conducted as interventions take place. A number of the inventories described in Chapter 1 of this book can be used during the assessment without interfering with the plan of the approach. This is something that could possibly have been considered here as well, in order to aid the therapist in developing a case conceptualization.*

An early intervention with the Bensons was the following:

THERAPIST: From what you're describing, it seems that you have been disappointed, but that you basically trust the other person's good intentions.

NANCY: That's right. Ben is as honest as the day is long, and he's a good person. *(Ben nodded affirmatively.)* [It would later emerge explicitly that Ben was more upset than Nancy and was beginning to mistrust her, feeling that she did not care about his feelings.]

THERAPIST: Perhaps some twinges of doubt occasionally, particularly when you don't know what the other is thinking or feeling.

NANCY: Well, Ben tends to keep things in, and I often don't know what he is thinking. I blow up quickly when something bothers me, but he puts it inside and—wham! It bursts out when I'm least expecting it. I'm devastated; I don't know where it is coming from.

THERAPIST: Sounds like you not only process things differently, but you also just approach the world differently. You have very different temperaments and energy levels. [This reaffirmed some of their earlier descriptions of Nancy as a "bundle of energy" and Ben as "laid back most of the time."] These temperament differences are not something you picked up in the last 3 years. They're something that you had long before you met each other. They're your automatic reactions to the world. They're neither good or bad, but just different. And they are requiring some understanding and adjustment on the part of each of you.

Working to elucidate the issues and to begin establishing some common bases of agreement, I focused on trying to explain the situation in "normal" terms, minimizing any nascent tendency toward blaming, and establishing their need for further clarification and understanding.†

> † *If this was desired, the therapist could also have drawn on the schemas that trickled down from each of their families of origin to convey how both spouses were affected by their previous environments. From a cognitive standpoint, this might have aided Ben and Nancy in beginning to reframe their view of each other and keep within the use of the genogram model.*

Marital Tasks and Interaction: The "Five C's"

The straightforward nature of Nancy's and Ben's presentation of their complaints and problems enabled me to sort out relationship issues and begin to form some hypotheses fairly readily as we moved through the first session. During a summary and feedback portion of the interview, I shared some of my impressions with them in a form that I thought would make sense to them, using a "five C's" framework. The "five C's" constitute a rule-of-thumb guideline for assessing major areas of interaction and potential problems in marital interaction. Nearly two decades ago, faced with a request to provide a framework that clients could understand and use to check how they were dealing with their joint tasks in their relationship, I formulated this set of categories after making a careful study of 100 consecutive marital therapy cases from my files; I have continued to refine it since then (Nichols & Everett, 1986; Nichols, 1988, 1996).

Commitment. Commitment, in brief, is concerned with the degree to which the spouses value the relationship and what their intentions are with regard to continuing it. During the past quarter century in particular, with the advent and spread of no-fault divorce, it has become much more crucial than formerly to ascertain at the outset the nature of the bond between the husband and wife in cases presenting with marital problems. Napier (1988) has appropriately called marriage "the fragile bond." Not only is marriage the lone voluntary relationship in a family, but, unlike other family relationships, it can be ended by either party, thus severing any formal relationship between the former spouses. The voluntary nature of the relationship and the accompanying fragility have significant implications for marital relationships and marital therapy. Many descriptions of marital cases focus on the presenting complaints and do not mention whether there is any question about whether one or both partners may be thinking of divorce. Answering this question—how the partners are joined, and whether and how they are committed to continuing the marriage—seems to me deserving of careful and explicit attention; continuity cannot be automatically assumed.

Heuristically, the partners may be "preambivalent," "ambivalent," or "postambivalent" in their commitment to the marriage (i.e., being positively committed and not having seriously considered leaving the marriage; being ambivalent about whether or not to continue; or having struggled over continuation and either decided to stay [postambivalent positive] or to leave [postambivalent negative]) (Nichols & Everett, 1986; Nichols, 1988, 1996). There are at least a half-dozen ways of exploring and assessing the commitment of marital partners (Nichols, 1996, p. 149).†

> † *One of these methods is to explore the spouses' conceptualization of what commitment means to them, and, using the cognitive model, to search in a collaborative manner for whether any aspects of this conceptualization are based on distorted or faulty thinking. It is also important to address any differences in the partners' conceptualization of the concept of commitment and how these may be affected by any of their cognitive distortions.*

Nancy and Ben were both strongly committed to the marriage and were preambivalent. Ben, as noted, was the more dissatisfied of the pair, but had not seriously considered ending the marriage.

Caring. What kind of emotional attachment exists between the partners? I use the more neutral term "care" instead of the popular term "love," because it is a synonym that taps into the same feelings as "love" without plunging into the romanticized ideology associated with "love" (e.g., "My feelings have changed; I don't love my spouse as I once did. Therefore, there is no basis for staying married—love is gone"). Caring involves the ability to be concerned with the welfare of the other, instead of being primarily focused on what one receives. From an object relations perspective, the issue is whether the partners are functioning at the need gratification level, in which the other is seen as a "service station" to provide what one desires, or at the "object constancy" (or "object love") level, in which the partner is valued for himself or herself whether fulfilling a wish or not.

Both their verbal statements and their other behaviors seemed to support the idea that Ben and Nancy basically cared for each other quite deeply.

Barriers to caring can include communication difficulties, lack of skill in coping with differences, incompatible expectations ("contracts"—see below), apprehensions regarding risking failure or rejection in a relationship, and various unresolved problems from the past (Nichols, 1996, p. 151).

Communication. How effectively do the partners communicate, both verbally and symbolically? What kinds of meanings do they share, and how effectively? To borrow from research terminology, communication appears to be a necessary although not a sufficient condition for successful interaction. However, as the semanticist S. I. Hayakawa pointed out four decades ago, communication is no panacea; people can communicate clearly and disagree absolutely. Hence, concern with communication readily slides over into the ways in which partners deal with their disagreements.†

> † *Cognitive-behavioral therapists view this issue very similarly, in that communication may not be sufficient to engage in successful interaction. A greater emphasis is placed on how partners deal with disagreements.*

Conflict and Compromise. Failures in agreement are inevitable in any intimate relationship. How well do the partners recognize their disagreements, and how effectively do they deal with them? I consider it important to recognize with clients that compromise is essential in marriage, that developing and maintaining a workable relationship typically require giving up some of what one desires, and that compromise is sometimes the only way to achieve a so-called "win–win" result.

Contract. Commitment to each other and to the marital relationship, and caring for each other, do not insure that the members of a couple will have similar expectations. Discrepancies between strong commitment and caring on the one hand, and the individual expectations and emotional "contract" that each partner carries can in fact create an ongoing combustible mixture of disappointment, disillusionment, discouragement, and disagreement. "Contract" is used here in the sense in which it is described by Sager (1976): Partners hold expectations and agreements— explicit, implied, presumed—which for each individual constitute a "contract" that the other is expected to fulfill. "When the other vows, 'I love you,' I think it means that [the other has] agreed to fulfill my wishes." These expectations may be conscious and verbalized, conscious but not verbalized, or outside of awareness.

Feedback and Discussion

"If I am interpreting what you are presenting accurately, it seems to me that both of you are pretty strongly committed to this relationship, to making a go of your marriage," I remarked to Ben and Nancy, after sketching the "five C's" framework. "You also seem to care a lot about each other, to respect each other, and to be frustrated and somewhat bewildered that things are not going as you had planned."

"That's right," they assented. Each of them asserted positive regard for the other, as well as determination and desire to make the marriage satisfying and fulfilling. Conjunctively, they expressed some of their disappointments and bewilderment. "I thought Nancy was ready to stop working—she had been working all of her adult life. But instead of staying home and doing things with me, she spends most of her time in volunteer work, just as if she were going to a job," Ben complained.

"Ben seemed to be a very social animal when I knew him before," responded Nancy. "He was the life of the party. He was active, joking around, full of good humor—really, a very attractive, active person. Now he doesn't seem to want to do anything except be with me. As I said, I need some breathing room."

Briefly and in a somewhat oversimplified fashion, they assessed their fulfillment of joint marital tasks essentially as follows:

Commitment: "Good. Solid."
Caring: "Good. Fine."

(Mutual respect was evident both in their nonverbal behaviors and in their words and declarations.)

Communication: "Good. Honest."

(Their techniques were rather good. No pathology was evident in their communication, and the communication was clear enough to expose some of their differences. Essentially, it revealed rather than concealed.)

Conflict and compromise: "It's upsetting how we handle differences.
     We don't seem to be able to solve problems."

(Ben and Nancy could delineate many of their apparent differences and problems, although this did not reach into their "contract" expectations. They did not, however, have effective ways of resolving even those differences of which they were aware.)

Contract: "I thought it would be different [disappointment]. I know
     what I wanted and thought I knew what [spouse] wanted."

(Ben had explicitly carried notions of delayed gratification. After retirement, "I looked forward to golfing and traveling with Nancy—all the things that I didn't have either the time or opportunity for before. I thought that was what she wanted, but she wanted to do her own thing—her club activities and so on." Nancy, on the other hand, pointed out that she was now able to do "all of the things with volunteer organizations that I was never able to do when I was a paid staff member, and this is much more important to me than I ever realized.")

The clients nodded in agreement as Sager's (1976) levels of expectations and their reactions of disappointment to the breaking of their assumed "contract" were sketched. The statement "Neither of you seems to have deliberately misled the other" produced an obviously sincere assent: "No, you're right. I remember what [spouse] said, but I thought it meant. . . . "†

> †A cognitive-behavioral therapist would label this response as an example of "unrealistic expectations" or the cognitive distortion of "mind reading." This might have been a very good spot for the therapist to introduce this couple to the list of cognitive distortions, particularly the notion of "mind reading," so that they could become more familiar with the common dysfunctional patterns that tend to lead to a violation of expectations. This would also have fallen into line with the notion of improved communication, which the therapist later addressed nicely. This could have been done directly in the session or assigned as a separate reading.

Ben and Nancy's reactions of disappointment were discussed in terms of normal processes in marriage. Typical actions of idealizing a new love (or a new teacher or other significant persons in one's life) were described as being followed by disillusionment after a period of time, under the impact of getting to know the person better and learning about his or her shortcomings under the strong light of reality.

Following this reinforcement of the idea that there had been no deliberate attempts to delude, we moved to a general agreement that the couple's commitment and caring seemed to be in pretty good shape, but that "As trite as it sounds, some work is needed on your communication, particularly with regard to improving your ability to be clear about your expectations. And we need to work on how you deal with differences—on conflict management."

Individual and Family-of-Origin Assessment

After the initial conjoint sessions, each spouse was seen for an individual session that focused on his or her individual history and family of origin.

Position in Family of Origin

One of the major patterns disclosed from Ben's background was his withdrawal in the face of difficulties that he could not overcome. From early in his adult life, as he recalled, when he "got enough," he would go away by himself until he recovered. He did the same thing in "mini-form" with disagreements now, pulling back into himself. As the youngest child in his family of origin, he had been accustomed to being approved and taken care of by his older siblings, especially his sisters, during his childhood. They had been supportive of his educational pursuits and business success, much as a group of aunts and uncles would have been. His ordinal position had prepared him for being appreciated and even catered to in the family. Ben's first wife had been very deferential to him and highly appreciative when he added to his business career what amounted to a "second career" of taking care of her during her extended illness and invalid role. He said he had become aware that he had an unconscious need to be needed, that Nancy knew this, and that it was not a problem.

Nancy also had been "adored and appreciated" by the males in her family. Although her family-of-origin sibling position would seem to indicate that she would be an ideal mate for Ben, she fit snugly into Toman's (1993) description of the oldest sister of brothers as being "independent and strong in an unobtrusive way" (p. 174). The strength of her independence and the fact that she came from a family in which achievement was highly valued combined to change the equation somewhat. Her continuing need to achieve even though she had retired, for example, restricted her availability to spend the time with Ben that he desired.

Family Life Cycle: Remarriage Issues

The Bensons were no exception to the widely accepted idea in family therapy that clients are significantly affected by how they deal with family life cycle issues. They were faced not only with the issues that individuals deal with during the post-child-rearing and later stages of the life cycle (Nichols & Pace-Nichols, 1993), but also with the tasks associated with a second or subsequent marriage. As we explored, we formed a consensus that they had dealt effectively with two of the major problems associated with remarriage: the presence of children, and issues of property, money, and inheritance. The third area, "ghosts from the past" (Nichols, 1996), continued to pose some problems. These ghosts were primarily in the form of "how we did it" in the earlier marriages.

Both Ben and Nancy carried some idealization of their first marriages. Nancy had been "adored" by her first husband. Losing him had been a major shock, a "terrible trauma." She had married her second husband in large measure, she said, because of the need for a "father" for her son. "There never was much between us, but he was a wonderful male model for my son; they still have a great relationship." She eventually divorced him after her son became an adolescent. Ben's first wife had simultaneously "catered to" him and needed him. As became evident, both Ben and Nancy had become accustomed to doing "what I wanted to do" in their marriage and home relationships. That is, each had set the pace and provided the guidelines in their earlier marital and domestic activities; they had both been in control.†

> †*One of the techniques of cognitive-behavioral therapy is to investigate both partners' concepts of change in their lives and what specifically it means to them. Often this uncovers faulty perceptions about how change will affect them, particularly with regard to control and satisfaction in their lives. In this particular case, it appeared that Ben and Nancy were operating under some of these misperceptions about change.*

Loss: Bereavement and Grief

Although Nancy and Ben certainly had been strongly attached to their first spouses, it seemed that time had enabled each of them to resolve feelings regarding loss of the person. What seemed more important was the loss of a pattern of living in which they were in control. In object relations terms, each desired to return to a former "model of relationship" that had met their relationship needs. A "good" mate for Nancy was a man who adored her and gave her adequate range and freedom to pursue her achievement needs. A "good" mate for Ben was a woman who demonstrated her dependence on him and "needed" him in ways that reassured him that he would not be abandoned, as he felt he had been with the death of his mother when he was in kindergarten. He wanted a mate who "catered to" him as his sisters had done following the mother's death.

There were what I have come to call "courage and risk in relationship" factors operating with Ben and Nancy. Both had lost significant persons in their lives. Ben found it hard to symbolically "let his spouse out of his sight" and tried to hold on to her too strongly. Nancy attempted to avoid suffering the pain of loss again by limiting her attachment and her overt indications of need and dependence. Each spouse was, however, functioning primarily at the "object constancy" or "object love" level (Blanck & Blanck, 1968), so that the other person rather than his or her own need was primary. The maturity of their object relations development both made their frustration clear and gave promise of keeping them at the task of trying to achieve the kind of relationship that they declared they desired.

Complementarity

Although there was a great deal of congruity in the values and sociocultural components of Nancy and Ben's relationship, there was not a smooth complementarity of needs between them. Their emotional needs and expectations did not form a good fit, in other words. They pulled against each other with their attempts to stay in control and thus, in my judgment, to avoid possible loss and pain.

FURTHER CONJOINT SESSIONS

The majority of the remaining sessions with the Bensons were conjoint meetings. Both expressed optimism and said that they were encouraged as we opened the fourth session. Some of the cloudiness that had been present at the beginning had been dispelled. They had a rather clear understanding that both of them were ethical, principled people who were committed to the marriage and cared about each other; that there was too much emotional conflict; and that control was a central issue. Their expressed goal was to meet each other's needs while retaining their own personal integrity.

Working on Communication

To state it briefly, we began to work on communication—on clarifying Nancy's and Ben's expectations and their messages to each other. Fortunately, their basic communication skills were rather good. Their ability to use humor, indicative of ego strength, was a decided asset. Our focus was on both process and content.

THERAPIST: We need some truth in advertising here. It's only fair to remind you that better communication may be hazardous to your tranquility. Clearing up communication may expose some differences that you typically leave unexposed.

NANCY: Meaning that things may get worse before they get better.

THERAPIST: Yes, I think so. I don't say it lightly, but that goes with the territory. As you probably remember from your conflict management training [at Nancy's job], the first step in solving a problem is generally considered to be deciding what the problem is. We need to do some more exploring of some of the things you have mentioned already, and to decide where we will try to focus our efforts. But we won't simply take a "Damn the torpedoes, full speed ahead!" approach. At the same time, we'll try to set a safe climate in which we can deal with things effectively.

In keeping with this promise, I engaged in a considerable amount of "midwiving" of the relationship as we proceeded (Nichols, 1996, pp. 155–157)—trying to sustain a general atmosphere of warmth and support, as well as serving as a go-between (Zuk, 1976). This sometimes took the form of active listening, sometimes that of actively guiding the direction and flow of the conversation (e.g., suggesting to one spouse, "Don't tell me, tell her [or him]"), and sometimes that of interpreting meanings. Thus we affirmed the positive elements that came forth, while working with the conflicts that emerged even more clearly as more effective communication and elucidation of their differences developed.

Working on Conflict and Compromise

We began to work out compromises between Ben and Nancy at an early stage in our contacts. These—as is normally the case with most couples— were not *quid pro quo* (Thibaut & Kelley, 1959), but rather "good-faith" contracts (Weiss, Hops, & Patterson, 1973) and "good-sense" actions. Rather than seeking to secure a *quid pro quo* contract, I attempted to help each of them take action on the basis of "volunteering"—doing something without the promise of immediate reward from the spouse, but because each of them cared about the spouse and the marriage. After we had discussed one of their practical, everyday problems, discovered what (if anything) they had attempted to do to solve it, and talked about some possibilities, I would ask one or both of them, "Do you suppose you could ... ?" or "What would make sense to you if you were approaching this from the kind of problem-solving approach that you have been taught in your work? What could you try?"

Occasionally, the Bensons were given homework assignments in which they were to try out some of the behaviors that we discussed. These were typically accompanied with the suggestion, "Well, why don't you try [whatever it was] and see how it goes?" When they reported what they had attempted and what had occurred, a "Pollyanna" tactic was used (Nichols & Everett, 1986, p. 309). This is a tactic in which the therapist helps the couple to recognize any positive effort or result that has taken place, rather than permitting the spouses to emphasize their failures or shortcomings.†

> †*This is quite consistent with the cognitive-behavioral approach, which places great emphasis on homework arrangements. Since a therapy session is usually limited to one 50- or 90-minute session per week, homework serves to strengthen the skills learned in therapy and serves as a training ground for trying them out and receiving feedback on the results from the therapist. It is also a major step toward helping the couple to make independent change.*

This use of what can be termed taking a reasonable, "civilized" approach to problem solving was possible with Ben and Nancy because of the nature of the "C's" and particularly because of Ben's desire for them to do as much as possible for themselves. This often took the form of starting with a general issue and proceeding to specifics of change.

THERAPIST: As I understand you, you agree that there is too much emotional conflict. You feel that as the struggle for control becomes stronger, you begin to mistrust each other. You feel like there is a lack of consideration of each other's feelings or position.

BEN: That's for sure!

THERAPIST: Tell us about a time that you intentionally meant to hurt the other, that you deliberately lied. . . . What about a time in which you feel the other deliberately tried to hurt you?

The partners agreed that they could not recite such instances, admitting that their reactions were "feelings" stemming from being disappointed, rather than conclusions based on accurate or demonstrable facts. As they cited times in which one spouse did feel hurt or upset by the actions or attitudes of the other, it was possible to help each put himself or herself in the place of the other. This process helped to remove the noxious effects of blaming, which is ubiquitous in present-day Western society and culture.

THERAPIST: And both of you have pointed out that for much of your life you were accustomed to doing what you wanted to do.

NANCY: Yes, I guess so.

BEN: *(Nodding in agreement)* And we can't now.

THERAPIST: Right, not if you are going to be fair, as you say you wish to be. I use the term "conflict and compromise" to emphasize that in a marriage nobody gets everything they want. It is not simply a matter of negotiating what you want. When both want the same thing, it is necessary to compromise.

This was stated as a reality, as a fact in this kind of intimate peer relationship. It was presented in a "dumb barter" fashion, meaning that it was simply laid down in front of the clients so that they could consider it and "pick it up" later if they wished. Nevertheless, we began to apply the concept to concrete situations.

Dealing with Time

Nancy emphasized that having personal time was very important to her. Ben pointed out again that he wanted "a lot of Nancy's time," but that he didn't feel that he was going to get any of it. Under examination, his resentment at staying home when Nancy was "on the go" turned out to be an expression of his fear that she did not wish to be with him.

THERAPIST: We can divide our time up into "private time" and "interactive time." Private time, of course, is the time that people spend by themselves, not dealing with other people. There are two kinds of interactive time: "shared time," in which a person is engaged in a high degree of interaction with somebody else, and "parallel time," in which a person is in the proximity of another person or persons but is not directly interacting with the other(s) at a very high level. For example, one person may be reading, and the other may be knitting, watching television, or doing something else. Or one may be mowing the lawn and the other working in the flower bed, or whatever. All of us seem to need some of each, and we need different amounts, and different amounts at different times. Let's look at what the needs and desires of each of you are.

As a part of this exploration, we also dealt with Nancy's need for "decompression time" when she came home in the afternoon. Ben understood the need to "decompress" or "gear down" at such times; he had little difficulty recalling his own need to be "left alone" when arriving home from work in years past. This work laid a basis for beginning to assure Nancy of some private time and for providing Ben with some realistic expectations of getting reasonable amounts of shared time. We structured in some time apart, some travel in which both were "fully present," and some parallel time and parallel pursuits, as well as shared activities.†

> † *In addition to this, the therapist might have found it helpful to reinforce the reframed cognitions of each partner and to monitor their new perceptions of their changed behavior in the relationship. This could have been done verbally or by using the reframing form introduced in Chapter 1.*

Ben took seriously the challenge of finding some pursuits outside the home without Nancy. After a few false starts, he discovered to his surprise that tennis was enjoyable. He had not played since college, but took some lessons to "get the rust off" and found a group of men in his age group with whom he played doubles a couple of times per week. Eventually he reported, "Well, I like it: it's not cutthroat and competitive, as it was when I played before. We set our own pace." He laughed. "Occasionally we get into volleying and get a little competitive. Mostly, though, it's just fun."†

> † *Again, this is another example of reframing of an old schema of what a situation may have been at one time.*

The "juggling" in this case involved not only moving among clarifying and improving communication between the partners, dealing with conflict and compromise, and increasing understanding and assisting them with changes in their daily living, but also shifting between a focus on their interaction and a focus on their individual concerns. When we got the situation between the partners settled down adequately, it seemed both necessary and appropriate to tackle some individual problems. I chose to work on Ben's major individual concerns, because he was the one who seemed to be hurting more and because we had already "given" something to Nancy in making the present environment safer for her. That is, we had provided greater opportunity for her to do what she wanted, and had lessened Ben's pressure on her for time. We could focus on her individual concerns later if that were deemed necessary. The approach taken was not necessarily "the only way" to proceed, or even "the best way." It was an effective way, as it turned out. The systems construct of equifinality undergirds therapists' confidence that they can use different ways to reach a desired goal.

Ben's Family-of-Origin Work

Both clients gave indications that they were carrying unresolved issues from their upbringing. As indicated, I made a tactical decision to deal with Ben's family-of-origin issues, because they seemed the more pressing; I would follow these with Nancy's if necessary. Over the years, I have used five major patterns of dealing with unresolved issues from clients' families of origin: conjoint marital therapy, individual psychotherapy, coaching a client on a trip home, therapy with members of a client's family of origin, and sessions with a client's total family of origin (Nichols, 1988, pp. 220–231).

In this case, I dealt with family-of-origin concerns of both clients in conjoint marital sessions, and also coached Ben on going home to take up some issues with his siblings. I introduced the latter point as follows: "Ben, it looks as if you've got to 'go home' one way or another, to try to deal with some of your issues about the loss of your mother. I'm raising this for you because of two things: One, we have to start somewhere on these old, unresolved issues; and, two, they appear to be causing you a considerable amount of pain and difficulty." He agreed, and we then explored what he recalled and what questions he had about what had occurred during his early years. He decided to discuss these things with his siblings. We worked out a list of questions that were especially important to him. With coaching, he felt ready to go.

After spending a weekend with his siblings, Ben returned with some answers. He said he realized "that I loved her very much and that I am sorry that she was taken from us." This was an obviously different idea from his childhood thought that she had abandoned him.†

> † *This would have been an excellent opportunity from a cognitive standpoint to investigate with Ben how his perception changed—that is what constituted the switch from his view of his mother's "abandoning" him to her "being taken from us." This would have been important to reinforce in his mind for future reference. It was important that he understand that it was a matter of how he chose to think about it.*

However, he still had a strong feeling that he needed to "bring some closure" on his feelings about his mother. "Why don't you try to do that?" I asked. "It sometimes helps to go to the cemetery and to say at the grave what you would like to say directly if you could say it in person. Some people find that doing that and then talking about the experience in therapy helps to bring closure." I then referred to the book *A Marital Puzzle,* by Norman and Betty Paul (1975), suggesting that Ben read it and discuss it in therapy.

Ben did this and then made the "graveyard" visit, returning with a taped recording of what he had said to his mother: "I wish I could have known you better. I actually don't remember much about you. You were warm and soft and smelled good. You were kind. You smiled a lot, even after you got sick." On the tape, his voice broke. "I'm sorry that I have been angry with you for leaving me. I know now that you couldn't help it. Then I didn't know how much pain you were in, what a relief dying must have been."

Explaining to Nancy and me what had happened as a result of the visit, Ben said, "A couple of days later [after going to the cemetery], it hit me! It was like I was back home as a child. The feelings just poured out of me: 'Don't die! Don't die!' I was begging my mother not to die, but there wasn't anything I could do about it. I remembered how scared I was." As we examined his feelings and processed his experiences, Ben was asked how he had dealt with the pain as a child. He recalled that he did not tell anybody. Now he thought it would have been much better if he had done so: "I have talked with both my sisters [since the "breakthrough" experience], and I know that they would have done the best they could to comfort me. I don't think I would have been so scared. And getting those feelings out is like having a pinprick that lets tension out, like [air out of] a balloon that has been punctured."

As Ben "loosened up," so did Nancy. Freed of the omnipresent concern that he wanted to be with her "24 hours a day," she reported that she was much more "present" when they were together than she had ever been previously. Ben confirmed that he was much more comfortable than he had been—that he did not "need to cling and demand and get upset, as I think I was doing." He worked out a plan in which, if he began to get upset because he was home alone, he would go somewhere and do something pleasurable rather than "staying at home and stewing." Thus, a behavior that he formerly used as running away was now used as a planned coping mechanism. Interestingly enough, Nancy's time away from the house began to lessen, not dramatically but perceptibly. She knew that she usually could depend on her "half hour of solitude" when she got home. Ben knew that he could rely on her to share with him afterwards. She seemed to secure more control over her "need for achievement," so that working as a volunteer was not marked by the driven quality that prevailed at the start of therapy.

During the later stages of therapy, the Bensons were using the "C's"—especially communication, conflict/compromise, and contract—as a gyroscope, a rough guideline for how they were faring. Sometimes they did so seriously and soberly, and sometimes they did it playfully. There were other indications that their learning, their coping, and their skill improvement were continuing. As they became more comfortable with their understanding of the dynamics that had nourished the tension in their relationship during the early years of their marriage, they became able to joke about their concerns. The following exchange, which first occurred in the therapy office with a heavy loading of feeling, was periodically used afterwards with a smile:

NANCY: I'm not going to leave you.

BEN: I'm not going to hobble you.

Conversely, Ben might joke, "I'm not going to leave you," and Nancy would respond, "I'm not going to hobble you."

SUMMARY

This report summarizes a case that was treated in an integrative fashion across the span of approximately 9 months. Initially, the clients were seen once weekly, but this soon moved into a biweekly or even less frequent pattern of sessions. The clients were in their 60s and 50s respectively, and were in a remarriage (a second marriage for the husband, who had been widowed, and a third marriage for the wife, who had been widowed and divorced). The presented complaints centered around "different needs"—his for more closeness and hers for more distance. This case illustrates interventions both with the marital system and with one client's extended family system (family of origin). The partners developed an increased basis of understanding of their relationship and themselves, an increased universe of discourse, and new and improved skills.†

> † *This was an excellent case of an older remarried couple displaying problems very typical of couples in this situation. The integrative approach to marital therapy is wide open for augmentation with cognitive-behavioral strategies, which may serve to enhance the already effective approach of the integrative modality.*

AUTHOR'S REPLY TO EDITOR'S COMMENTS

The techniques and strategies proposed by Dr. Dattilio do augment my treatment modality. As noted in the chapter, the focus in integrative marital therapy is on integration of theory, not integration of techniques, as in eclectic therapy or technical integration (see p. 234). Also as noted in the chapter (see p. 251), the systems construct of equifinality—combined with research and clinical observation—strongly supports the notion that a desired goal can be reached in many different ways. As Alan Gurman has pointed out, all approaches demonstrate some success with some clients. Hence, I recognize that a number of different approaches can be used with my integrative approach. As noted throughout the chapter, I attempt to tailor my interventions in accordance with my assessment of the needs of the situation (including the needs of the client[s]) and my perceptions of my own skills. Other therapists following such an integrative approach can use different forms of intervention than I might use in a particular case, and can do so successfully.

I certainly do consider cognitive-behavioral techniques and strategies to be integratable with my integrative marital therapy approach. The approach, in fact, explicitly acknowledges and attempts to include a social learning aspect. My conclusion from observation, supervision, and case consultation is that many therapists—and I suspect most—actually use cognitive-behavioral methods in working with clients, whether or not they acknowledge or even recognize what they are doing. Some, of course, do it with explicit intention and do so more effectively than others. As Dr. Dattilio notes in the editorial comments, "The integrative approach to marital therapy is wide open for augmentation with cognitive-behavioral strategies. . . . "

REFERENCES

Blanck, R., & Blanck, G. (1968). *Marriage and personal development.* New York: Columbia University Press.

Boszormenyi-Nagy, I. (1996). From family therapy to a psychology of relationships: Fictions of the individual and fictions of the family. *Comprehensive Psychiatry, 7,* 408–423.

Boszormenyi-Nagy, I., & Krasner, B. R. (1986). *Between give and take: A clinical guide to contextual therapy.* New York: Brunner/Mazel.

Dicks, H. V. (1963). Object relations theory and marital studies. *British Journal of Medical Psychology, 36,* 125–129.

Dicks, H. V. (1967). *Marital tensions.* New York: Basic Books.

Fairbairn, W. R. D. (1952). *Psychoanalytic studies of the personality.* London: Routledge & Kegan Paul.

Fairbairn, W. R. D. (1954). *An object-relations theory of the personality.* New York: Basic Books.

Fairbairn, W. R. D. (1963). Synopsis of an object-relations theory of the personality. *International Journal of Psycho-Analysis, 44,* 224–225.

Feldman, L. B. (1979). Marital conflict and marital intimacy: An integrative interpersonal and intrapsychic approach. *Family Process, 18,* 69–78.

Feldman, L. B. (1992). *Integrating individual and family therapy.* New York: Brunner/Mazel.

Feldman, L. B., & Pinsof, W. M. (1982). Problem maintenance in family systems: An integrative model. *Journal of Marital and Family Therapy, 8,* 295–308.

Framo, J. L. (1992). *Family-of-origin therapy: An intergenerational approach.* New York: Brunner/Mazel.

Napier, A. Y. (1988). *The fragile bond: In search of an equal, intimate, and enduring marriage.* New York: Harper & Row.

Nichols, W. C. (1985). A differentiating couple: Some transgenerational issues in marital therapy. In A. S. Gurman (Ed.), *Casebook of marital therapy* (pp. 199–229). New York: Guilford Press.

Nichols, W. C. (1988). *Marital therapy: An integrative approach.* New York: Guilford Press.

Nichols, W. C. (1996). *Treating people in families: An integrative approach.* New York: Guilford Press.

Nichols, W. C., & Everett, C. A. (1986). *Systemic family therapy: An integrative approach.* New York: Guilford Press.

Nichols, W. C., & Pace-Nichols, M. A. (1993). Developmental perspectives and family therapy: The marital life cycle. *Contemporary Family Therapy, 15,* 299–315.

Paul, N. L., & Paul, B. B. (1975). *A marital puzzle: Transgenerational analysis in marriage counseling.* New York: Norton.

Sager, C. J. (1976). *Marriage contracts and couples therapy.* New York: Norton.

Sullivan, H. S. (1953a). *Conceptions of modern psychiatry.* New York: Norton.

Sullivan, H. S. (1953b). *The interpersonal theory of psychiatry.* New York: Norton.

Sullivan, H. S. (1954). *The psychiatric interview.* New York: Norton.

Thibaut, J. W., & Kelley, H. H. (1959). *The social psychology of groups.* New York: Wiley.

Toman, W. (1993). *Family constellation: Its effect on personality and social behavior* (4th ed.). New York: Springer.

Weiss, R. L., Hops, H., & Patterson, G. R. (1973). A framework for conceptualizing marital conflict, a technology for altering it, some data for evaluating it. In L. A. Hamerlynck, L. C. Handy, & E. J. Mash (Eds.), *Behavior change: Methodology, concepts, and practice* (pp. 309–342). Champaign, IL: Research Press.

Williamson, D. S. (1991). *The intimacy paradox: Personal authority in the family system.* New York: Guilford Press.

Zuk, G. H. (1976). Family therapy: Clinical hodgepodge or clinical science? *Journal of Marriage and Family Counseling, 2,* 299–303.

SUGGESTED READINGS

Feldman, L. B., & Pinsof, W. M. (1982). Problem maintenance in family systems: An integrative model. *Journal of Marital and Family Therapy, 8,* 295–308.

Framo, J. L. (1992). *Family-of-origin therapy: An intergenerational approach.* New York: Brunner/Mazel.

Nichols, W. C. (1985). A differentiating couple: Some transgenerational issues in marital therapy. In A. S. Gurman (Ed.), *Casebook of marital therapy* (pp. 199–229). New York: Guilford Press.

Nichols, W. C. (1988). *Marital therapy: An integrative approach*. New York: Guilford Press.

Nichols, W. C. (1996). *Treating people in families: An integrative approach*. New York: Guilford Press.

Nichols, W. C., & Pace-Nichols, M. A. (1993). Developmental perspectives and family therapy: The marital life cycle. *Contemporary Family Therapy, 15,* 299–315.

Chapter 11

Transgenerational Family Therapy

LAURA GIAT ROBERTO

Transgenerational therapies, based chiefly on the founding theories of Carl Whitaker, Murray Bowen, Norman Paul, and Ivan Boszormenyi-Nagy, stress the importance of family relational patterns over decades. The patterns studied and addressed in the process of therapy include both explicit interactional and behavioral patterns, and implicit, value-laden patterns formed gradually during periods of family upheaval. Family process as it is viewed in the transgenerational model "feeds forward" in a chronological or spiraling fashion from emotionally influential events in the lives of great-grandparents, through those in the lives of grandparents and parents, into the lifetimes of their children; it does so via unique variations in attachments, in management of intimacy and power, in specific identifications and in conflicts, and other relational events that distinguish one family from another (Boszormenyi-Nagy & Krasner, 1986).

Although the passage of events in this model is systemic, it is not completely "circular." Unresolved issues in families of origin have their outlet, albeit one that is greatly mediated later, in the symptoms of offspring for generations (Kerr & Bowen, 1988; Roberto, 1992). The case study that follows describes the therapy of a young woman, her marriage, and her family of origin, as it took place in two segments over a period of 4 years. Although the therapy was at first undertaken to treat a dangerous medical disorder—anorexia nervosa with purging—the course of treatment utilized a wider lens of 40 years in the client's family history. This was done in order to construct the frame of reference of dreams cherished, mistakes

257

made, deep emotions moved, anxieties played out, angers unleashed, moments survived, and lessons taken—all of which found their way into the needs and wishes of a young girl on her way to adulthood.

CASE BACKGROUND: STARVATION AND SELF-DENIAL

Katherine was first referred to me at the age of 18 by her primary care physician. A college freshman, she was unable to concentrate on her schoolwork; was failing her courses; had lost 20 pounds (her weight was currently an emaciated 90 pounds); and was secretly swallowing 15 Ex-Lax tablets daily, which caused severe diarrhea, pain and cramping, insomnia, dehydration, and colonic bleeding. Although she was single and had free time, she had only one or two female friends. In her isolation, she had told no one of her fasts or daily purging (even the physician had to diagnose it on the basis of his own suspicions).

When she reached 90 pounds, she saw her physician because she developed a throat infection that would not improve, due to her weakness and compromised immune system. The family practice physician recommended to Katherine that she seek counseling "to try to work out her problem with eating," but didn't place any demands on her regarding her weight, or tell her when to return for the next checkup. Neither did the patient ask; she demurely agreed, and did not inquire into his view of the situation. Katherine arrived for her initial consultation very ill. She was depressed, dehydrated, ashamed of her purging, exhausted from sleep deprivation, and mentally distracted by obsessive wishes to binge and purge. She admitted having recurrent thoughts about ending her life with pills. It was difficult to engage her attention long enough to review all of her medical symptoms and mood problems. She felt she was in grave trouble, but focused instead on her school performance. Her health and every other personal concern were distant second priorities.

Katherine's emaciated physical state made it necessary to admit her to the hospital for several weeks to rehydrate her, guard her life, and clear her mind. As I prefer to do when inpatient care is used, I took a "consultant" rather than an "expert" position with Katherine. I explained to her that hospitalization is an unusual way to start therapy, and that I wanted her to make the decision for admission because she could "accidentally" enter into a critical state as a result of purging. Confused and passive, she clearly required a significant other to aid in the admission and approve the cost, but she only had one member of her family present in the area (her father). She informed me fearfully that her father and stepmother could be notified and could attend the admission with her, but her father would be furious and disappointed with her, since "*he's* the one who expects me to do well in school and pays the bills." Her mother, who had lived with her "spoiled younger brother" since the parental divorce years earlier, was described as "very nervous and self-conscious" and "likely to get embarrassed and upset about what the neighbors would think" if she received bad news.

Thus, it was clear in the first interview that Katherine was essentially without a trustworthy, intimate connection to her family. She also experienced great shame and disregard for herself and her care, and had little emotional strength or motivation left to concentrate on her studies. In addition, Katherine harbored a deep sense of isolation; envied and resented those who kept their health, such as her younger brother; and saw herself, at 18, as basically alone in her world. She was now, on top of all the emotional problems, suffering from a life-threatening disorder. If left adrift any longer, Katherine could easily collapse from heart failure at any time, appearing as another sad entry in the local newspapers. Yet she had been using selective inattention for a long time to screen out frightened or shocked comments from friends, which surely would have challenged her behavior.

Because the treatment center where I work uses a collaborative health care model, I placed a telephone call to her referring physician to share our findings. He confided that he feared that her condition would quickly deteriorate, and that she should be hospitalized for her medical safety. He agreed to an admission to a psychiatric floor with an eating disorders program; this would enable us to refeed her, begin a weight gain protocol, and watch over her purging. The hospital internist was to assume care of her until she was stable and ready to return to outpatient medical follow-up.

TRANSGENERATIONAL THERAPY AND THE THERAPEUTIC ALLIANCE

Transgenerational family therapy uses a "wide-angle lens" to view the symptom bearer in the unique setting of his or her marriage or family. When two to three generations are viewed in therapy, the dysfunctional patterns that surround the problem—its context—can be discussed and altered *as part of the therapy*. At first, the transgenerational therapist works with the complaint most clear to the family, which is almost always the presenting symptom. However, in this model the family of origin is the focus, not simply the distressed member. If the patterns of relating that center around a client can also be altered, the contextual pressures that underlie a symptom can be eliminated. In the case of eating disorders, the therapist starts with the illness as the problem definition. The diagnosis of anorexia nervosa, bulimia nervosa, or compulsive overeating conveys a concrete and dramatic sense to other family members that the ill member is out of control and needs their help.

However, the transgenerational therapist walks a fine line to insure that a diagnosis is not used as an explanatory tool by a family. Transgenerational therapists are careful not to reify symptoms, elevate them as explanations, or allow them to be used to blame distressed clients. Reifying symptoms leads client to see themselves as afflicted ("I am a problem"), instead of focusing on the relational patterns that support them, or on solutions ("We have a problem"; Whitaker & Keith, 1981). Asking the spouse or family to be involved in therapy is the first step in treatment. Pulling one or two more generations onto the stage can immediately show the therapist many problematic behavior patterns and beliefs. This is referred to as "constructing a transgenerational frame" and is paramount in this treatment approach (Roberto, 1992).

In the earliest stages of care, family members are asked to comment on their observations of the problem, their theories or explanation of the problem, and their past and current responses. In this way, the interactional patterns surrounding the illness become clear, as well as many implicit beliefs and values underlying these patterns. Obtaining multiple descriptions of family history—a hallmark of all systemic therapies—has the additional advantage of creating a therapeutic alliance with the entire family that is also multiple in nature. Relatives who are consulted feel important and dedicate more to the tasks requested of them. At the end of this inquiry phase, an attitude of concern and heightened self-awareness has been created in other family members, to underpin the treatment plan.

In extended family interviews, the transgenerational family therapist uses a stance of "multidimensional partiality" (Boszormenyi-Nagy & Krasner, 1986). If the realities in a family are multiple, then family life is "multidimensional"; that is, it looks and feels different from the position of different family members. Katherine's younger brother experienced the fear of losing Katherine differently from her mother, who worried for her; her father, who mistrusted her; her stepmother, who felt rejected by her; and her grandparents, who watched disapprovingly from a distance. The therapist aims to ally with each family member from his or her vantage point, rather than trying to ally with the client alone or with the family unit as if it were some huge monolith. In addition, multidimensional partiality includes working in a *personal* way—using open expressions of empathy for the concerns of each member—rather than taking a more formal and distant or impersonal "neutral" stance.

EARLY-STAGE THERAPY: A WOUNDED FAMILY

In the hospital, Katherine withdrew almost completely—dutifully eating her meals on trays, asking to use the locked bathrooms when needed, and generally being a "good girl." She did not raise her own concerns except when explicitly encouraged by her individual therapist (myself), and took a lone and watchful position in milieu groups, in which she listened to the feelings of others and expressed empathy for their hardships. Although her father and stepmother visited only weekly for family therapy, her mother and brother came into town almost at once, staying with friends and visiting daily for a week. When not sitting silently with her mother and brother, she did schoolwork constantly and obsessed about her test grades.

In individual therapy, I focused on helping Katherine to identify the intense anger, hurt, mistrust, and fear that prompted her to withdraw, and established with her that these were also the cues that triggered fasting and purging when she was at home. I assigned her a daily journal in which she entered the time when she had severe impulses to purge, and any emotions or events she was aware of within the preceding hour. Events were easier for Katherine to describe than her own emotions. At times, she could not identify any internal responses except to say that she "felt good" (usually when an a morning weighing showed that her weight had plateaued) or "felt bad" (when it increased or when she had a family visit).†

> † *Dr. Roberto nicely portrays the difficulty that Katherine experienced in expressing her internal responses; such difficulty is not uncommon with eating-disordered individuals. At this point, a cognitive-behavioral therapist might have begun trying to help Katherine gain access to her automatic thoughts (i.e., the spontaneous thoughts associated with her descriptions of "feeling good" and "feeling bad"). This might have enhanced the next step that Dr. Roberto so appropriately addressed, regarding internal pressures and trigger points. This would also have led the therapist to the core schemas governing Katherine's beliefs about her eating habits.*

Along with the identification and verbalization of affect, therapy focused on exploring what internal pressures and what relationship problems were triggering her misery and her self-abusive purging. This was confusing for Katherine, whose laxative abuse, constant stomach pain, and weight obsession had long obscured any connection between her thoughts and the events in her daily life. She described how her parents' marriage had disintegrated into a vengefully handled divorce. She recalled fleeing to the basement as her enraged father exploded and smashed family belongings; she remembered withdrawing or "numbing out" for long periods of time in the basement. She began to recognize that these "numbing-out" periods still occurred when she was hurt or angered by loved ones, dating partners, or friends, or when she did not receive an A on an examination. She also began to recognize that the "numbing-out" (dissociative) process was so ingrained that she had forgotten how to read and utilize emotional responses in making decisions and expressing herself. She began to characterize food and laxatives as "her best friends." At this time, the end of the first week of hospitalization, she concluded that one persistent source of anxiety and sadness was her mother's defensiveness when she confided to her about having problems.

Family therapy for Katherine meant holding sessions with each branch of her remarried, binuclear family. I structured each meeting with her and one family, to force a dialogue among the family members about her illness and watch each person's reactions. My goals at this time included clarifying each relative's approach to Katherine, assessing the emotional tensions that made them each keep their distance, and insuring that each person had a safe environment to express his or her needs and wishes. Sessions with the father and stepmother were difficult to arrange because of their frequent business traveling (obviously another source of the disconnection Katherine had felt since her parents' divorce). She struggled to admit to them that she felt distant, reacted with shame to their discomfort, and feared that her father would become enraged and stop his college tuition payments. In meetings that her mother traveled to attend, Katherine also tended to become lost in feelings of anger—a belief that she had only a conditional place in her family's life, and was "putting Mother out" by requiring her to come to meetings. With a great deal of encouragement, Katherine admitted her anger about past attempts to ask for help from her mother, which had derailed into her mother's own emotions. She had to combat verbal challenges such as "Are you saying I wasn't a good mother?" This was quite frightening to Katherine, and led at least once to food refusal and weight loss.†

> † A significant area of focus in the cognitive-behavioral approach to family issues is addressing schemas that individuals develop about themselves and their family relationships (Dattilio, 1993, 1994). This may also include schemas about the relationship between two or more family members. In this case, Katherine had obviously developed specific schemas about her mother, and these had already triggered the emotion of anger. Again, these schemas night have been an area worth pursuing, especially in respect to testing the likelihood of any cognitive distortions that Katherine might have developed during her upbringing. (Such distortions are described) very effectively by Dr. Roberto later in this segment.) In addition to cognitive restructuring or challenging of automatic thoughts, behavioral exercises might also have been used here with regard to considering alternative behaviors to use in lieu of food refusal or other life-threatening experiences. For example, the therapist could have collaboratively developed a plan with Katherine for choosing an alternative behavior that she felt she could live with in place of bingeing and purging.

Katherine was pained by each parent's somewhat competitive comments about the other's part in the parental divorce, and was frequently too confused by these "triangling" patterns to stick to her topic. Her brother, who had a distant and timid relationship with his moody elder sister, was able to participate as she described her self-abuse, and to contribute by expressing concern. This change created the beginning of the first alliance between brother and sister in their memories, and seemed to reduce their sense of isolation and improve their self-esteem. As a transgenerational therapist, I was eager to rebuild the little subsystem of brother and sister, since I look forward into the future and consider how to help members of an extended family preserve their relational resources for the long term, after the parents decline and eventually depart from their children.

When Katherine had increased her weight to 95 pounds (which required 2 weeks of hospitalization), she returned to her apartment and her roommate near the college campus and resumed classes. Many of the family patterns addressed in the hospital quickly became peripheral to Katherine, and her own mood took center stage as her impulses to fast and purge intensified rapidly. Although she spoke with her mother and brother weekly now (mostly at the mother's urging), Katherine returned to sporadic and staged phone calls to her father, in which she gave academic progress reports and whitewashed how she was doing. In weekly individual therapy sessions, she began to tackle her intensely negative body image, competitiveness with other women, and resulting lack of friendships and dates. Although Katherine was beginning to understand, for the first time, the interactional context in which her poor self-esteem had taken shape, she still did not realize that her self-esteem was poor. To her, criticism, mistrust, and dismissal were so internalized that they now "felt normal," in Katherine's words.

Therapy sessions maintained a continuity and focus for her, in which I repeatedly examined and discussed Katherine's urges to binge and purge and the intermittent relapses in which she followed through on her impulses. Crisis intervention techniques were also used to separate her from binge food and make sure she wasn't alone to binge. These included unplanned walks around the block to get away from her pantry; calls to "check in" with a friend; and locking up cash in the car and parking it down the street so that she was penniless during store hours. Efforts to help her identify the events and ideas that drove her impulses also became a major focus of treatment.†

> † *This was an excellent move, and one that is used commonly in a cognitive-behavioral approach to eating disorders. It allows for direct intervention with and arresting of the mechanisms that propel the restricted intake of food. In addition, it is essential for the therapist to focus on the schema-driven content of the behaviors in order to address the behaviors. It is both the cognitive and behavioral components of treatment that may facilitate this change.*

Katherine, at this stage (some 12 sessions into care), was unable to control herself when she became obsessional, or to use the structure of her daily life to combat her urges. Instead, on bad days she isolated herself and turned off the telephone. She also closed the blinds and hid in her room, weeping for hours or gorging herself on loaves of bread and leftover rice.

MIDPHASE THERAPY: FROM WOUNDED DAUGHTER TO YOUNG FIANCÉE

In the middle of the spring semester, Katherine announced that she had met the man she was going to marry. To her surprise, her love interest—Timothy, a graduating senior—was courting her seriously despite her health problems. Now 19, Katherine felt lonely and disconnected from her two families, despite the increasing contacts. She had few interests outside of her classwork and felt little pride in her accomplishments. She still perceived herself as "sick," "weird," and "a failure." Although in therapy she acknowledged that it was important to give herself more credit when she was doing well, instead she sought approval from Timothy, who had become lover, fiancé, advisor, and father figure all rolled into one. The young partners quickly fused together. Katherine had a sense of relief that now "I can have my own family," and Timothy took great pride in the idea that he was ready for a wife, a home of their own, and a career.

On the one hand, Katherine was beginning to make her own choices for the first time. She could accept her sexuality and express it, pursue an intimate relationship, and treat herself like a competent adult rather than a problem child. On the other hand, she was quickly submerging most of her questions about self-acceptance and self-respect by turning to her fiancé for reassurance. In therapy sessions, I walked a thin line between acknowledging her right and ability to make her own choices, and pointing out to her her pitfalls of focusing too much on the views of her fiancé. For example, she had amassed a small amount of money from working nights and weekends at a veterinary clinic nearby; she badly needed this money to pay for living expenses. These savings were the first attempt she had made to provide for herself instead of having to ask her father for money every week. Earning pay was truly an important step in taking care of herself. Yet when Timothy announced his intention to take a summer course to prepare for entrance to law school, and expected financial support, she immediately offered it to him. I saw a big impasse in my treatment plan coming. It became clear that beneath his loving and protective behavior, Timothy felt entitled to take whatever he needed from her. At this stage of therapy, Katherine still had no self-protective instincts, outside of the old patterns of acting sick and physically withdrawing from the world. When I gently tried to question what she felt she would gain from supporting her fiancé financially, she was aware only of concern for his welfare and a desire to help.

Katherine's thoughts were still almost always focused on the needs and expectations of her significant others. In fact, when I was not extremely careful to be neutral in my own position on couple issues, she easily became suspicious about my expectations of her. On at least one occasion, Katherine canceled a meeting "in order to go to work," but later confessed that she was feeling guilty and afraid that I would not approve of a decision she had made. This phase of therapy was fraught with self-defeating actions, persistent overfocusing on what her loved ones wanted, self-denial, and a great deal of underlying contempt for herself that she just did not notice.†

> † Once again, focusing on Katherine's automatic thoughts and uncov-
> ering the schemas behind these emotions and behaviors might have
> helped the therapist to understand what it meant to Katherine to
> violate the expectations of a loved one or to deprive herself of her
> own needs. An important focus here might have been on the rationale
> behind Katherine's self-deprivation. What was its purpose, and what
> might have been the secondary gain? A schema-focused approach
> would have brought this out directly, so that it could be addressed
> in treatment and in her relationships.

Yet now, 4 months into treatment, Katherine was only binge-eating and purging once or twice a week; in between, she was able to use the meal plan sent home with her from the hospital to eat at normal 4-hour intervals. She affirmed that with her food spread out into three meals and two snacks throughout the day, more foods "felt safe," and she could eat them without either starving or bingeing and trying to purge. She was moving toward her target weight of 115 pounds, hovering at 105, although this made her quite anxious and she "felt fat."

TRANSGENERATIONAL THERAPY AND
THE THERAPIST'S ROLE

In transgenerational family therapy, the therapist assumes a *consultant* role when old patterns of behavior reappear. Even when presenting symptoms have improved, clients and their intimates frequently ignore their own growing competence and retreat into self-defeating, worn-out doubts and helplessness (Waters & Lawrence, 1993). This is especially true in the middle phase of therapy, when using newfound understandings and new solutions takes great effort. During this period, for example, Katherine would frequently announce a choice she made that went against her own self-interest, such as giving her savings to Timothy, and then look at me out of the corner of her eye to see whether I looked approving. The transgenerational therapist strives not to accept a client's bids for direction—to coach and advise, rather than to take over for the client (Roberto, 1992). Directing the client and assigning therapeutic tasks have their place in early-stage therapy, but later they can come to replicate the dynamic of the idealized parent and the inadequate, reactive child.†

> † *The therapist's aim as described by Dr. Roberto is identical to that in cognitive-behavioral therapy—particularly that in the approach proposed by Beck (1967), which involves a "collaborative empiricism" in therapy that allows the therapist to work in a consultant's role (as opposed to the more "directive" role taken by the therapist in Ellis's rational–emotive behavior therapy). In Katherine's case, this effectively deparentifies the therapist, creating more of a collaborative relationship.*

Transgenerational therapies hold that by their 40s, adults should be able to shift their relationship with parents onto a peer level, and to take on "personal authority" (Williamson, 1981, 1982), or strong personal agency, in caring for themselves. Interventions in the middle phase of therapy are therefore best aimed at strengthening the client's own resources and sense of authority, as a good coach would do. Family sessions, or family subgroups, are convened in middle-stage therapy for consultations on progress and continued discussion of earlier themes. The use of subgroups helps a client to focus on relational changes in one or two relationships—for example, a meeting with client and mother only, or a sibling meeting. These family consultations are conducted in a manner that elevates the client to peer status, improve self-confidence, and promotes empathy between the client and other family members.

A MARRIAGE, A COLLAPSE, AND A CONFRONTATION

The summer after her freshman year, Katherine went to work for her stepmother full time. Her day-to-day life revolved around adjusting to her soon-to-be father-in-law, Chris, and his conflictual relationship with Timothy. She was worried about being accepted by Chris, a practicing Mormon who looked down on her newfound socializing, love of parties and dances, and social drinking. Although Timothy had seemed to distance himself from his father's expectations during his courtship, as the August wedding approached he became increasingly tense, serious, work-oriented, and impatient with her.

Rather than looking at these tensions as expressions of Timothy's own divided loyalties, Katherine felt guilty, unworthy, intimidated by Chris, and more depressed. She could not purge easily while busy with wedding plans, and felt that Chris viewed her as emotionally disturbed and questionable as a daughter-in-law already. She withdrew from Timothy, lost her sexual desire, and became angrier and angrier at herself for having been hospitalized and underweight. During this period (the sixth month of treatment), therapy often focused on squabbles with Timothy over such logistical issues as his getting to the dinner table on time, her fatigue from running errands for the wedding, and his lack of time off from his own full-time clerking job in a law office. Katherine couldn't, or didn't want to, acknowledge that she was exceedingly uncomfortable with Chris's religiously observant home and Timothy's increasingly obvious workhorse mentality. She did not ask her father or stepmother for support, despite the increased understanding her father had shown over the passing months. Still prone to inappropriate guilt and a tendency to criticize herself, Katherine felt she had forfeited the right to ask for his support, since she was not taking summer school classes "like Daddy would want."

Shortly before the wedding, Katherine announced that she "felt ready to take a break from counseling and try things on her own." She planned to work for her stepmother until the week before the wedding, take a short honeymoon with Timothy, take a year off from college, and return to work when Timothy began law school nearby. She seemed cheerful about the loss of school, where she had been earning top marks in the spring; the loss of her identity as a successful student; the likelihood that her stepmother's pastry shop would not satisfy her intellect; and the loss of time with school friends. I congratulated her on her marriage, but added my concern about the way she still could be too hard on herself. I reminded her that marriage and family life call for joy as well as hard work, and urged her to continue to take care of her own health and well-being.

It was during the following Thanksgiving, almost a year after Katherine was first referred to me, that I received a call from a staff therapist at an eating disorders hospital outside Philadelphia. Katherine had been admitted there 2 weeks earlier for food restriction, laxative purging, and dehydration. The hospital personnel felt that, after "drying out" from her purging and some refeeding, she was ready to return home to outpatient follow-up. She had asked them to contact me to set up an appointment, and they went along with her somewhat helpless request. I asked them to have her call when she arrived in town.

The following week, a wan, thinner, defeated-looking Katherine arrived at my office. Guardedly, she told me about her relapse, and about her intense feelings of shame and depression during and after her wedding. Although the minister and both families had been upbeat and cooperative, Katherine could not control frightening thoughts that she was "just being tolerated" by her parents and Timothy's. When I asked her about the events of the honeymoon, the return home, and the early fall, she expressed confusion, depressed feelings, fears of her relationship with Timothy, and frustration that she wasn't enjoying her work more.†

† *At this point, the therapist could have considered the use of the "downward arrow" technique (see Chapter 1) in order to trace Katherine's automatic thoughts to their core beliefs, particularly with regard to what she anticipated to be the worst possible outcome if her fears were to come true.*

Although she had never claimed to be in love with Timothy, or satisfied by her work, or comfortable with his father, she seemed to expect that after the wedding these feelings would magically appear. It was as if Katherine were trying to squeeze herself into some internalized image of a wife, and then was shocked that she wasn't happy that way. The images that guided her did resemble her stepmother and mother, but had no relevance to her own life. It was painful to watch this proverbial "good girl" contorting herself into some idealized notion of marriage that just wasn't her. I interpreted to her the fact that her crisis must mean that her plan of action wasn't working (i.e., it wasn't good for her). Katherine spoke to me like a sleepwalker. She had no awareness that she was pressuring herself unrealistically. She stated that she felt "numb" and didn't really want to live; she also couldn't assure me that she was safe at home and wouldn't hurt herself again. At this point, I recommended that Timothy accompany her to therapy to get his assistance with Katherine's severe depressive episode, since conjoint therapy is my treatment of choice when marital stress is involved in a depression (Prince & Jacobson, 1995). Katherine made a verbal contract with her husband and myself in a marital session, to call him or me at work if she felt she were in danger of harming herself with laxatives.†

† *Once again, the approach Dr. Roberto took here is identical to the cognitive-behavioral approach. The notion in both modalities is that couple therapy occurs only with both partners present, and is indicated particularly when the problem is deemed to be a relationship issue.*

In the several marital sessions that followed, Timothy showed himself to be attentive and responsive to his wife and family—in fact, overconcerned, where the family was involved. He seemed to be a male version of Katherine, exemplifying the long-held clinical observation that women with eating disorders either marry fatherly or brotherly men. He said that he loved Katherine and was worried for her, but that he was equally worried about his father, who felt that the new daughter-in-law was not religiously observant enough and was leading Timothy astray. This marital session confirmed Katherine's sense that she was once again disapproved of by a parent—and that her intuitions were not far off the mark. Just as Katherine had been encouraged to express herself to her own family a year earlier, and to set her own direction, now Timothy had to be encouraged as well.

The couple was mired in several anxiety-provoking quandaries, one of which was pressure from Chris to have children right away. Since Katherine had never returned to work after her second hospitalization, she seized on this fact to find fault with herself: "I should start having children—I'm not even bringing in an income." Rather than using the opportunity to reexamine where to work, or whether to continue school, she seemed to want to defer to yet another set of answers from someone else—her father-in-law. Therapy sessions moved back and forth from urging Katherine to create her own goals, to challenging Timothy to set a boundary with his father so that the marital dyad could become stronger.†

> † *The notion of "challenging" self-defeating beliefs or self-statements is very important, particularly when individuals base important behaviors on strong beliefs about what others may say and do. In this case, Dr. Roberto encouraged the challenging of perceived boundaries in order to improve the marital relationship. This is an excellent method to begin helping clients to reframe their perceptions with firsthand information derived from reality.*

When Katherine would take a stand, such as suggesting that they move into their own apartment before starting a family (they had remained with Katherine's roommate), Timothy would backstep and spend more time attending to his father. I confined myself to supporting any expression of personal wishes from Katherine, and to pointing out the need for an emotional boundary around the marriage. Finally, Timothy confronted his father on their religious differences openly, and admitted to both his father and himself that he had married Katherine because he himself shared her values. This confrontation made life much harder with Chris, who openly blamed Katherine for "putting these ideas into Timothy's head." Clearly, this young wife from an emotionally distant family was not going to find compensation in her in-laws.

The young couple struggled along this way until Easter, with Timothy plugging away at his studies, and Katherine keeping house for themselves and her roommate while she agonized about what to do with her time. Some weeks she did not purge, and ate meals at regular intervals without too much trouble. We called this healthier routine "using her food for fuel." Other weeks, especially when she felt dissatisfied with her progress or was lonely or depressed, she skipped meals and purged by either vomiting or abusing laxatives. Her weight seesawed up and down the same 5-pound range, like a barometer registering weather changes. I shared this metaphor with her, which helped her to bypass her old defensive feelings about admitting her purging. Therapy sessions were structured with four goals in mind: to push Katherine to stop harming her body with purging; to challenge her whenever she told herself that she was incompetent or unworthy; to refuse her invitations to control her; and to increase her awareness of how she used submissive and self-critical behavior to get the love and attention she felt she had always missed.

USE OF SELF AND INTIMACY IN THERAPY

Transgenerational therapists work with mandates, family myths, and internalized images of the self that have been passed on by family interaction over the course of a client's lifetime. These long-term, implicit emotional processes are rooted in identification, family projections, and selective alliances, and thus carry enormous power to restrain clients from changing (see, e.g., Paul's papers on grief, mourning, and parental directives; Paul, 1970, 1982). A family "mandate" is an unspoken directive that is passed to particular members because of their position in the family, usually over at least two generations. For example, many adults whose parents became poor during the Depression feel a certain "pull," or mandate, to make money and restore the family to a better economic class. One variation of this process is the deathbed mandate, in which a parent or grandparent voices wishes or regrets to loved ones, who then feel obligated to make choices accordingly (such as leaving a career to take over the family business).

A family "myth" is more explicit than a mandate. Myths are the explanations that family members are given for events in the past, especially tragedies and challenges. They often don't contain much factual information, but are emotion-laden stories that help families to come to terms with losses or to restore self-esteem. For example, a common family myth in the last generation was that when a man left his marriage and did not visit his children often, he was a bad person who had deserted his family. It's easy to see that therapeutic feedback, although it carries a certain power to heal, simply doesn't carry the weight of years of family needs and struggles.

There is one source of influence that therapists can add to increase influence: therapeutic "use of self" (Napier & Whitaker, 1978; Roberto, 1991, 1992; Whitaker & Keith, 1981; Whitaker & Bumberry, 1988). Use of self is a key technique of symbolic-experiential family therapy. Like psychoanalytic therapists who make interpretations, transgenerational therapists use personal metaphors and images to help guide the therapeutic relationship. Use of self is difficult to define in empirical terms, but can be described in this way (Whitaker & Bumberry, 1988):

> Therapists really don't have the power to inflict growth on a family. You can't tell them how to be more real. Your impact can really only come from the personal process you participate in with them. . . . If you lose yourself and fail to be both caring and tough, no one will stand to gain. (p. 38)

To put it another way, a therapist can promote clients' understanding of problems by using carefully chosen images and learnings drawn from his or her own life experience. For example, a therapist may observe that if he or she were in the client's shoes, he or she might feel the same way. Or the therapist may reflect on a therapy impasse and recount a similar situation with another family in treatment, along with the solution the other family found. Such reflections can refocus clients who are having repetitive, helpless reactions to chronic family problems.†

> † *Images and internal dialogues are extremely important aspects of cognitive-behavioral therapy. They are often used effectively to uncover hidden beliefs that may lead to disturbing emotions. Anything that may jog individuals' memories as to what may have contributed to their beliefs or emotions can be extremely helpful, such as the techniques Dr. Roberto used with Katherine and Timothy.*

A therapist can also tell a personal story with material that has been understood and emotionally integrated, such as a story of how a falling out with a loved one was resolved in the past. This type of well-integrated personal story is also called a "teaching story." Personal stories using parent–child experiences can be extremely powerful in empowering clients with poor self-worth; for example, a therapist can describe the day he or she "beat Dad at tennis for the first time" (C. A. Whitaker, personal communication, 1979). Such stories demonstrate to demoralized clients that personal authority and self-respect evolve over time and are always difficult to achieve. Teaching stories have been adopted extensively by narrative therapists as a central technique of change in the past decade (Roberts, 1994).

"Therapeutic metaphors," in contrast to teaching stories, are less narrative. They involve creating pictures or scenarios of change, with rich descriptive phrases. Personal metaphors also carry the weight of deep emotion. For example, one of my favorite metaphors, loosely adapted from Ernest Hemingway, is that "life breaks everyone—and afterward, we can come out stronger in the broken places." Therapeutic metaphor is a central technique of symbolic-experiential family therapy (Whitaker & Keith, 1981). A more recent use of therapeutic metaphor, developed in systemic therapies, is the creation of therapy metaphors using the words of both therapist and client drawn from events in the therapy. For example, one couple in treatment for a sexual dysfunction came to realize that the husband hid his desire out of fear that he did not deserve his wife. The husband used certain words to describe his problem, such as "loneliness," "needing to be strong," and "hiding." The therapist referred to the husband's "strong suit of armor," which hid deep loneliness and sad memories, and the couple then used this metaphor whenever a problem of distancing occurred.†

† *This is similar to the types of collaborative examples used by cognitive-behavioral therapists who are attempting to help members of couples think on the same wavelength. This type of collaborative definition is important in developing cohesiveness in a relationship.*

Use of self, whether in teaching stories, personal metaphors, personal observations, or associations within the session, mimics the process of emotional identification that ordinarily goes on in marriages and families. Such expressive talk is much more intimate than other types of conversation. Memorable and evocative images add momentum to a treatment plan and move the heart.

TAKING MATTERS INTO HER OWN HANDS

As summer approached—the second summer in our therapy relationship—Katherine shifted her attitude toward her parents and in-laws. She suddenly began to see the rigidity of her father-in-law's religious life, as well as the disadvantages that her mother and stepmother suffered by not having gotten a college education. It was as if all my comments, and all the dialogues in my office, were emerging from a place within her that had been invisibly storing them up. She told Timothy that she wanted to resume individual meetings with me and to invite him along only when marital decisions were necessary. She also found an apartment about half an hour away from their old home, nearer to the university. Katherine was surprised to see that when she took more initiative, Timothy agreed enthusiastically. He, in turn, became more attentive as Katherine took action to create a home away from relatives.

Katherine began to revisit the issue of whether to return to school to complete her degree. Because I was unwilling to step in as the advisor (part of the old pattern in Katherine's relationships), I assumed a listening position as she debated the pros and cons of conceiving a child in the spring versus planning a second year of college. It was difficult to watch this bright young woman juggle her future with such ambivalence, since she seemed to keep shortchanging the education side of the equation. I was tempted to give her advice leading her toward finishing her education. However, I knew that the only right answer for Katherine's future would be the answer she came to herself. As I often do in later-stage therapy, I shared with her part of my thinking, posing the question of whether people need both family and meaningful work. Although Katherine struggled over this concept, she seemed to gain self-respect and confidence as she considered both possibilities more seriously. She did not collapse into helplessness this time.†

†*A possible exercise for reinforcing this new change might have been to review the new internal dialogue that Katherine was using to fortify her disposition. A common cognitive-behavioral inquiry is to ask, "What are you saying to yourself that has allowed you to change your disposition in this matter? And, most importantly, how much do you believe in what you are telling yourself?"*

Katherine was able to explore her decision that fall by talking with her husband as an equal instead of asking for his approval. Timothy, who'd previously acted insensitive and self-righteous, showed increasing respect for her new thoughtfulness. Katherine was amazed that he didn't tell her what to do! However, Timothy's self-righteousness was really quite reactive to her confusion, based partly on his fear that he would have to get all the right answers alone. She now saw, without hearing it from me, that he really did not know any better than she did what was right. She began to make major decisions without criticizing herself or asking permission.

For example, she decided that for the upcoming Christmas holiday she wanted to visit her mother with Timothy, to get to know her mother better and ask her about her early married life. When she approached him, Timothy showed his new responsiveness by putting aside his own traditions and telling Chris that they would not "be home this year for Christmas." Almost casually, Katherine told me just before the holiday that she had not binged or purged for a month. Although she was eating smaller meals, out of anxiety over her weight, she was maintaining her weight at 105 pounds. She also informed me that she would be taking classes when she returned after New Year's. When I asked what classes she had chosen, she told me that she had been thinking for some time about the ministry and might pursue training as a Methodist minister. Katherine and I used the occasion of this first long family visit to make several plans. One plan was that she would continue to ally herself with her brother, talk to him about her self-esteem problems following their parents' divorce, and ask for more time with him. A second plan was that Katherine would find out more about her mother's experience of her own distant marriage and bitter divorce.†

†*Dr. Roberto used a common strategy here—one that is implemented also by cognitive-behavioral therapists who are helping patients to reframe their recollections and beliefs about events that occurred within their families of origin. Cognitive-behavioral theory contends that often schemas are developed in part from information that is passed down either directly or in more subtle fashions through families of origin. These, combined with individuals' own personal life experience, constitute how they view themselves, their world, and in this case their intimate relationships.*

When Katherine returned after that New Year's, she told me that she had asked her mother many questions: why she had chosen a volatile husband like her father, how the divorce occurred, and why her mother had allowed her father to act violent in the house without taking her and her brother away. She learned that although her mother was a "social butterfly" on the surface, she too had low self-esteem. Her mother told Katherine how her own parents had passed her over in favor of an elder brother who "they thought had hung the moon and stars." She admitted to Katherine that she had graduated from high school convinced that the only way to get respect was by marrying a successful husband. She also admitted that she had deliberately denied herself a supportive and warm partner, and that she had given up her own interests to "play the wife and mother." Finally, Katherine's mother told her that it had been a mistake not to get job training, which made her feel trapped and unwilling to risk life without a husband to support the family. She hoped that Katherine would do a better job of looking out for herself.†

> †*As a result of the discussion with her mother, Katherine now saw that she had a choice as to how to conduct herself and what role to play in her relationship. She seemed to want to restructure this into her thinking and to develop her own identity in her relationship with Timothy.*

Armed with these confidences, Katherine seemed much stronger on her return. She was not purging at all. I pointed out that Katherine deserved credit for this powerful encouragement from her mother, because she had chosen to make the trip and to ask about long-hidden family problems. After this session, I used the metaphor of "playing the wife and mother" whenever Katherine criticized herself for putting off pregnancy or for setting personal goals that differed from the family's. I also encouraged Katherine to go to her father and stepmother at this point, armed with her new self-confidence, and let them know that she had harbored fears of being unwanted since her parents' divorce.†

> †*From a cognitive-behavioral standpoint, this might have been an excellent opportunity for Katherine to challenge some of her distorted beliefs or expectations by gathering new information about her father's and stepmother's anticipated reactions. Depending on what she encountered, this might have aided her in restructuring some of her automatic thoughts, and thus in changing her schemas about herself and her current situation.*

Katherine contacted her father during the spring semester in a most interesting way. She waited until Timothy came to her about a paper he needed to write for law school about real estate. Since Katherine's father worked in a large real estate corporation, she now used this happenstance to arrange a visit with him and her stepmother. It was as if she felt she needed her husband and his agenda to lean on in order to approach her father face to face. During the visit, she plucked up her courage and told her father about her childhood memories—the household objects smashed, the storming rages, and her sense of abandonment the night he left their home. He apologized. Although he did not show a great deal of affection, Katherine came away heartened by his apology and by the warm reception she had received from her stepmother. The confession, and the apology, seemed to ease a great rift in her soul.

Toward the end of spring semester, she told me that she liked herself and was looking forward to the summer with Timothy. She had remained purge-free since her Christmas vacation, and her weight had gone up in ½-pound increments to 114. Although this was 2 pounds below her target weight, Katherine said she knew what to do: "I'm not afraid of my target weight, and I don't worry about my figure much any more." She stayed busy with schoolwork and several close women friends, visited her father at holidays, and went out with Timothy often. Katherine also acknowledged that she had belittled her own wishes in much the same way that her mother had, and that she now knew that it was an important part of health to give oneself approval rather than seeking it elsewhere. She transferred to a small Methodist seminary in the area to begin her religious training, and managed to communicate to Chris and Timothy that she loved and respected her chosen denomination as they did their own. To her final session of therapy, which she attended with Timothy, she brought a needlepointed plaque she had made that read, "This is the day the Lord has made." As a threesome, we discussed the burdens of being ill and the advantages of being well again, and we wished one another well. Katherine emerged from therapy whole.†

> †*This was a very interesting case, in which many techniques similar to cognitive-behavioral strategies were used. The transgenerational approach that Dr. Roberto describes seems to lend itself well to the use of cognitive-behavioral therapy as a complement to this approach, particularly with regard to restructuring old schemas passed down from the family of origin. It is my distinct impression that the cognitive-behavioral approach would nicely augment the transgenerational approach, especially in cases such as Katherine's.*

AUTHOR'S REPLY TO EDITOR'S COMMENTS

Dr. Dattilio's excellent suggestions about cognitive-behavioral interventions indicate that these can be combined with transgenerational therapy in a generally compatible way. Added to such symptom-modifying techniques, a transgenerational framework allows clients to study themselves in the context of family relationships in a way that has enduring power to transform thought.

A more contextual definition of self not only alters clients' roles and habitual ways of relating, but adds a "meta-" layer of observations that can change the meaning of behaviors in clients' eyes. Contextualizing the meaning of behaviors, both in intimate relationships and toward the self, makes it more possible to weigh them, change them, and make choices in the direction of health.

I do wish to make a specific comment about Dr. Dattilio's remarks on page 262, concerning the possible development of alternative behaviors for food refusal and the like.

At this point in therapy, a client is unlikely to commit to an alternative behavior because the current symptoms are "driven" by underlying relationship pressures (i.e., to be the ill family member). Although finding alternatives to purging is an important short-term goal, transgenerational therapists focus more heavily on the short-term goal of challenging enmeshed and avoidant behaviors with the family. We expect that a later commitment to combat purging will have to go hand in hand with assertive and direct communication.

REFERENCES

Beck, A. T. (1967). *Depression: Clinical, experimental, and theoretical aspects.* New York: Harper & Row.

Boszormenyi-Nagy, I., & Krasner, B. R. (1986). *Between give and take: A critical guide to contextual therapy.* New York: Brunner/Mazel.

Boszormenyi-Nagy, I., & Spark, G. M. (1973). *Invisible loyalties: Reciprocity in intergenerational family therapy.* New York: Brunner/Mazel.

Dattilio, F. M. (1993). Cognitive techniques with couples and families. *The Family Journal, 1*(1), 51–65.

Dattilio, F. M. (1994). Families in crisis. In F. M. Dattilio & A. Freeman (Eds.), *Cognitive-behavioral strategies in crisis interventions* (pp. 278–301). New York: Guilford Press.

Kerr, M. E., & Bowen, M. (1988). *Family evaluation.* New York: Norton.

Napier, A. Y., with Whitaker, C. A. (1978). *The family crucible: The intense experience of family therapy.* New York: Harper & Row.

Paul, N. L. (1970). Parental empathy. In E. J. Anthony & T. Benedek (Eds.), *Parenthood: Its psychology and psychopathology* (pp. 337–352). Boston: Little, Brown.

Paul, N. L. (1982). *The paradoxical nature of the grief experience.* Paper presented at an international conference, Department of Basic Psychoanalytic Research and Family Therapy, University of Heidelberg.

Prince, S. E., & Jacobson, N. S. (1995). A review and evaluation of marital and family therapies for affective disorder. *Journal of Marital and Family Therapy, 21,* 377–401.

Roberto, L. G. (1991). Symbolic-experiential family therapy. In A. S. Gurman & D. P. Kniskern (Eds.), *Handbook of family therapy* (pp. 444–478). New York: Brunner/Mazel.

Roberto, L. G. (1992). *Transgenerational family therapies.* New York: Guilford Press.

Roberts, J. (1994). *Tales and transformations: Stories in families and family therapy*. New York: Norton.

Waters, D. B., & Lawrence, E. C. (1993). *Competence, courage, and change: An approach to family therapy*. New York: Norton.

Whitaker, C. A., & Bumberry, W. M. (1988). *Dancing with the family: A symbolic-experiential approach*. New York: Brunner/Mazel.

Whitaker, C. A., & Keith, D. V. (1981). Symbolic-experiential family therapy. In A. S. Gurman & D. P. Kniskern (Eds.), *Handbook of family therapy* (Vol. 1, pp. 187–226). New York: Brunner/Mazel.

Williamson, D. S. (1981). Personal authority via termination of the intergenerational hierarchical boundary: A "new" stage in the family life cycle. *Journal of Marital and Family Therapy, 7*, 441–452.

Williamson, D. S. (1982). Personal authority in family experience via termination of the intergenerational hierarchical boundary: Part III. Personal authority defined, and the power of play in the change process. *Journal of Marital and Family Therapy, 8*, 309–323.

SUGGESTED READINGS

Boszormenyi-Nagy, I., & Krasner, B. R. (1986). *Between give and take: A critical guide to contextual therapy*. New York: Brunner/Mazel.

Carter, B., & McGoldrick, M. (1988). *The changing family life cycle: A framework for family therapy* (2nd ed.). New York: Gardner Press.

Framo, J. L. (1992). *Family-of-origin therapy: An intergenerational approach*. New York: Brunner/Mazel.

Kerr, M. E., & Bowen, M. (1988). *Family evaluation*. New York: Norton.

McGoldrick, M. (1995). *You can go home again*. New York: Norton.

Napier, A. Y., with Whitaker, C. A. (1978). *The family crucible: The intense experience of family therapy*. New York: Harper & Row.

Roberto, L. G. (1986). Bulimia: The transgenerational view. *Journal of Marital and Family Therapy, 12*, 231–240.

Roberto, L. G. (1992). *Transgenerational family therapies*. New York: Guilford Press.

Whitaker, C. A., & Ryan, M. O. (1989). *Midnight musings of a family therapist*. New York: Norton.

Chapter 12

Cross-Cultural Couple Therapy

PAULA HANSON-KAHN
LUCIANO L'ABATE

The purpose of this chapter is to show how an Asian husband and wife were (and are still being) treated in their native language by one of us (Paula Hanson-Kahn) under the supervision of the other (Luciano L'Abate). This example suggests how important it is to know about the culture as well as the language of individuals, couples, and families who seek professional psychological help. It would have been impossible to conduct therapy in English with this couple because of the limited language skills of the identified patient, the husband. Even though his wife was more fluent in English, the nuances of the identified patient's thinking would have been completely lost.

The therapeutic approach used with this couple consisted of a combination of straightforward and paradoxical techniques. Once the straightforward techniques (directives, homework assignments, rehearsals, and suggestions) used from the outset of therapy were found to be both futile and frustrating to the couple and to the therapist, it was necessary to switch to more paradoxical techniques, such as positive interpretation of the symptomatic behavior, prescription of the symptom, a "one-down" position for the therapist, and prescription of no change (Weeks & L'Abate, 1982). This therapeutic approach took place (and is still taking place) within the context and confines of a relational and contextual theory of interpersonal competence that makes the family the primary and most salient context for personality socialization (L'Abate, 1986, 1994; L'Abate & Baggett, 1997, in preparation). Links between the theory and the course of therapy from the viewpoint of this theory are considered at the end of this chapter.

CASE EXAMPLE

This couple voluntarily signed an informed consent form for us to discuss this case here, provided it was sufficiently disguised to guarantee anonymity.

Background

The couple was referred by a local psychiatric hospital for outpatient aftercare at the time of the identified patient's discharge from a 2-week voluntary hospitalization. The husband, the identified patient, named K. C., was a 42-year-old Asian male who had lived in the United States ever since his parents' immigration 20 years earlier. He completed high school in his country of origin, but admitted that he was never a good student. For most of his working life, he had been employed in his family's business. Despite lengthy residence in the United States, he hardly understood or spoke any English. He lived with his wife, Pat, who was 40 years old; their home was not far from his parents' home and only a short distance from the business. Five years after coming to the United States, K. C. returned to his native land to marry his former neighbor and elementary schoolmate, Pat, with whom he had kept in touch through letters, telephone calls, and several visits to his country of origin. They had no children because of K. C.'s low sperm count. They eventually decided against adoption as well as against artificial insemination.

After their wedding, the couple lived apart for 4 years. K. C. returned to his job in his father's business, while Pat continued living with her mother while they worked on her immigration papers. On their fourth wedding anniversary, she finally flew to the United States, clutching the long-awaited immigration visa in her hand. During those weeks and up to the day prior to her arrival in the United States, there were many trans-Pacific telephone conversations full of happy, exciting plans between the couple. Pat was looking forward to beginning her married life.

Upon her arrival, Pat was met by a sister-in-law who informed her that K. C. had just attempted suicide by setting himself aflame after dousing himself with gasoline at a local filling station. Pat dismissed this as a joke in very poor taste until she was taken to the hospital, where K. C. was being treated for third-degree burns. It was subsequently assumed, from his few responses to his siblings' many questions, that K. C. had tried to kill himself because he was afraid that he might give his wife a sexually transmitted disease. Subsequent medical tests found no such disease, and the matter was never mentioned again.

Five years after Pat's arrival in the United States, the couple borrowed capital from family and friends (both locally and abroad) to start their own business, but the business failed. After 1 year, the couple returned to work for K. C.'s father in semimanagerial (K. C.) and clerical (Pat) positions. Ten years later, the couple had almost paid off the debt from this business loss. It was at this point K. C. started again to make ambitious plans.

Presenting Problem

Three months before his hospitalization, K. C. became obsessed with the notion that the Asian community in the United States should be more cohesive, and that Asian businesses in particular should be more cooperative. Their business was and is intensely competitive and at times cutthroat; family members can slave away for up to 80 hours a week to make a meager income. In their business, competitors are known to call the Immigration and Naturalization Service if there is the possibility of illegal immigrants on the premises, or even to set fire to a competitor's establishment. Asian gangs sometimes extort money from businesses as payoffs to prevent unpleasant consequences. K. C. complained bitterly about the price-cutting practices he said Asian business owners were employing against each other. He also criticized U.S. immigration laws for being too lax. K. C. felt that these laws should be tightened to "keep out social parasites" to insure the continued growth of the U.S. economy. Beset by these concerns, he wrote many articles promulgating tighter immigration rules for "quality control," as well as Asian unity and cooperation for mutual benefit. He kept extensive files of all articles and editorials he found on these themes, and he submitted some of his own writings to Asian newspapers both locally and in his country of origin. Even though there was no indication of any of these writings' being accepted for publication, they grew in fervor and profusion. His zeal for the project grew to such a pitch that he was staying up all night to write, despite his working at the family business till nearly midnight 6 days a week.

Highly energized by these expectations, K. C. compiled an impressive dossier of his writings and news clippings as the basis for his proposal for an ambitious "New Asia Town" development. He took several days off from work in order to present his proposal to meetings of Asian civic groups and to potential investors among leaders of the local Asian community. The response was not encouraging. Deflated at last, K. C. discarded his project and became his usual taciturn self; over the next few days, he alternated between locking himself in his room and disappearing for the whole day. He lost his energy, and with it all apparent interest in anything. He felt humiliated. He made such comments to Pat as "I've lost my confidence," "I'm a big loser in the eyes of others," and "I feel like I'm dying." He also fretted about his father's upcoming birthday dinner, which he was reluctant to attend. He complained to Pat that he was feeling restless and distraught. It appeared to calm him when Pat agreed to attend the birthday dinner alone and make excuses for him. (His extended family, incidentally, was glad that he was "finally over his crazy phase," as various family members had made unsuccessful attempts to discourage him from badgering people about his ideas.)

Despite her acquiescence to his decision regarding his father's birthday celebration, Pat was surprised to see K. C. getting dressed for the occasion. When asked, he answered, "I might as well go." Again she acquiesced. At the birthday dinner, surrounded by his large three-generational family, Pat noted that K. C. didn't utter a single word to anyone the entire evening, not even to wish his father "Happy Birthday." Fearing that he might become more agitated and disturbed, she began their leavetaking as soon as the birthday song was sung and the cake had been cut.

K. C. did not appear to be disturbed in any way when he retired for the night. The following morning, Pat awoke first. After getting dressed, she woke K. C. with the remark that she was going downstairs to make breakfast. He answered, "Come here and let me give you a kiss." She sat down again on her side of the bed and leaned back toward her husband. To her horror, she felt his hands around her throat strangling her. On the verge of passing out, she managed a gurgled plea, whereupon K. C. loosened his grip momentarily. That momentary lapse was sufficient for her to twist her body to grab the metal alarm clock from the night stand. With the little strength she had left, she clubbed him over the head with it. Stunned by the blow, K. C. released her. She jumped off the bed beyond his reach, and stood up to adjust her clothes while he attempted in vain to grasp her. When he failed, he then covered his face with his arms.

Pat left K. C. in the bedroom; still in shock, she went downstairs to the kitchen to make tea. However, as soon as she reached the kitchen, she began to feel dizzy and to have blurred vision and severe pain in her eyes. She telephoned her brother-in-law, trying to convince him that this incident was real and that he should inform his father. After 15 minutes without any contact from her in-laws, Pat decided that her brother-in-law must not have believed her. Pat decided to call her father-in-law herself. When he answered the telephone, Pat asked if he had "heard anything" and he answered in the affirmative, whereupon she burst into tears and told him she needed to go to a doctor. He promised to be there in a few minutes.

While Pat was waiting for her father-in-law, K. C. came downstairs. He was dressed. He did not look at or say anything to her. When he reached for the car keys hanging on the hook, she asked him where he was going. She objected to his leaving on the ground that she was feeling sick and needed to go to the doctor. (She reported later that she was dimly aware of the need not to let him go out on his own at that point.) K. C. looked at her for the first time, and what he saw convinced him. Unbeknownst to herself, Pat's eyes were bloody and bulging. K. C. helped her into the car and drove to the doctor's. When they arrived, he told her to go in on her own. Pat insisted that he accompany her, as she was unable to make it on her own. K. C. reluctantly agreed.

After 2 minutes in the waiting room, K. C. became agitated and said that he couldn't wait. He got up and left. Pat followed him and got into the car with him. He drove around the neighborhood for a bit, and Pat began to be afraid. She asked again to be taken to the doctor, whereupon K. C. immediately stopped the car about four blocks away from the doctor's office and insisted that she walk to the doctor's clinic on her own. He seemed quite serious and started shoving her. Pat got out of the car, walking the four blocks to the clinic, where it was discovered that she had burst capillaries in both eyes and bruises on her neck. The doctor indicated that if K. C. did not see a mental health professional immediately, he was going to have to report the assault to the police.

Pat's father- and brother-in-law picked her up from the clinic and spent a couple of hours cruising the area in an attempt to find K. C. When all efforts failed, they decided to return to the house to wait for him. They were surprised and relieved to find him home and apparently calm. Upon his family's insistence and the doctor's ultimatum, K. C. agreed to see a counselor at the local psychiatric hospital 2 days later, where he was admitted for inpatient treatment and given a diagnosis of major depression with psychotic features. Because of his poor English, he was able to communicate with the hospital staff only through his wife or through one of his siblings during his 2 weeks in the hospital. He was lethargic and unresponsive; he had trouble answering direct questions, and his answers were vague and at times irrelevant. His condition was stabilized through the use of medication. After 2 weeks he was discharged for outpatient psychotherapy. The discharge diagnosis was atypical psychosis.

Individual, Family, and Social Context

"A man of very few words," K. C. was known to have hardly any friends. Pat recalled that he was not one for conversation, except during times of excitement such as that surrounding the "New Asia Town" project. He would go for months without saying a word to anybody, except for such exchanges as might be essential in the course of their restaurant business. Occasionally, when he was "in a really good mood," he would chat with his wife. He was in the habit of reading many Asian newspapers, magazines, and books. He would make an almost daily trip to the Asian news agency or bookstore and return with the papers, magazines, and a few books each time, even if he still had unread books at home. He had no other hobbies or interests.

K. C. was the oldest of five children and one of three sons. His father, Kao (71 years old) had immigrated to the United States with his entire family 20 years earlier, as noted above. Kao was minimally educated; his wife of 47 years, Fei, a 66-year-old housewife, was totally uneducated, but with strong and loud opinions about how the business should be run and how to play her favorite game of cards. Her dominance was in sharp contrast to her husband's passivity and subservience to her opinions and wishes. Kao started their small family business when he first came to the United States. Although the three younger children (including the two younger sons) were given opportunities for technical, high school, and college education, respectively, the five children worked in the family's business. The business survived despite its small size and its less-than-ideal location, due in part to some regular Asian patrons who remained loyal to them, especially for their tendency to talk in the same dialect used by the family and their ties to the common province in their country of origin.

Kao was described by both K. C. and Pat as "a man of few words," like K. C., himself. Pat remembered how it took her some time to get used to the lack of conversation between K. C. and his father. Both K. C. and Pat indicated that Kao was that way with all his children except for Yue (aged 32), his fifth child and middle son, who was an accountant. Yue was the first in the family to make something of himself; conversely, the youngest daughter (aged 22) had dropped out of college after her sophomore year, moved away, and shunned all contact with the family for about a year. Sibling rivalry was denied by both K. C. and Pat. However, both recalled with resentment in their words and voices that although Kao expressed appreciation at the time, he did not subsequently wear the $100 sandals they had given him for his birthday, but Yue was often seen wearing them. When asked whether he had found the style, fit, or color unsuitable to him, Kao had assured Pat that everything was just fine. When asked how they felt about Kao's giving their costly gift to Yue, the couple denied any resentment.

When asked about the communication between himself and his father, K. C. denied that there was any problem. Pat disputed that denial by describing an incident that left a very deep impression on her. K. C. had a minor disagreement with Kao about the business a couple of weeks prior to his father's birthday. Subsequently, in conversation with an elderly Asian neighbor (a man about Kao's age), K. C. broke down and wept uncontrollably, complaining that "the old man does not understand me." Pat was quite struck by the incident because in all their 15 years of marriage, she had never before known her husband to cry even in private, much less in front of somebody outside the family.

Pat and K. C. indicated that they had different values from K. C.'s parents and often "got into trouble" with them because of these differences. On several occasions, K. C. had thrown away materials that, though not exactly outdated, were nevertheless irrelevant to the present business. His parents had been violently angry at what they considered his lack of common sense and business acumen. They contended that most of their customers would not have even noticed the outdatedness of these materials. Pat confessed that K. C., and occasionally she herself, had nevertheless continued discarding materials when they were no longer relevant, except that they now took great care not to get caught. On the occasions when they were caught, they were soundly scolded. Still, the couple agreed that despite his parents' displeasure, it was better to have a smaller profit margin in order to give their customers good-quality materials and insure their loyalty. They also felt strongly that to do otherwise would be dishonest, and, in the long haul, unwise.

Fei was described as an obese, loud-mouthed, irritable dowager who ruled the roost with her ready and acid tongue, lashing out at members of the family when anything even minimally diminished her sense of well-being. She had a gambling addiction, which she vociferously denied, on the grounds that "having lived such a hard life," it was her "right to have some pleasure in life." She made frequent trips to a nearby casino city to lose substantial sums of their hard-earned money, and hosted weekly high-stakes, all-night mah-jongg games in her home. She glibly applies the same argument about "her right to enjoyment in life" when resisting the family's efforts to help her comply with the dietary restrictions necessitated by her diabetes.

Pat described a recent occasion several months ago when K. C. had gently urged Fei not to make such frequent trips to the casino, since she often lost large sums of money. Her harsh response was "You wretched son, why do you presume to deprive me of my enjoyment of life when it's not your money I gamble with!" She similarly asserted her rights whenever she was reminded to cut down on her sugar intake. Pat indicated with a mixture of pride and exasperation in her voice that K. C. was the only person who was still "pig-headed enough" to venture to say anything about her lack of discipline in her diet; everybody else had learned to leave her to her own devices.

Pat observed ruefully that as the wife of the eldest son, she was the designated bearer of all blame insofar as her mother-in-law was concerned. It was her fault that K. C. was not doing well and that he was not recovering quickly; she was also blamed for whatever Fei happened to be upset about at any given moment.

K. C. usually did not talk to his brothers and sisters or their spouses at all. Apart from birthday presents for his parents, the only other expressions of affection consisted of gifts for the nieces and nephews at Christmas ("a nice fashion we picked up from the Westerners") and auspicious red envelopes containing money, mandated by Asian tradition for the same nieces and nephews on the lunar New Year's Day. Bright and early on the morning of the latter occasion, K. C. and Pat would go as required by tradition to his parents' house, and, kneeling before them, would formally deliver the usual ceremonial New Year's greetings. In return, they would each receive a formal blessing as well as a substantial red envelope with money. This was their extent of any exchange of affection with other members of the family. Intimacy was foreign to them, save in the most limited conjugal physical sense.

The basic tenet of this family seemed to be that life is about winning or losing; if there is no advantage to oneself or one's immediate family, then action is irrelevant. A brother-in-law suggested that K. C. had tried to strangle Pat in order to benefit from her life insurance. Various members of the family decried K. C.'s psychotherapy as a waste of money and a "loss of face." In the words of his mother, K. C. needed to just "snap out of it and buckle down to life" and quit being such a damper on the family's sense of well-being. Pat revealed that on several occasions when K. C. had been out of earshot, Fei had expressed her resentment against K. C. for being "afflicted with his condition."

Pat, by contrast, came from a more close-knit family. The oldest of three daughters of a widowed mother, Pat spoke very warmly of her own family of origin. Her mother, aged 70, was in ill health, having suffered from tuberculosis for years. Pat telephoned her mother and one of her sisters at least once every other week. She also talked to her other sister, who was living in another part of the United States, weekly. Every other year, Pat returned to her country of origin in Asia for a 2-week stay with her mother. K. C. never accompanied her, since he had to work at the business. Pat admitted that the pleasure of each of her trips to the home country was lessened by the recurring thought that it might be the very last time she saw her mother alive. Pat's eyes filled with tears whenever she considered this eventuality: "I love my mother more than anything in the world, and the thought of her dying just makes me very sad. I hope she lives for a long time so I can keep showing her my filial piety." She derived great strength and emotional support from these regular contacts with her family, as well as a small handful of friends and classmates, with whom she still maintained regular if somewhat limited contact. She recalled how K. C. used to derive much vicarious pleasure from all such contacts of hers. Although he would not talk to her mother, sisters, or friends himself, he would eagerly pump her for a full and detailed report of everything that was said. He wanted to hear every scrap of news or gossip. Pat admitted becoming impatient with him at times, because he would keep pestering her for more details when she had told him everything that had transpired: "But what were you laughing about just now?"

Whenever Pat compared her family with K. C.'s, her husband would declare that his family was just fine. He would say that they did care about each other and that their communication was all right, but not frequent. Pat disputed this denial by pointing out how he coveted the obvious intimacy between his third sister's husband and the latter's father: "That father-and-son duo are always so happy to see each other. They hug whenever they get together even after a brief absence, and they can talk about everything under the sun."

Treatment Goals and Therapeutic Plan

Among the goals that we (the therapist and supervisor) developed were the following: (1) reduction of risks for any suicidal or homicidal behavior; (2)

stabilization and improvement of K. C.'s mood (with a reduction of his depression, particularly his hopelessness and helplessness, and his anxiety, particularly his restlessness, agitation, and inability to concentrate); (3) reorganization and reintegration of K. C.'s thinking, feeling, and behavior; (4) improvement in K. C.'s sense of self—self-understanding, self-esteem, and self-agency; (5) improvement in his interpersonal relationships, especially the expression and experience of intimacy in the marital relationship, and renegotiation of relationships with his father, mother, and other members of his family; (6) development of realistic occupational goals; and (7) improvement in the couple's social life (e.g., enlarging the number of friends outside the family, and expanding leisure-time activities to include more active pursuits than just window shopping). To decrease the complexity of so many goals for the couple, only the most concrete and immediate goals were presented and discussed with the couple—namely, the first, second, and third. The other goals were seen as being farther down the line of treatment.

The couple agreed to meet weekly for supportive–expressive psychotherapy. (Later in the treatment, sessions were held every other week, because without health insurance the couple was paying the therapist out of pocket.) Treatment was directed at (1) helping K. C. confront his denial in various areas; (2) exploring the history of K. C.'s suicidal/homicidal ideation, intent, and attempts, and securing a suicide/homicide contract; (3) examining K. C.'s core conflictual relationships (father? mother? siblings?); (4) helping K. C. develop a stronger sense of self; (5) guiding both clients into the dialogue of feelings; and, therefore, (6) developing relational intimacy, especially within the marriage.

Treatment Process

The First Part of Treatment: Straightforward Interventions

Part of treatment was continuing cooperation and contact with a psychiatrist, who at different times administered a whole armamentarium of medications (sertraline, amitriptyline, fluoxetine, trifluoperazine, benztropine, and alprazolam). In the psychotherapy, treatment was hindered by K. C.'s initial reluctance to talk to or even look at the therapist. Consequently, most of the therapeutic discourse took place through Pat, at least initially.

The extended family (the father, mother, and one brother) were seen only once. They made it clear that they saw K. C.'s problems as not having anything to do with them. They were not interested in seeing the therapist again, since they believed that nothing useful would come out of it. Eventually K. C. started to become more open, even though treatment could be characterized as a continual approach–avoidance dance, coming and going. K. C. usually failed to admit to his own denial; his moods would vary from being completely unresponsive to being agitated and restless. He would question the need for psychotherapy and would not perform any homework assignment given to the couple, as discussed later.

This resistance was seen as an expression of oppositionality that colored most of K. C.'s responses. If he was supposed or even required to talk, then he would not talk. If he was required to do something, even having to go to work every day, then he would not go. If he had to attend his father's birthday party, then he would not go (in this instance, he only reversed himself at the last minute, bowing to external pressures from his family). Hence, again, most of the treatment (at least during the first half of the process, lasting at least 6 months) consisted of the therapist's talking with Pat, and only occasionally and very briefly of K. C.'s participation. Sessions were held in a clinic located in the basement of a church located in the midst of a mostly Asian community.

As therapy went on, it became more evident that K. C. was subject to a continual pattern of discounting—not only from his wife, who became more and more manipulative, but also from his family. During the one family session, for instance, he was rarely given a chance to talk; when he did, either his father, mother, or brother would disagree with him and put down whatever he had said as being either irrelevant or unimportant. His wife, on the other hand, suggested that K. C. said whatever was most expedient to say at the moment. For instance, during one marital session when he appeared agitated and confused, the therapist suggested that he should see the psychiatrist for changes in the medication. He refused to go, but when the therapist called the psychiatrist on the phone to report on his obvious restlessness and agitation, Pat prodded him to say whatever it was necessary to get the psychiatrist "off his back."†

> † At this point, the therapist could have inquired into K. C.'s automatic thoughts and his conceptualization of the therapist's role in helping him. From a cognitive-behavioral standpoint, it would have been important to understand why K. C. wanted to get the psychiatrist "off his back."

The major pattern of coping for K. C. was direct and immediate denial of any unpleasantness or painfulness. For instance, even if he was obviously agitated and upset, he would deny it. The second pattern was an inconsistent and persistent pattern of going from one absolute or extreme way of thinking to the other extreme (e.g., from black to white, from true to false, from right to wrong). As a result, therapy was difficult because he would go from one extreme of feeling "good" to the other of feeling "bad." At the beginning of therapy, K. C. was refusing his meals, just lying in bed or on the couch all day long, apart from the few hours a week that he would work.

Pat reported (when K. C. was asked) that he had been unable to follow the therapist's suggestions from the first session (regular marital meetings, completion of written homework assignments, regular intake of medication). He had shown some improvement by working an entire shift (4 hours of continuous stir-fry!) the day after his first therapy session, but he had been restless and lethargic the rest of the week. He worked 1 hour on two subsequent days and 2 hours on another day (after his wife had reacted to his refusal to work by saying that she was also going to stay home). His response to her telling him to go to work with her was "Don't push me."†

> † *Once again, it might have been extremely helpful to follow an affective response by inquiring into K. C.'s cognitions regarding his wife's "pushiness." In examining what thoughts were going through his mind, the therapist might have been able to uncover K. C.'s schemas about his relationship with his wife and others, and then to explore with K. C. whether or not his perceptions were distorted.*

Pat and K. C. had planned to go window shopping (a pasttime they had previously enjoyed together on a weekly basis) instead of working one day, but on their way out of the house, he said, "It's dangerous out there. . . . I am afraid of what I might do. . . . It was safe in the hospital," whereupon his wife asked if she should call his psychiatrist. He responded, "No, let me see the therapist first." Instead of going out that day, he slept the whole day and through that night.

During a directed "sharing of hurts" exercise (L'Abate & Baggett, 1997), consisting of the partners' closing their eyes, holding each other's hands, concentrating on their hurts, and expressing the feelings of hurt kept inside ("I hurt"), Pat reported that she felt pain whenever she returned to her country for her 2-week visit with her mother because she had to leave again. K. C. insisted that he could not think of any pain. After several minutes, his wife pointed out that he could be a very emotional person, such as when he wept bitterly at the grand opening of a local Asian hotel. At this point, he reported suicidal ideation (jumping off some building or throwing himself in front of an oncoming train). A "suicide contract" was then negotiated and agreed upon with K. C.†

> † *This might have been a perfect time to introduce the Dysfunctional Thought Record (see Chapter 1), as well as some depression and suicide inventories, such as the Beck Depression Inventory, the Beck Hopelessness Scale, and the Beck Suicide Scale (again, see Chapter 1). These inventories were designed not only to provide a clinician with an index measure of a client's level of distress, but also to provide insight into the sequence of the client's thinking and, more importantly, the way the client's thinking affects his or her moods.*

Later, Pat called in a panic because K. C. had taken a slight overdose of his medication (trifluoperazine and benztropine). When confronted, he said that he was only trying to feel better. When the psychiatrist was consulted on this matter, he said that this dosage was nonlethal. Pat, however, was advised by the therapist to remove the medication from easy access when K. C. was home alone. Over many therapy sessions, the importance of communication and the need to be proactive in this area and other areas were discussed. The therapist also suggested that weekly family meetings might be held. Pat objected strongly to this suggestion: "It cannot be done—K. C.'s mom and sister go regularly to [the casino city] to gamble. Any mention of their missing a weekend is met with obstreperous chastisement and/or very rude rebuttals." Other possible ways to communicate with family members were suggested, but Pat remained loudly unconvinced. K. C. remained silent, appearing thoughtful.

On another occasion, the therapist assigned both partners to write down a list of all the hurts and traumas they had ever experienced, as far back as they could recall. They were instructed to set an appointed time each day and write for 15 minutes each day for 4 days in a row (Pennebaker, 1990). Both K. C. and Pat failed to follow through with this and other written homework assignments. "We have no time or are too tired. We are not the kind of people who write very much," according to Pat. In spite of this resistance, a definite time was set up with the couple for completing written homework assignments, in addition, a daily behavioral chart was agreed upon by both partners.† These efforts, however, met only with further resistance.

> † *Charts such as these are usually very helpful in order to monitor daily activities and to introduce behavioral exercises. K. C. apparently required a great deal of structure in his life. Perhaps the chart would also have served to engage him and his wife in a conjoint exercise on a daily basis.*

Gradually, however, K. C. began to appear more alert. His eyes were more open and less dull; he made more eye contact with the therapist; he preceded his wife into the therapist's office instead of trailing way behind her; and his speech became less restricted. As therapy went on, K. C. started to volunteer some information about his own state of mind: "I feel very tense, a great tightness in my head like a headache. . . . I feel myself to be very frail. . . . I feel fearful, lacking in confidence, and anxious about everything." He reported that he had been this way for 2 weeks now, and that it was getting worse: "I feel so tense and anxious I wish I were dead."†

> † *If K. C. could have been persuaded to use the Dysfunctional Thought Record, the therapist would have had a daily monitoring of his moods and distorted thoughts. This might also have been a good time to have him begin to weigh some of the alternative modes of thinking as introduced in Chapter 1.*

Pat reported that K. C.'s emotions were improving slowly. He was now working steadily, despite bouts of intense agitation. When informed of the agitation, the psychiatrist added alprazolam (0.5 mg), to K. C.'s medication. Despite this reported and observed symptom, K. C. was less withdrawn, brighter in countenance, more open in expression, and less flat in affect. However, when asked about the noticeable trembling of his hands and knees (especially the very marked tremors of his right hand), he looked at his limbs but denied seeing any tremors.

During one session, the therapist guided K. C. through some breathing and relaxation exercises, at the end of which he claimed that he was not helped to relax. Pat reported that K. C.'s father intended to engage some Asian Taoist monks to exorcise demons from K. C. K. C. indicated that he did not believe in demon possession and did not wish to be subjected to such proceedings. At the therapist's suggestion, K. C. agreed to communicate his position to his father. Pat volunteered that communication between K. C. and his father had improved, since both parties had begun taking the initiative to begin conversation unrelated to their business.

K. C. had also been eating better since Pat had begun making nutritious soups each night for his consumption the following morning. However, he still refused to eat the dinners that his mother prepared each evening for the family. His mother still cooked each day for the family members who worked at the family business. When asked whether he would eat dinner if Pat cooked it for him, K. C. nodded and answered, "Yes." Pat laughingly objected: "I would have a hard time persuading him to eat my cooking if he would not eat his mom's cooking. She's a very good cook, and I cannot cook at all!" Asked if that was the case, K. C. shook his head vigorously "No." Asked whether he was certain he would eat dinner cooked by Pat, he nodded distinctly "Yes." It was suggested that Pat try cooking for the two of them.

When the therapist tried to explore how his family expressed intimacy, K. C. answered, "Don't know." When he was pushed for specifics, he responded, "By being filial, by respecting them," but admitted that he and his parents had "nothing to talk about, unlike my third sister's husband and his dad." As far as his siblings were concerned, annual Christmas gifts for each nephew or niece to those siblings with children was enough intimacy, as noted earlier. In regard to intimacy with his wife, he responded, "Holding hands, hug, sex," but did not mention verbal communication.

Pat elaborated that K. C.'s mother was harsh in both her words and her tone. Also, since she was uneducated, she had very few topics of conversation. "She likes folks to talk to her, but there is no subject on which you can really hold any conversation with her. Also, she is often unintentionally hurtful in her speech but is generally unaware of it." Asked how he dealt with his mother's hurtful speech, K. C. answered, "Tell myself she's not educated."†

† *Obviously, a characteristic that had trickled down for several generations in K. C.'s family was the use of nonverbal communication. In many ways, K. C. was operating within the tradition that was established in his family of origin. His schema about communication within the family was being upheld. Interestingly, K. C. was already using a technique known as "internal dialogue" when he accounted for the sharpness of his mother's words by telling himself that "she's not educated." This apparently mediated his emotions successfully, at least in this situation. This leaves me wondering whether he could have applied the same technique elsewhere.*

The therapist discussed sharing "hurts and joys" as a means to intimacy, closeness, and wholeness. She then said, "Since you have not done your homework, we are going to do it now. Write down all your hurts." The couple wrote for 10 minutes, K. C. very reluctantly. Pat shared her "dislike of living in the U.S., sadness at seeing mother's failing health, feeling like the end of the world to witness K. C. becoming sick and yet my surviving [his attack]." K. C. wrote: "Since childhood, father's going overseas to work long distance because of infrequent contact. A three-foot iceberg is not the result of a single night's frost; family problems are usually a result of accumulation of small things." The therapist complimented him on this conclusion.

Despite their failure to cooperate with homework assignments, K. C. was displaying further evidence of improvement. In addition to appearing more alert and maintaining eye contact, he initiated greetings at the beginning of sessions, and muttered thanks and good-byes when leaving. His wife reported evidence of his progress at home and in his workplace. He even initiated conversation with his parents from time to time. Nevertheless, despite the therapist's observations (at times communicated to him in congratulation), and despite his wife's narrating all the signs of his progress in his presence, K. C. consistently reported that he was not getting better: "Very moody and depressed," "Absolutely no self-confidence to do anything."†

† *Perhaps at this point a daily activity schedule might have been helpful if someone could have gotten K. C. to use it. It appeared that the less he did, the more withdrawn and depressed he became.*

At this point in treatment, the therapist was hospitalized for an emergency operation, and a couple of sessions had to be canceled. Upon the therapist's return, Pat reported that K. C. had felt such frustration one day that he had raised his fists and said he wanted to hit her. Although he did not touch her, the family members had held a meeting, with his knowledge but not with his participation. After he had calmed down from his emotional outburst, K. C. had wanted his family to admit him to the hospital, where he felt "safer," but his mother and a brother had dissuaded him. During the family meeting, one of his brothers-in-law (a sister's husband) had erupted: "We should just lock him up. Then there will be less hassles for the rest of us." K. C.'s youngest sister had earnestly suggested to Pat, "Since this outburst, Eldest Brother appeared to feel that being married to you is so stressful. Why don't you go ahead and leave him and run away?" Her idea, ostensibly, was for her parents (Pat's in-laws) to shelter Pat and keep the fact from K. C., so that he might realize he could not do without Pat. Pat declared that she could not bring herself to do it because she was afraid that K. C. might take his own life if he thought she had left him. When Pat described all of this in the session, K. C. showed no indication of any emotion, even though it was apparently the first time he was privy to the proceedings of that meeting.

K. C. had admitted suicidal ideation to Pat when she questioned him, and K. C. now admitted to the therapist that he was still entertaining suicidal thoughts. He was reminded of the "suicide contract" he had previously signed.†

> † *This idea of a contract against any suicidal gestures or behaviors is an excellent idea. However, K. C. needed some cognitive-behavioral tools to utilize while dealing with his depression and suicidal thoughts. Even though K. C. appeared to be extremely resistant to interventions, he might still have felt "safer," as he would say, if such techniques as thought stopping or a mechanism for weighing alternatives had been made available to him.*

K. C. was also required to see his psychiatrist immediately. He refused, saying that all he needed was for the therapist to tell his wife and parents that he "needed to rest from work at home for 2 days." Pat objected strongly, saying that all he would be doing for the 2 days would be to "lie on the sofa and shut his eyes tightly until he gets fed at mealtimes." K. C. became agitated and burst out, "You are forcing me, putting too much pressure on me!" He was obviously angry—stomping his feet, raising his voice, and glaring at his wife, while refusing eye contact with the therapist.†

> † *Granted, K. C. was a very explosive individual who at times appeared to be quite volatile. However, one aspect that the therapist might have focused on in this situation with Pat and K. C. could have been helping Pat identify, with K. C.'s assistance, those topics that seemed to inflame him or aggravate him. Perhaps from a behavioral communications approach, Pat could have been taught via modeling to approach K. C. in a different manner—one that he might have felt less threatened by.*

At the therapist's insistence, the psychiatrist was contacted and an appointment set up for that afternoon. Meanwhile, K. C. wanted to go home to rest; however, Pat angrily insisted that he attend work with her, since *she* had to work and there would be nobody to carry out the therapist's charge that K. C. not be left unaccompanied until he had seen the psychiatrist and received the latter's instructions. The therapist suggested a compromise—that they call the restaurant and take 2 or 3 hours off for the morning so that Pat could accompany K. C. home to rest, and that they then go in together to work in the afternoon. They both agreed.

K. C. kept reiterating his lack of confidence and weakness; he seemed to be really invested in showing that he was really not well. The therapist excused Pat from this session and discussed with K. C. the paradox of the "weak one"—that is, the fact that the one who is sick has a lot of power. She pointed out that there might be a limit to his wife's being strong for him, and pointed out signs of her fatigue.

After the psychiatrist threatened to stop seeing him, K. C. finally went to see an internist for diabetes screening. He was found to be a borderline diabetic, and was advised to reduce his sugar intake. Despite his being the one in the family who continually chided his mother for disregarding her physician's instructions about her sugar intake, K. C. used his mother's arguments against his wife's entreaties to reduce his own sugar intake. K. C. also complained bitterly that Pat was trying to restrict him and rob him of any enjoyment in life: Pat had told him to limit himself to drinking Diet Coke or just one regular Coke a day.

The couple admitted to not having any leisure activities, having hardly any friends, not talking very much at all to anyone or with each other, and rarely laughing or having any fun. An assignment was given to them to develop a new hobby of collecting jokes and sharing them with each other. K. C. did not follow through with this assignment: "Can't concentrate enough to read anything." Pat was very proud of the one joke she had cut from the Chinese newspaper and shared with K. C.: "He didn't even smile, though he finally said it was funny when I pressed him for a response." The therapist then attempted to introduce some levity during the session by blindfolding K. C. to see whether K. C. was able to differentiate between the taste of Diet Coke and regular Coke. He correctly picked out his preferred beverage on each of three tests. The exercise served to bring some smiles to the couple, a glow of triumph to K. C.'s face, and surprised admiration from his wife. She muttered that she had really thought he was just giving her a hard time.

K. C. appeared less restless and more alert than at previous sessions, yet he reported that he was tired. His sleep patterns were all right, but he was tired because he had to get up half an hour earlier in order to come for therapy before starting work at the business. He said he had felt OK last week; indeed, he had played mah-jongg with his family (after the mother's birthday dinner). He'd feared he would lack the confidence to do that, so he'd asked Pat to sit by him while he played. He "felt OK and confident enough." Pat added with a pleased expression that she was doing much for him, awakening early each morning to make his tea and venturing out in search of fresh bread for him.

Thus, K. C. was continuing to improve, despite his occasional complaints of "nerves" and/or "moodiness." Pat was also very pleased about his improved appetite. However, Pat revealed that she had fears of being strangled again. She also feared that K. C. might commit suicide by jumping from one of the tall apartment buildings in her native city, if and when they returned there for a vacation together.†

> †*Even though K. C. did have a history of violent behaviors, it might have been important for the therapist to investigate the validity of Pat's fears about K. C.'s repeating this behavior. This might perhaps have been a distortion of her own that she was projecting onto the situation, and hence could have elicited a negative reaction from K. C.*

The couple indicated that no such travel plans were anticipated in the foreseeable future. Still, K. C. continued to protest that he was not getting any better, enumerating his getting nervous easily, his inability to concentrate, his lack of confidence, and so on. It was remarkable that although K. C. was listing negative things, he was communicating effectively and doing so with appropriate affect.

The Shift from a Straightforward to a Paradoxical Approach

Tired of K. C.'s rather negative attitude, the therapist put limits on the relationship by requiring completion of written homework assignments as a prerequisite for continued treatment. This requirement was coupled with a contract: "I will try to write down my thoughts every day for 20 minutes. I will start at 2 P.M. and call Paula [the therapist] to let her know when I have finished my homework each day." Both partners signed this contract, since Pat was also required to complete written homework assignments.†

> †*This was an excellent idea, and one that was likely to provide K. C. with the type of structure he needed at this point.*

The therapist's threat of terminating treatment unless greater involvement in the process was demonstrated was followed by a surprise request by K. C. to his wife that she should ask the psychiatrist about his problems with increasing impotence. This was the first time that K. C. had been able to admit to any concern about himself. As a result, the therapist received a note from the psychiatrist (delivered by the couple) to this effect:

> Please try to get some sexual history from Mr. K. C., who complains of recent impotence in regard to morning erections. Does he have them?

Reassure him that occasional impotence is nothing to worry about for men in their 40s. But if it continues, we need to get further medical examinations. Be sure to call me, please, before you terminate with him. I think it is helpful to have the monitoring of him even if he does not do homework. The language barrier is so bad, I need you to help me know what is going on—even if we can't get any long-term changes. Thank you.

At a subsequent session, K. C. discounted his wife's report of his improvement. Pat observed that K. C.'s appetite had recently improved since his mother had begun preparing all his favorite dishes for him. K. C. denied both of her assertions—about his appetite, as well as his mother's efforts. He also again disregarded the therapist's perception of tremors in his hands and knees, and so on. It was pointed out to K. C. that just as others discounted him, he in turn discounted others. The therapist felt that it was opportune at this point to use a written homework assignment suggested by her supervisor. K. C. and Pat were asked to keep written track, over the course of 4 days, of their answers to the following questions: (1) Who denies my importance? How? (2) Whose importance do I deny? How? (3) Who affirms my importance? How? (4) Whose importance do I affirm? How?

They were further instructed to call the therapist daily to report that they had each completed the assignment. K. C. protested that it would be a difficult assignment. The therapist acknowledged that it might be difficult, and invited him to write also about how difficult it was for him. However, since both K. C. and Pat had signed an agreement to complete the written homework assigned, they were informed that for each session that they failed to complete the assignments, they would be charged the therapist's full fee instead of the current discounted fee. The supervisor expressed consternation at such coercion, which was derived from the therapist's own frustration in obtaining desired changes. He suggested instead the use of paradox (Weeks & L'Abate, 1982) to circumvent K. C.'s oppositional character, as well as to gain therapeutic control over the therapy sessions and prevent therapist burnout.†

> †*Paradoxical procedures are often used as cognitive-behavioral strategies, especially with clients who prove to have rigid cognitions that are impervious to change. When a therapist repeatedly encounters obstacles with rigid cognitions, an alternative may be to prescribe a paradoxical behavior, such as the therapist attempted in this case with K. C. and Pat.*

During the following week, the couple duly reported to the therapist by telephone each day. They came for their next session with their written assignments. Among K. C.'s responses were the following: (1) Who denies my importance? "Paula." How? "She said I'm uncooperative." (4) Whose importance do I affirm? "Pat." How? "I will say she's working very hard to help me recover." Using his responses as a stepping stone to implement her supervisor's recommendation, the therapist apologized to K. C. for coercing him to do any homework assignment, for demanding that he change, and thereby for causing too much anxiety for him: "The best thing is for you to do exactly as you have been doing. Do absolutely nothing to change. I'm sorry I went by your words [that you wish to get better] instead of going by your behavior [that you wish to avoid change]. I realize I didn't accept you unconditionally—making demands on you and penalizing you with the threat to raise my fees. I thought if I had expectations of you, you were going to perform. I've been wrong. From now on, go ahead and do exactly as you have been doing: Do not exercise, refuse to eat if you feel like it, sleep in late if you wish, go home in the afternoon and vegetate. Do absolutely nothing. If you want, do not talk to anyone, defeat everyone. . . . "

To Pat, the therapist explained that K. C.'s condition was one that will resist change at all cost. She was to understand that the thought of any change created extreme anxiety in him. Also, he would not allow anyone to win with him, even if defeating others meant that he would be defeating himself at the same time. Pat was to make no demands on him, as he would only feel compelled to do just the opposite of whatever she asked, just as he had been doing all along: "It is his own life and he's the only one who is in charge, who has the right to decide how he wants to live it. No one should deny his importance by trying to dictate to him about his life. He does not need to get better if he does not want to—that is his independent choice." Pat was requested to continue the last assignment for the coming weeks if she wished, as it might help her to become more self-aware if she wanted to do so.

At the second session after the paradox was established, Pat complained bitterly about the disappointment she felt when K. C., who had agreed to go with her on a 4-day vacation to another city, abruptly changed his mind 10 days later. For the ensuing 6 weeks, these comments were reiterated in one way or another. When K. C. reported that he was "the same, no improvement, as down as ever," the therapist responded: "That's right, you just remain the same. Keep it up. Don't do anything different. Don't make plans or travel, just follow routine. Just go on doing the opposite of what anyone suggests."

The therapist turned to Pat and explained to her that going on vacation constituted too much change and that K. C. could not possibly take such pressure: "Let me explain to you how he operates." Turning to K. C., she said, "You correct me if I'm wrong." Then to Pat again: "He has to follow his routine as much as possible. He can't tolerate change. A new place, meeting new people, would be too much for him. He does not want to enjoy life, and that is his prerogative. This position eventually will lead to long-term hospitalization. Hopefully the medication will keep him out, but if he chooses to live this way—to defeat anyone who has anything to do with him—no one can win with him."

The following week the couple went for an appointment with K. C.'s psychiatrist, who happened to explain to Pat about K. C.'s resistance to change as a feature of his illness. That appeared to set her mind at ease about the paradoxical tenor of our sessions.

At the next session, Pat was very upset because after K. C.'s had accepted his young nephew's offer (a week before his birthday) to give him a puppy for his birthday, he had then stated (on the day before his birthday): "I don't want a puppy!" His mother and sister were going to give them a trip to the casino city, and Pat really wanted to get away for a break, but K. C. would not have any of it. She demanded to know why he kept doing things like that. The therapist told them the fable of the scorpion and the frog by way of explanation: "K. C., you just keep right on defeating everybody, including yourself. This is the only way you keep from changing."†

> †*I also suspect that this was K. C.'s way of avoiding intimacy, as well as his manipulative way of controlling others—something he probably learned early in his life. Uncovering his early maladaptive schemas of survival would clearly have provided further insight into his perceptions and mechanisms of operation.*

It was pointed out again to Pat that all people, including K. C. and herself, have the freedom and the right to choose how they wish to handle their lives. In her case, she had the freedom to choose to go on the trip by herself if she wanted. She had other choices about everything else as well.

After the start of the paradoxical intervention, K. C. began to appear more alert, brighter, and more open in countenance; to maintain more eye contact with the therapist; to be more communicative; and, very occasionally, even to initiate conversation. His wife reported from week to week that he had been improving—working more normal hours, eating with the family, going window shopping with her or even by himself, scanning the newspapers, purchasing an Asian newsmagazine, sharing with her that he was looking forward to therapy sessions, and actually getting up early and getting ready to leave for the counseling center on his own initiative. By his self-report, however, he was remaining "just the same, no improvement, even getting worse . . . used to be just a quiet, moody person, but now depressed, agitated, and anxious." The therapist assured him that she appreciated him for doing the best that he could, and she repeated that he did not need to change. In fact, he was going "too fast, too soon," and should "slow down." At this writing, therapy is continuing in this manner.

THEORETICAL CONSIDERATIONS

The theoretical framework for understanding this couple in its cultural context consists of a relational and contextual theory of personality socialization that makes the ability to love and the ability to negotiate the two cornerstones of health and functionality (L'Abate, 1994; L'Abate & Baggett, 1997, in preparation). The ability to love consists of two resources: the attribution of importance to self and significant others, and intimacy. These resources are universal and operate in all human beings, regardless of their culture. They are continually exchanged among intimates, usually family members and very close friends. "Intimacy" is defined as the sharing of joys, hurts, and fears. This couple seemed able to love, to the extent that Pat did things for K. C. However, their relationship lacked reciprocity and intimacy. As shown throughout this chapter, they were unable to become intimate and share their hurts and fears of being hurt because of K. C.'s strong and repeated denial of feeling any hurt.

Within the many models used by the theory, three stand out in the case presented in this chapter. The first model is circular and relates to Emotionality–Rationality–Activity–Awareness–Context *(ERAAwC)*. *E* covers the range of experiencing feelings and expressing emotions. Deficits in *E* derail the entire process of displaying and sharing love, as well as intimacy (Goleman, 1995). K. C.'s definite deficits in experiencing feelings as well as in expressing them derived developmentally from the family's orientation toward *Activity* rather than experiencing and expressing emotions *(E)*. As a result, the rest of his personality, *RAAwC,* was skewed and inappropriate. His *R, A,* and *Aw* were concrete and limited because of a very negative familial *Context* that demanded uncritical loyalty and allegiance, with very little leeway for personal variance, self-determination, discussion, or negotiation.

The second model, *ARC,* refers to relational styles within the family context: (1) Abusive–Apathetic (neglectful), (2) Reactive–Repetitive, and (3) Conductive–Creative. The *AA* style, most dysfunctional style, is the one that was essentially prominent in K. C.'s family context, as shown by gambling and smoking addictions. Also in evidence between K. C. and Pat, as well as within the family as a whole, were *RR* ways of relating to each other. The most functional style, *CC,* where intimacy is prominent was essentially absent both in this couple and in K. C.'s family. K. C. was exhibiting the *AA* style of relating with his wife, his family, and the therapist. No one could win with him, and, by the same token, he was not winning either, even though one could interpret his oppositionality as the only way he knew how to survive. He was unable to love either himself or anybody else; nor was he able to negotiate, because both love and negotiation were impaired in his family of origin. His inability to speak English after 20 years of residence in the United States, for instance, indicates a high level of passive isolation. The same was true, to a lesser extent, of his family: Even though most of his family members were able to speak acceptable English, their most frequent interactions took place within the family, and only seldom did they venture outside of it.

Unless some change for the better occurs in the continuing therapy,

K. C. will continue to be dependent on his wife and on his family for economic and emotional support. However, in his "no-self" personality (see below), K. C.'s propensity to be oppositional, contradictory, and inconsistent with his intimates has been quite evident. As described above, his frequent, overt denials of disturbance and covert denials of dependence were coupled with his extreme dependence and his inability to carry on without the constant help and support of his wife.

The third model describes how importance is attributed to self and to relevant others (partner, children, parents, relatives, friends). Once the attribution of importance is accepted as the major resource exchanged among intimates as well as nonintimates, four personality propensities can be seen to develop within the family context, as well as in school/work and leisure activities: (1) "Selfulness," when importance is attributed to self and significant others to the point that everybody wins; (2) "selfishness," when importance is attributed to self but not to others, leading to "I win—you lose" interpersonal sequences; (3) "selflessness," when importance is attributed to others and not to self, leading to "I lose—you win" interpersonal sequences; and (4) "no-self," when importance is denied both to self and to others, leading to "We both lose" interpersonal sequences. The first personality propensity is the most functional; the second and third are intermediate in functionality; and the fourth is the most dysfunctional, as shown in K. C.'s case. Either importance in K. C.'s family was completely denied, or else there were definite selfish or selfless personality propensities present in family members. For instance, K. C.'s mother was apparently quite selfish, while the father seemed rather selfless. The relational style in no-self is *AA*, while in selfishness and selflessness the relational style is mostly *RR*. The relational style of selfulness is *CC*, but it was not present in this couple or in K. C.'s family.

Consequently, within these models, it is possible to view therapeutic interventions as consisting of ways and means (1) to increase the positive values of all five *ERAAwC* components to increase interpersonal competence; (2) to help a couple change from *AA* and *RR* styles of relating to mostly a *CC* style; and (3) to help a couple move away from selfish–selfless polarizations and no-self personality propensities to selful ones. One way to increase these changes, in addition to prolonged professional contact, would be through written homework assignments (L'Abate, 1986, 1992), such as the ones attempted from time to time with K. C. and Pat.

CONCLUSION

Any treatment approach developed in the United States, whether straightforward or paradoxical, needs to be adapted to cultures other than U.S. culture. In the case of Pat and K. C., once linear, straightforward approaches (whether emotive, cognitive, or behavioral) seemed ineffective, a more circular (i.e., paradoxical) approach was initiated. In spite of the immediate results, the therapist is very cautious about claiming any therapeutic progress. Again, at this writing, therapy with this couple is still ongoing; perhaps the paradoxical approach may not even work. However, it has given the therapist a more positive outlook by helping her feel in greater control than she ever felt before. There is now less frustration, since no requirements for change are indicated. Thus, there is less chance of burnout on the part of the therapist, and it is hoped that the paradoxical effects may serve to motivate K. C. in a different direction.

AUTHORS' REPLY TO EDITOR'S COMMENTS

Any comments that help to expand the repertoire of a therapist are always welcome. We would have no trouble implementing any cognitive-behavioral techniques and strategies if the patients were always able to respond to them. The writing medium, which the therapist tried to implement unsuccessfully in the case of K. C. and Pat, is, after all, a cognitive interpretation. Even though we are not exclusively cognitive in our approach, we recognize its value. However, we feel that at the bottom of human existence there are feelings of hurt and fears of being hurt that are universal, and that people need to share these with the ones they love and who love them. Unless we deal with these feelings (even cognitively!), we are going to miss an important chunk of our own and our clients' experience (L'Abate & Baggett, 1997). In this case, we see K. C. as a very hurt human being who was unable to break out of a cage constructed around his deep feelings of being hurt and of having been hurt. All of his behavior could be interpreted as avoidance of feelings he was unable and unwilling to share with anybody, because this sharing was frowned upon by his family.

Some specific replies to Dr. Dattilio's comment follow.

Page 287: Asking K. C. about his conceptualization of the therapist's role in helping him would have been met (at least at that point in the therapy process) by a noncommittal admission of puzzlement and ignorance. It was clear that K. C.'s oppositionality was directed toward anybody who required something of him—family members, the therapist, or the psychiatrist.

Page 288 (top): The therapist did ask K. C. about his wife's pushiness. His reply, as usual, was a noncommittal "Nothing—no thoughts." That K. C.'s perceptions were distorted, there was no doubt. How and whether these perceptions could be corrected was the question. At a recent point in therapy (after completion of this chapter), the therapist was in the process of explaining K. C. to Pat in terms of his resistance to change and to demands made of him. He was asked not to speak, but to listen (if he wanted) to the therapist's "explanation" of his oppositionality to Pat in terms of his having had to meet family demands for "blind and unquestioned obedience" since childhood. He was not allowed nor was he able to develop self-determination. When he exercised it, either he was criticized and put down, or he failed miserably, fulfilling all of the negative prophecies made of him. As K. C. left the session in which this "explanation" took place, he turned to the therapist and warmly said, "Thanks." This was the first time he had ever expressed any appreciation.

Page 288 (bottom): True. However, it is clear from everything we know about K. C. that he would have resisted any demands made of him by the therapist, as is abundantly clear from his resistance to all the homework assignments.

Page 289 (top): Again, K. C. consistently resisted any homework assignment. We doubt very strongly whether he would have started, let alone completed, any daily chart or logging of his behavior. We must remember that this couple had very little time and energy for anything except eating, sleeping, and working.

Page 289 (bottom): Possibly so. However, we doubt once again whether he would have followed any instructions to complete daily charts. The therapist has become aware, more recently, that some of K. C.'s moods are related to the amount of business done at work; if business is slow, he will be in a foul mood. Suggestions of alternative ways of thinking would have been met by resistance because they would have been perceived as additional demands made of him. At present, we feel that indirection and paradox may be the most useful ways of helping him, through talking with his wife. As the saying goes, "You can bring a mule to the water, but you cannot make it drink."

Page 291 (top): That K. C. does have an internal dialogue, there is no question. The basic issue here is to have him share this dialogue with someone—his wife as well as the therapist.

Page 291 (bottom): We doubt very seriously whether K. C. would be able to complete a daily activity schedule. His wife Pat would, but if she were to complete one, this would be something else that would deprive him of his self-determination (as he sees it).

Page 292 (top): We doubt whether any suggestion of this kind would have been followed up by K. C. We are constantly reminded of his strong opposition to any suggestion.

Page 292 (bottom): This is an excellent suggestion, and we will implement it in the near future.

Page 294 (top): We do not see much distortion in Pat's thinking and recollections of the attempted strangulation. This is too much of an emotional issue to confront as yet. This does not mean, of course, that this issue should not be confronted before therapy is terminated.

Page 294 (bottom): Thank you.

Page 295: Thank you for your support of such techniques.

Page 297: We agree completely with this statement. Obtaining any information about K. C.'s early life and childhood has been extremely difficult. Isolation of affect, nonresponsiveness, oppositionality, and passive–aggressive behaviors were apparently his major coping strategies. How could he become intimate emotionally with Pat if he had never experienced intimacy in his family of origin? Sharing hurts or fears of being hurt was unacceptable behavior in his family of origin. In marrying Pat, he at least sought someone who might have some potential for reaching intimacy. Even though Pat may possess such potential, we question whether she is just as afraid of it as he is.

REFERENCES

Goleman, D. (1995). *Emotional intelligence: Why it matters more than IQ.* New York: Bantam Books.

L'Abate, L. (1986). *Systemic family therapy.* New York: Brunner/Mazel.

L'Abate, L. (1992). *Programmed writing: A self-administered approach for interventions with individuals, couples, and families.* Pacific Grove, CA: Brooks/Cole.

L'Abate, L. (1994). *A theory of personality development.* New York: Wiley.

L'Abate, L., & Baggett, M. S. (1997). *The self in the family: Toward a classification of personality, criminality, and psychopathology.* New York: Wiley.

L'Abate, L., & Baggett, M. S. (in preparation). *Personality socialization within the family and other contexts.*

Pennebaker, J. W. (1990). *Opening up: The healing power of expressing emotions.* New York: Morrow.

Weeks, G. R., & L'Abate, L. (1982). *Paradoxical psychotherapy: Theory and practice with individuals, couples, and families.* New York: Brunner/Mazel.

SUGGESTED READINGS

Aries, E. (1996). *Men and women in interaction: Reconsidering the differences.* New York: Oxford University Press.

Boszormenyi-Nagy, I., Grunebaum, J., & Ulrich, D. (1991). Contextual therapy. In A. S. Gurman & D. P. Kniskern (Eds.), *Handbook of family therapy* (Vol. 2, pp. 200–238). New York: Brunner/Mazel.

Bowen, M. (1978). *Family therapy in clinical practice.* New York: Jason Aronson.

Comas-Díaz, L., & Griffith, E. H. E. (Eds.). (1994). *Clinical guidelines in cross-cultural mental health.* New York: Wiley.

Feeney, J., & Noller, P. (1996). *Adult attachment.* Thousand Oaks, CA: Sage.

Hafner, R. J. (1986). *Marriage and mental illness: A sex roles perspective.* New York: Guilford Press.

Odell, M., Shelling, G., Young, K. S., Hewitt, D. H., & L'Abate, L. (1994). The skills of the marriage and family therapist in straddling multicultural issues. *American Journal of Family Therapy, 22,* 145–154.

Prager, K. J. (1996). *The psychology of intimacy.* New York: Guilford Press.

Sue, S., Zane, N., & Young, K. (1994). Research on psychotherapy with culturally diverse populations. In A. E. Bergin & S. L. Garfield (Eds.), *Handbook of psychotherapy and behavior change* (4th ed., pp. 783–817). New York: Wiley.

Chapter 13

Social Constructionist/ Narrative Couple Therapy

TERRY MacCORMACK
KARL TOMM

The approach to couple therapy described in this chapter is informed by the assumption that mental phenomena may be regarded as fundamentally social or interpersonal, and as only secondarily psychological or intrapersonal (Gergen, 1985). The significance or meaning of any particular behavior or event is seen to arise through social interaction and is constantly being negotiated in relationships. Conversation is regarded as the major means by which the social construction of realities takes place. The process of giving meaning is extremely complicated, as the plasticity of the human nervous system allows people to internalize and retain prior conversations and anticipate future ones, both of which also influence the meanings being generated in the present.

Before describing this approach to couple therapy in more detail, or describing the case we have chosen to illustrate it, we feel that a word about our construction of the chapter may be in order. Each of us—Karl Tomm, the therapist in the case, and Terry MacCormack, who conducted the videotape therapy reviews that were an important aspect of the case as part of his doctoral studies—wrote sections of the chapter; to preserve our particular perspectives, each of us narrates his section as "I." Shifts from one of us to the other are introduced as "I (Karl)" or "I (Terry)."

A SOCIAL CONSTRUCTIONIST/NARRATIVE APPROACH

I (Karl, the therapist) find it useful to think of the mind as social, as it orients me to look at patterns of interaction between persons as the locus for my therapeutic response. Much of my work revolves and evolves around the careful use of language to co-construct the kind of awareness that supports movement in a direction of healing and wellness. I use Maturana's definition of "language" or "languaging" as "the consensual coordination of the consensual coordination of action" to inform my initiatives in therapy (Maturana & Varela, 1987). The use of words in talking constitutes social actions that serve to coordinate people's interaction and their relationships. However, there is much more to conversation than languaging. An ongoing process of "emotioning"—the coupling of emotional dynamics of the interactants—becomes braided with the languaging during the conversation; it influences the meaning that specific utterances are given both during the conversation and afterward. I assume that an emotioning process of mutual caring and respect greatly enhances the possibilities for greater consensuality in the coordination of action to generate preferred meanings through the use of words. Thus, in my relationship as a therapist with a couple, I strive to create an emotional dynamic of respectfulness and safety with the couple, as well as between the partners.

To concretize and implement my view of mental phenomena as mainly social, I have developed a simple typology of interaction patterns between persons that generate and/or promote pathology, healing, or wellness in one or both of the individuals who are interacting (Tomm, 1991). For instance, a pervasive pattern of acts of "dominance and control" by one person, coupled with acts of "submission and compliance" by the partner, would be a "pathologizing interpersonal pattern" (PIP). The person who enacts the dominating aspect of the pattern may be living a so-called "pathology" of an "aggressive personality disorder," while the person enacting the submissive aspect of it may be living a "pathology" often defined as "depression." For me, the fundamental pathology exists primarily in the disembodied interaction pattern between the interactants, rather than in the persons who have drifted into the pattern through their interaction. In contrast to this PIP, I might look for and identify a pattern of "protesting the dominance" coupled with "listening and acknowledging the injustice" as a "healing interpersonal pattern" (HIP). An egalitarian pattern of mutual affirmation and respect would be seen as a "wellness interpersonal pattern" (WIP).

Much of my therapeutic initiative is oriented toward replacing the PIPs with HIPs and WIPs. When the PIPs are conceived of as disembodied and located between persons rather than inherently within them, space is opened to "externalize" and separate these patterns from the persons who engage in them. The externalizing process takes place through the selective use of language in the therapeutic conversation and is a common practice in narrative therapy (Freedman & Combs, 1996; White, 1993; White & Epston, 1990; Zimmerman & Dickerson, 1996). For instance, instead of describing one person as a "complainer" and another as "withdrawn," I describe them as under the influence of a "complaining habit" and a "shutting-down habit." In my use of externalizing conversation, I point out how these habits become coupled with each other in a repetitive and recurrent pattern. The therapeutic conversation itself should constitute a "transforming interpersonal pattern" (TIP), which includes a therapist's asking about clients' experiences, coupled with clients' disclosures of relevant experiences. TIPs also include patterns of a therapist's offering alternative meanings and/or new connections, coupled with clients' entertaining these new meanings and connections.

To take the interpersonal focus further, I think of the individual "self" as made up of a history of prior relationships, including the conversations in which they are embedded. I regard the self as constituted by an internalized community, which includes all the individuals a person has been in relationship with or has even only heard about. It is then easier for me to interview any member of that internalized community as an "internalized other." In couple work, this can be implemented by interviewing each partner as an internalized other within the other partner to clarify previously internalized PIPs, to bring forth preferred HIPs and WIPs, and to begin influencing these internalized patterns as well as the external interpersonal patterns in a preferred direction. To engage partners in such an interview process is to invite them to move into the interpersonal space where meanings are generated and negotiated.

The patterns in a relationship are usually more easily recognized by an outside observer than by those who are actually participating in the pattern. However, if this observer shares his or her observations with the participants, they are invited into a position of reflecting upon themselves and their interaction, to become more aware of the pattern in which they are immersed. Much of the therapist's work has to do with being able to make relevant observations, to language them, and to invite clients into increased reflection. As such, clients are invited into a second-order perspective of looking at their looking to see what they are seeing, and listening to their listening to hear what they are hearing, by seeing and hearing themselves and their relationships through the eyes and ears of the therapist.

Another aspect of my therapy entails the use of this reflective stance to identify alternatives to patterns of giving meaning or taking action. It is important to bring forth an awareness not only of the problematic aspects of certain behaviors and patterns, but of alternatives that may be employed at a problematic point in an interaction pattern. Alternatives can be sought in clients' preexisting knowledge or introduced directly. For instance, a therapist can juxtapose contrasting distinctions or actions (obedience vs. initiative, or confrontational demands vs. requests for kindness) to highlight alternatives. These can then open space for the clients to move in a direction they prefer.

Finally, this therapy includes a procedure called "doubling" (Lee, 1986; Roth & Chasin, 1994), to offer clients some actual practice in enacting a preferred pattern of interaction. In this, I move my chair to sit behind one or the other partner and offer that partner words, phrases, sentences or questions to consider using as he or she tries to engage in an alternative pattern of interaction. I feel it is sometimes useful to create conditions for clients actually to do something new rather than just speculate about doing it. Having a therapist available as a guide or coach to enable the new doing is a resource in the social construction of new patterns of interaction, conversation, and relationship.

BACKGROUND INFORMATION ABOUT THE COUPLE AND THE VIDEOTAPE REVIEWS

Jim and Sue were referred for marital therapy following their meeting with a colleague who specializes in sexual issues. Initially, they felt their problem was sexual incompatibility, with Jim initiating the search for help. According to Jim, over the past few years Sue had become cold, distant, and uninterested in sexual relations. He threatened to leave if things didn't change. Sue agreed that she had withdrawn sexually from Jim, but attributed this to his constant criticism of her, which led her to feel blamed, inadequate, and worthless. As a result, she found herself responding to his advances out of defensiveness, becoming either aloof or openly hostile. The spouses felt that if they could resolve their sexual difficulties, their relations might then improve. During their initial consultation for the treatment of their sexual incompatibility, however, Sue and Jim agreed that it might make more sense to address their marital concerns before their sexual problems could be resolved; hence the referral for marital therapy.

Prior to their first marital session, I (Terry) asked Sue and Jim whether they would like to participate in a research study that I was conducting to explore the experience of couple therapy from the participants' perspective. This would entail my videotaping their sessions with the therapist (Karl) and then meeting with them to go over the tape of their initial interview, as well as those of two other interviews that they and Karl agreed felt especially significant or meaningful in some way. I explained that I was looking for their uncensored, "play-by-play" descriptions of what they were each thinking and feeling during the course of therapy. I also assured Jim and Sue that what each partner shared with me would stay confidential and would not be discussed with the other partner or with Karl. (For details of this procedure, "interpersonal process recall" [IPR], see Elliott, 1986.)

SESSION 1: ASSESSMENT AND AN
INTERNALIZED-OTHER INTERVIEW

Jim, 30, and Sue, 28, had known each other since high school. They had lived together for 8 years before getting married 5 years prior to treatment. They had a 5-year-old daughter, Shelly, who accompanied them to the first interview. Jim earned what little he could as an unskilled laborer, but said that his ambition was to develop a career as a musician and to attend a university to study performing arts. Sue described herself as a housewife who had recently finished a course in dental hygiene and was now seeking a job where she could fulfill her apprenticeship requirements. Both partners talked openly about coming from backgrounds in which there had been substantial drug and alcohol use. Jim described himself as an addict who grew up in a dysfunctional family, although he noted that he had been "clean and sober" for the past 2½ years. Sue had been Jim's companion in drug and alcohol involvement throughout most of their relationship, but she too had decided to "kick the habit" simultaneously with Jim. She also described herself as coming from a problematic family; in hers, she was the sole adopted child and the youngest of six. Furthermore, Sue revealed that she had been sexually abused by an older brother in grade school, and that it was he who had introduced her to a life of rebelliousness and drugs during her teenage years.

Both Sue and Jim described experiencing good relations up until the birth of Shelly. They shared common interests and did things together, including the use of drugs. At some point, however, their sexual interests diverged, and a feeling of incompatibility began to cloud their relationship. However, according to Jim, things worsened after he discontinued his drug use and began attending therapy for his substance-related problems. He earnestly followed the Twelve-Step program of Alcoholics Anonymous. According to his perception, Sue hadn't lived up to her promise to "work the program" with him. As a result, she had failed to take advantage of the therapy that had been offered to them, and thus they'd failed to "grow" to the extent that Jim anticipated. As Jim added, he was disappointed that although Sue knew that she had to work the program in order to make changes in her life, up until now he had seen no action on her part.

In the interview, Jim presented as forceful, demanding, and critical with Sue. This seemed due to the numerous unmet expectations he had of her. Sue appeared tentative and withdrawn, presenting herself as someone who, unless spoken to, would offer little regarding what she thought or felt. It was also apparent that the partners had received extensive therapy during their efforts to remain substance-free. This was especially the case with Jim, who admitted that he had told his story many times before; it was less so with Sue, who said that her sexual abuse had never been directly addressed in therapy.

As a result of their history of extensive prior therapy, Karl decided midway through the first session to try an "internalized-other interview" with the couple—something that he believed would be a novel experience for them. The internalized-other interview was presented to Sue and Jim as an opportunity for them to experience each other differently, as well as to help both of them gain a better sense of their interactions as a couple.

KARL: One of the things I'm often interested in is how much each member of a couple is in touch with the experience of the other, rather than just having an idea about the other person's experience. How I'd like to explore this is to interview "Sue" within you, Jim, as an "internalized other," and then "Jim" within you, Sue, while you each listen. Afterwards, I'd like to give each of you a chance to respond to what you've heard the other say, so you'll each have an opportunity to clarify and say whether you agree or disagree with what you've heard the other say. *(The couple consented to proceed.)* Which of you would like to go first?

JIM: I will.

KARL: OK, Jim, I'm going to talk to you as if you were actually "Sue." What I'd like you to do is to speak from your experience of Sue's experience—from your inside picture of her. I want you to try to speak from that place within you. Don't role-play her in terms of her surface behavior, but your internalized view of her. Speak from what you feel might be going on deep inside Sue, and even say the things she might not say but that you think or expect she's feeling inside. *(To Sue)* And while he's answering, Sue, you can take notes on this pad that reflect the things you feel pleased about or that you may have answered differently. Later we can talk about your notes in more detail.

COUPLE: *(In unison)* OK.

KARL: *(To Jim)* So let me start by talking to you as Sue and ask you, "Sue," how did you feel about coming to this meeting today?

JIM: A little bit nervous about it, but looking forward to it as being helpful.

KARL: What are you hoping for, "Sue," in your relationship?

JIM: Just to be happy.

KARL: What would make you happy, "Sue"?

JIM: For us to get along and not argue and work through the difficulties we've had.

KARL: OK. "Sue," I'm also interested in what you find attractive about Jim.

At first Jim couldn't answer this question. Karl expanded it by inviting "Sue" to think about what she'd found attractive in Jim when they first met, and what had led her to get back together with him after a brief separation. Gradually "Sue" was able to convey some of Jim's more positive qualities. Karl then asked "Sue" about changes that she would most value and appreciate seeing in the relationship and in Jim. To this, "Sue" said she would like for Jim to decrease his sexual desire, to let her be "the way I am," and to change his "seeming interest in other women."

KARL: Does this interest in other women bother you a lot, "Sue"?

JIM: I feel it demeans me—that I'm not appreciated or wanted, or I'm being compared.

KARL: Are you worried that he's going to leave you for another woman, "Sue?"

JIM: Yes!

KARL: How come you're so worried about that, "Sue"?

JIM: He's had affairs in the past, and when we were separated he saw someone.

KARL: Are you hurting a lot because of those things, "Sue"?

JIM: I guess so.

KARL: What hurts you the most about that, "Sue"?

JIM: *(Sighing)* 'Cause I just want things to get better and to have a happy relationship and a happy family. And I guess it hurts the most to have that disintegrate.

To end this part of the interview, Karl asked whether there were other things he might ask to help him understand their relationship better. "Sue" added that she would like for Jim to take the lead in their relationship, but not to be the boss. Speaking to Jim as Jim, Karl then asked how difficult it was to do the interview, and what percentage of his responses he thought Sue would have answered in the same way. Jim said about 90%, whereas Sue actually agreed with about 75% to 80% of what Jim had said as "Sue." Karl next asked Sue which of Jim's responses surprised or pleased her. She cited Jim's comment about her nervousness coming to the interview as being "right on."

Karl then asked whether Jim would be interested in hearing about the 20% to 25% that Sue would have answered differently, and whether she would be willing to share this with Jim. Sue clarified that she wasn't asking for Jim's sexual appetite to *decrease,* but for their desires to be the same. She also mentioned that she wanted more of a role in the house, but that sometimes she didn't know "what to do to help, or how to do things." Finally, Sue said that she wanted for Jim to show her more respect and not to be so cold to her.

Karl next turned to Sue and began by asking "Jim" how he felt about coming to the session. Karl wondered what "Jim" liked about Sue and what drew him to her. "Jim" said that Sue was a good homemaker and mother, and that he liked how she cared for Shelly. "Jim" also said that he was sexually attracted to Sue. Asked about changes he would value and appreciate in the relationship and in Sue, "Jim" noted that he would like for her to take more initiative in their relations and to be more willing to work on personal change. Here Karl tried to clarify with "Jim" whether he was asking Sue to be more obedient to his wishes, or to take more initiative even if he disagreed with what that initiative might lead her to do. "Jim" struggled with this.

KARL: I guess you probably realize, "Jim," that if you tell Sue to take initiative, then she's not taking initiative, she's obeying you. You understand that, "Jim"?

SUE: The difference between taking initiative and obeying . . . ?

KARL: Yeah. If you tell Sue, "Listen, I want you to take initiative," then she's in a bind. If she takes initiative, then she's obeying you and not taking initiative. So I'm curious whether you really want her to take initiative, or whether you want her to be obedient.

SUE: *(Pause)* I don't know . . .

KARL: The "I don't know." Is that "Jim" speaking now, or Sue?

SUE: Both. I don't know . . . it keeps bouncing back and forth.

Karl ended this part of the internalized-other interview by asking "Jim" whether there was anything else that would help him get a better picture of their relationship. As they debriefed, Sue said that about 50% to 60% of her answers were how Jim would have responded, while Jim said that Sue was 75% accurate, "maybe even a little higher." As they discussed the obedience–initiative issue that arose, Sue noted that there was the "Jim of the past," who she felt still wanted obedience from her, and the "Jim of the present," who wanted her to take initiative even if it meant doing something he might disagree with. Sue said, "I go back and forth. I'm confused."

INTERPERSONAL PROCESS RECALL
REVIEWS OF SESSION 1

Over the next 5 days, I conducted separate IPR interviews with Karl, Sue, and Jim, who shared with me their impressions of the initial session.

Karl's Perspective

For Karl, the flatness of the partners and of how they told their story stood out. "Sometimes couples come in with one member being depressed, but seldom is it the case when both are like this—impoverished and under the influence of 'the heaviness of life.' " Also striking was Jim's "complaining habit" and its oppressive influence on Sue. "It appears that she devalues herself because she feels he devalues her, but Jim seems quite blind to this."

KARL: He can't see his own actions feeding her sense of worthlessness. He can be compassionate about her pain, but he can't see how his complaining fuels her low sense of self-worth. He sees her lack of self-worth as emerging out of her lack of initiative.

TERRY: Understandably, then, his answer is for her to take more initiative.

KARL: Yes. Which I try to frame positively as a desire to improve things.

TERRY: And she becomes tearful at that point. You explore this with him.

KARL: Yeah, and he softens somewhat. [On the tape, Jim motioned for Shelly to give Sue a hug.] What I would have liked for him to say is "I'm sorry, Sue, I had no idea that I was making you feel so worthless. I'm really sorry, because what I want is for us to feel good together and enjoy ourselves." But he can't say it just yet. In my work I'll be trying to co-construct something along those lines, to bring that forth.†

> † *It might have been interesting here to compare the schemas both partners held of themselves and each other as they got more in touch with their internalized others. I might also have suggested that the expectations about "improvements" in their relationship be more defined, as they seemed to have varying perceptions of what these improvements might be.*

Given the couple's flatness, along with his sense of Jim's being out of touch with a significant part of Sue's experience, Karl turned to the internalized-other interview with them. "I thought maybe if Jim could experience her experience, he might then get it—you know, why she's not wildly enthusiastic about his demands for some kind of initiative on her part, sexual or otherwise. Plus it was all a little bit flat, and I wanted to liven it up." Karl also hoped that the interview might serve as a medium for change.

TERRY: And what do you think Jim took away from this session?

KARL: He's probably a bit more curious about what draws Sue to him and what she likes in him. I think it's novel for him, to think that she's attracted to him—something he knows at some level but doesn't think about. Also, by asking his internalized "Sue" what changes she'd value and appreciate in Jim, it's a nonblaming manner of stating things. I can help him see the possibility of him taking initiative in the direction that she values, and that's good for their relationship. Also, I sidestep the pervasive pattern here of mutual complaint. If I criticize his criticizing, I get caught in that pattern as well.

TERRY: And Sue? What do you think she carried away from the experience?

KARL: I think she was probably able to enter into her own experiences more easily while I was asking him the questions, because then she didn't have to answer. She could reflect more. Probably [it] also helped her get in touch with some of her feelings more easily, and to articulate or make sense of them in a way she hadn't before. She probably ended up wondering about some things she might not have wondered about previously.

TERRY: She seemed to struggle with the obedience–initiative issue in the interview.

KARL: I've experienced this before, where people slip out of their internalized other back into themselves. What this says to me is that this is an undifferentiated, undeveloped area of awareness. That makes it harder to be the other, and so she slips back into herself. This tells me that this is an issue that's not clear to Sue yet.†

> † This was apparently an area of real confusion for Jim and Sue, especially as it is natural for spouses to flip between roles. A remedy might have been to make hand-held signs or flags with each spouse's name; Jim and Sue would each have had two flags, one marked "Jim" and the other marked "Sue." As Jim was speaking as his internalized "Sue," he could have held up that sign so that everyone, including himself, would know to whom he was referring. This could have decreased confusion and the therapist's repeated need to ask them whom they were representing.

TERRY: So the internalized-other interview kind of invites struggle . . .

KARL: Yes. I'm inviting people to stretch themselves in quite novel ways. But you have to be careful, as it can be violating for some people. When I use it to bring forth positive possibilities and affirming certain types of dynamics, I feel good. I feel like I'm co-constructing wellness, or facilitating it because it already exists potentially, but I need to open space for it to emerge.

Finally, Karl felt that the session gave him a picture of the couple's predominant PIP. This emerged as he noticed Jim falling under the influence of the "complaining habit," while Sue responded with a "shutting-down habit." He noted, "Early on, I wanted to externalize the complaining and shutting-down habits from them. I was aware of myself thinking of Jim, for example, as a kind of persistent complainer. Now, I could choose to see him as that, or as coming under the influence of the complaining habit. My preference is to see him as under the influence of something external to himself, and then to invite him to liberate himself from that [see Tomm, 1989]. By opening space for Sue to speak up, I also invite her to get the better of the shutting-down habit." Using this as his framework, Karl noted that his intent in subsequent sessions would be to bring forth or co-construct a HIP as an antidote to this particular PIP.

Sue's Perspective

Sue said she was upset and nervous about coming to the interview: "I felt like everything was going to be thrown at me and that I'm the cause of it all." The session was not a pleasant experience for her at first, but later "it felt good to get things out in the open and the problems we've been having." Sue also expected that "the focus was going to be all on me." But as the session unfolded, she felt relieved that it was on Jim too. "Karl was also looking at Jim and the role that he played in our problems. That made me feel a lot better."

TERRY: And did you feel as though Karl understood your position?

SUE: I think so. I think that was an example of Karl having a little bit of compassion for me . . . feeling all of these things coming at me and then maybe turning it a little bit at Jim. But none of it in a negative or cruel way.

TERRY: Kind of like challenging Jim, but in a respectful way?

SUE: Not pointing the finger at him, like, "You're the bad guy." Not locking horns with him like other counselors, who kept supporting me and coming down hard on Jim and blaming him for different things. They might've made me feel good, but it wasn't helping our relationship very much. With Karl, it was like he was on our side—mine and Jim's.

Because Jim had stated at the outset that divorce was their only option if therapy didn't work out, it was especially important to Sue for Jim not to feel alienated in the process. In this respect, the first session had been encouraging. Along with a sense of fairness, however, a feeling of safety was also vitally important to Sue. At one point during the session, for example, Sue had touched on the couple's very difficult financial situation and her preference for staying home so that she could care for Shelly.

TERRY: This is one of those sensitive issues you were saying you can't talk about?

SUE: Yeah, and I can feel him [Jim] sitting there beside me, stewing and getting angry but not saying anything. The anger building and the tension—I can just feel it.

TERRY: And you're aware—I mean, bringing up this issue and knowing how Jim will probably react, but you touch on it anyway? You're taking a risk here . . .

SUE: Yeah, but feeling safe because of the environment we're in. Because of where we are and because of a mediator being there.

TERRY: So it's like, "OK, I can run the risk of Jim getting upset, angry, and stewing and maybe saying things out of anger, but Karl is here and it feels safe to do this."

SUE: Right. And Jim probably won't react the same way here, being with Dr. Tomm, as he would if we were talking about this at home. So I'm not really that worried.

TERRY: So at home you'd be less likely to bring it up? But it's safe to bring it up here.

SUE: Yeah, because at home it'd just lead into an argument, and neither of us would get anywhere. But here maybe we can talk.

TERRY: And the feeling of safety—that comes from where?

SUE: Some of the things he says. He tries to understand and look at the positives, and that helps me and Jim to see one another differently. Like, I was adopted, and he said that I was special because I was chosen. That felt good. And then he said about all we've been through and the changes we've already made together.

Sue noted that she felt especially anxious when Karl invited them to do the internalized-other interview. The process stirred up difficult and painful feelings for her. She referred, for example, to what she was experiencing while Jim's internalized "Sue" spoke to Karl of her hurt and jealousy over Jim's interest in other women.

SUE: A lot of the hurts and things I've just stuffed away and maybe thought that I've dealt with them. But then, coming to a session like this, they come back. I wasn't expecting any of this at all, the hurt and upset . . .

TERRY: So it touched something within you. . . . Are you wishing this hadn't happened?

SUE: No, I think it's good because it's telling me that the things I've gotten upset about haven't been dealt with adequately. And it's also letting Jim and Karl see that.

TERRY: This process, then, sort of raises new issues for you?

SUE: Uh-huh. Things I might not have been thinking about or feeling. When Karl asked me as "Jim" about the obedience thing, I hadn't thought of it like that before. Is it obedience or is it initiative Jim wants? I don't know. I'm still confused.

In closing, Sue said she felt relieved as the session ended. It was helpful, for example, to hear Karl explain the difference between Jim's intent to improve their relations and the effect this had on her. "It made me let loose a little, where everything wasn't focused so much on me and my feelings. And Karl was saying it was part of a pattern that maybe we didn't know how to break. And it felt good when Jim owned up to it and said we have to work on that."

Jim's Perspective

Like Sue, Jim was pleased that the focus had been on both of them more or less equally in the session. There was no sense that he and Karl were "rubbing one another the wrong way, like we're adversaries or something."

JIM: Everyone always picks me to start with. Maybe 'cause I'm the one who talks the most and Sue's so quiet. And I'm just getting a little tired of that. I've made major changes in the last few years, and I want to see some changes in Sue as well.

TERRY: So for you, then, was it like Karl kind of challenged Sue, or ... ?

JIM: I saw Karl making the effort to engage with Sue and giving her the message that this is about the both of us, not just me. So I'm really pleased about that. And then also hearing him say that my criticism—and I know I criticize, right?—but like he said, it's because I want to improve things between Sue and myself.

TERRY: Were you feeling supported by Karl saying that?

JIM: Yeah. Feeling quite joyous about the fact that, like, we're not sitting here and we've got another counselor saying, "OK, Jim, let's take a look at you and what you need to change." With Karl, I hear him saying, "Let's look at the relationship. We're going to help you grow and change, Jim, but we're also going to help Sue grow and change." So I felt this is a good place for us to be.

Jim also liked the fact that Karl gave Sue the space to talk, so that he got to hear what she was thinking and feeling. "It's like she never lets me know what's going on inside her head." Jim admitted, however, that despite trying to be open and honest, he held back much of his anger and frustration with Sue. At various times in the session, Jim was "fuming mad," "steaming," or "ready to jump down Sue's throat." Rather than expressing this, however, he found himself "holding back" or "tender-footing" around Sue, feeling his words would be experienced as "cruel, vindictive, and hurting her feelings," which would "not get us anywhere or do much good." Jim also revealed that he held back some of his more vulnerable feelings as well.†

†*Had Jim revealed this in his therapy session, it would have been an excellent opportunity to introduce the Dysfunctional Thought Record (see Chapter 1) to help both partners capture their specific automatic thoughts and link them with their emotions. This could have been done by first asking, "Jim, you just said you were fuming mad, steaming, and ready to jump down Sue's throat. What specific thoughts went through your mind as you experienced these emotions?" The idea here would have been to cut to the core of Jim's underlying schema. This might have uncovered distortions and misperceptions or a basic belief about Sue that led to his unjustified anger and resentment. The same could have been done with Sue, preferably in Jim's presence, so that both could have seen how automatic thoughts and schemas are uncovered and how the cognitive restructuring process begins.*

JIM: My biggest problem with our sexual relationship is my need to be wanted. That's the feeling I'm searching for in our relationship, which hasn't been there for six years. I don't feel she really wants me. And the fact that I always have to take the lead in things really bothers me. I come across as always in control and knowing what I'm doing, but she doesn't see inwardly that I'm a mess 'cause I just can't deal with some of this stuff.

TERRY: I'm noticing that you don't really mention this in the session . . .

JIM: Sue's not in the room here with us, so I can say things to you that might be hurtful to her, or that she'd be surprised to hear. But I couldn't say them there.

TERRY: Is that a function of Karl somehow, your own discomfort, or . . . ?

JIM: No, I feel confident in Karl's abilities and expertise to deal with my anger and so on. So in the future, I know I'll have time to discuss some of these things with him.

Although Jim noted that the internalized-other interview "met my expectation," he later said that he also felt nervous and off balance: "This is a struggle; it's really difficult to do." He appreciated being offered something different, however, and felt that the interview helped Karl to get to know them better. Speaking as "Sue" also allowed Jim to convey that he understood her "far more than she thought I did. She's always saying I don't understand her. Now she knows I do." Jim also said that "talking about things we appreciate and value in one another and in our relationship helped me see things differently." Furthermore, it left Jim with "an interesting paradox that really got me thinking. I tell Sue to take initiative, right? So if she takes initiative, is that taking initiative, or is that obeying? That messed me up. Yeah, what do I want?"

SESSIONS 2 THROUGH 6

In subsequent sessions, I (Karl) attempted to delineate more clearly with Jim his complaining habit, which he reluctantly began to acknowledge as a problem in his relationship with Sue. We then explored ways in which Jim might get out from under such a habit. Initially, he had difficulty imagining himself living a lifestyle of gratitude and unconditional loving, rather than one of chronic frustration and complaint. Sue, meanwhile, had been noticing Jim's efforts to be more appreciative of her, but wondered whether he was making these efforts out of love or a desire for more sex. This led to a touching exchange in which Jim initiated a potential HIP by expressing to Sue how much he genuinely appreciated her, and she began to weep. As we then explored Sue's experience of this, I was able to draw attention to the positive effect Jim's affirmations seemed to have on her.

The complaining habit persisted, however, in trying to dominate Jim. Whenever this became active in a session, I would interrupt it by drawing attention to my own experience of it. At the same time, I was careful to validate the intent behind Jim's complaining, and I also pointed out Sue's tendency to shut down in the face of it. I then asked whether they noticed how the complaining and shutting-down habits were "married" to one another, and how the pattern dominated their relationship. As they acknowledged this PIP, Jim and Sue began to focus more clearly on bringing forth a healing antidote or a HIP. In this, Jim offered to be more affirming and appreciative of Sue, while she offered to be more open and disclosing with Jim and more willing to take initiative with him. To solidify their awareness of this pattern as an alternative that, if enacted, would preclude the PIP, I invited Jim and Sue to talk to each other and enact the healing pattern in my presence, while I guided them in being selective in what and how they spoke to each other.

As the couple worked at getting the better of the PIP we had identified and replacing it with a HIP, Sue took more responsibility for her part in the relationship. Following a significant breakthrough in which she resonated strongly with something she had read, Sue acknowledged that Jim had made a lot of changes in his life according to her desires, but that she had not responded in kind. Curious about how Sue had come to recognize this, I explored with her and Jim how they had each contributed to create conditions in their relationship in which this realization could be brought forth. I invited them to elaborate on how they were able to be constructive, and invited them to identify more strongly with these aspects of themselves. Framing their breakthrough as a kind of victory over the PIP that had been dominating them, I then invited the spouses to find a way to celebrate this—by toasting each other with a glass of water, for example.

In addition to focusing on their relationship, Jim and Sue used their sessions to raise individual issues that had been concerning them. This gave me a chance to consolidate their HIP further by inviting them to talk about ways in which they could help and support each other in their respective areas of self-improvement. They agreed that this would not be easy, as they tended to engage in confrontational demands and arguments, which made it difficult for them to support each other. I pointed out, however, that the desire to support each other was there. Perhaps we had to find a way to build a pattern that differed from their confrontational expectations. To this end, Sue suggested that maybe if they made requests with kindness, they might not come across as confrontational demands. Jim agreed that they would try to notice how they made requests that were experienced as kind and gentle, so that they could strengthen their ability to "package" more of their requests in this manner.

By session 6, Jim and Sue were continuing in a constructive direction, despite some ups and downs. Together we explored how they had accomplished this, and gave credit to both of them for their achievements. We also touched on various gender and cultural issues and the patterns that these invite males and females into in North American society. I also congratulated the partners on the ways they had found to break the patterns of relating that had dominated their respective families of origin.† I then suggested that we break for a few weeks, and asked Jim and Sue whether they would be interested in a session in which we would invite others in to observe our work.

> † The need to address behavioral patterns that have been carried over from the partners' respective families of origin seems to be a common one with couples. Often these patterns follow ingrained beliefs that need to be restructured. Again, cognitive-behavioral therapy can be of great benefit in this restructuring process by helping the partners to consider alternative behaviors.

SESSION 7

Session 7 was used to affirm the partners' progress, and to give them a new experience of a reflecting team reflecting back to them from behind a one-way mirror what they heard and saw (Andersen, 1991). Jim and Sue agreed to take turns in another internalized-other interview. Because Karl and the couple considered this to be an especially meaningful meeting, I (Terry) later reviewed the tape of the session with each of them. (In this section, excerpts from these IPR interviews are interspersed with excerpts from the actual session.)

In his comments on the session, Karl noted being struck not only by Sue's willingness at the very beginning of the meeting to take the lead in their conversation, but by Jim's ability to keep from interjecting and to do a lot more listening instead. As their talk got under way, Karl asked, "How are things going with the two of you?" Jim replied, "Pretty good," while

Sue said, "I'm really happy lately." Karl then expressed his pleasure with this and wondered, "How do you account for that? What do you see as things that you're doing and Jim's doing that are contributing to that?"†

> †*This was an excellent and extremely important question, as it is essential for spouses or families to have a clear understanding of why change has occurred and how they can link their efforts to these changes. Too often change seems to occur by chance, so that spouses and families dismiss it too easily and do not recognize how their specific efforts contributed to the outcome.*

TERRY: You seemed to direct your question more towards her than to Jim.

KARL: Yes, that was deliberate. He's been so dominant in previous sessions. But when she seemed so participatory at the beginning of the interview, I began actively listening more to Sue than to Jim. I wanted to open space for her and sort of blow on those embers—like her speaking and being heard and so forth.

Although Sue said that initially she was very nervous because of the reflecting team's presence, she felt comfortable and safe with Karl's directing the dialogue toward her. Indeed, as they continued talking, she felt confident about opening up a sensitive issue that she hadn't really thought about until then. This occurred as Karl asked Sue whether their improved relations had led her and Jim to be more encouraging toward each other.

SUE: You mean like giving compliments and supporting one another? *(Karl nodded affirmatively.)* I don't know. Sometimes I try to, but something holds me back.

KARL: Like something blocking you? *(Sue nodded.)* Do you have a sense of what that is?

SUE: I'm not too sure. I think because of the past, and something to tie in with sex, where if I was nice and said nice, sweet things, then that might give Jim an idea of us getting together sexually. I think that might have something to do with it. But things have changed a lot now, and I don't feel so burdened by that any more.

KARL: You mean in terms of sexuality?

SUE: Yeah. I feel better about it now, more comfortable, and I don't have the old ideas of him just using me for sexual gratification. I used to feel that's all I was good for.

KARL: And how do you see it now that makes a difference for you?

SUE: I see and feel a lot of love from him, and caring, and I think more respect for me now than I felt before. But still—going back to what we were talking about, having ideas or thinking of saying things to him to compliment him or whatever. It's hard to just spit it out. I think them, but then I just push them away.

KARL: Afraid he might take it as a come-on, but that's not what you had in mind?

SUE: Yeah.

As Sue explained, prior to verbalizing this thought, she did not realize she was holding back compliments from Jim. Talking about it, however, helped her to clarify why she did this: "I was kind of figuring it out as we were talking. It's like something's lingering in the back of my mind there, and then just piecing it together brings it to a better description. Because when I started, I said, 'I think it has something to do with sex.' Because in the back of my head was 'Giving him compliments and saying nice, kind, sweet things to him—sex!' Right? And so, yeah, as I talked through it, then it all came out." Sue said that it was also important to her that Jim was there to hear her. "Sometimes I'll become aware of something and think it's important to share it with Jim. But then I can't get it out properly and it comes out wrong. He misinterprets or misunderstands, and then it's like it ends up hurting him or something. So I think, 'Why bother?' But here, Karl's there to help. And he's there to help Jim understand."

TERRY: And how was this for you? You talked for a fair length of time here.

SUE: *(Laughing)* Unusual! But I feel I did so well and we carried it on for so long, just between the two of us, and we actually got somewhere.

TERRY: And it felt good for you . . . ?

SUE: Yeah, and it was something within me. Something that I can contribute by trying to change it. Not just Jim trying and making changes, but me too.

Jim, meanwhile, was pleased that Sue had taken up so much conversational space. "I went dead quiet so she could talk. Like, I'm usually the one who hogs the conversation. But here I chose to just kind of drift back and let Sue go first. With other counselors, it's been like Sue doesn't say much. I like that with Karl. You know, he prompts her, right? He gives her space to talk. So here I want to give her equal time." Jim also said it was helpful for him to hear what Sue had to say.

JIM: I'm just sort of sitting there listening, just trying to hear how she perceives that things are going better. I'm hearing things here that are helping me understand. . . .

TERRY: And when she was talking about holding back compliments from you . . . ?

JIM: This is something we'll have to talk about, because obviously that's a habit that needs to be nurtured in her . . . in both of us, right? So we can make things better for the future. Probably for the last 5 years there's been lots of things we've wanted to say to each other that would've made today a lot better than it is.

Although this exchange was like "work" for Sue, and to some extent for Jim, I wondered whether it felt like work for Karl. He noted: "The only work I was doing was opening space for her to speak. I mean, she was just laying it out. I might have added a positive spin to things. For instance, when she invited me into negative conversation about being used, I could have gone with that. That would have dug a deeper hole. So I asked her how she saw things differently now, and she started articulating that. That's all I'm doing. I'm just giving her the space to speak in terms of healing and wellness rather than in a pathologizing pattern." To keep this momentum going, it then occurred to Karl to use the internalized-other interview. He began with Jim, asking his internalized "Sue" what it was like to come to this session.

JIM: Pleased to come, 'cause it seems to be really helping. I've noticed some real changes happening and a happier atmosphere in our relationship together.

KARL: What have you been most pleased about in our work together, "Sue"?

JIM: We've been able to shed light on new ways of thinking and of approaching issues and talking with each other with more kindness. Sort of encouraging more positive ways of thinking about things and making loving requests.†

> † *It is always nice to hear partners make such statements, particularly when they can link their improved emotional exchange to the changes they have made in how they perceive each other and the situation at hand. Because the therapist had done so well with this couple, it was important to solidify this to insure that the change in the relationship would be permanent.*

KARL: "Sue," one of the things you mentioned was that you feel more comfortable responding sexually to Jim now, because you experience him as loving you more. Can you tell me, "Sue," in what way have you experienced Jim differently?

JIM: No easy ones, eh? Uh—hmmm. I guess he's been more loving with me, and I just feel more loving towards him, closer and more in love with him.

KARL: How is he showing his love to you, "Sue"? What's Jim doing?

JIM: I feel a lot less pressure from him.

KARL: What's he giving you instead of pressure, "Sue"?

JIM: Freedom. Freedom to choose, as opposed to "This is what I want." And if I decide to go against what he wants, he doesn't turn around and treat me poorly.

KARL: So he's giving you more space. What else would you say has been an important change in Jim that you really appreciate and value, "Sue"?

JIM: I guess maybe just talking more in a conversation sense.

KARL: Ahhh, sharing . . .

JIM: Sharing, talking more about the relationship and just being kinder, more loving.

KARL: Do you wish sometimes, "Sue," that Jim would talk to you about some of the things that he talks to Lynn [Jim's individual counselor] about?

JIM: Well, I guess he talks to me about some of those things. But the things that he talks about with Lynn are more about his own personal development.

KARL: So you want to respect that, "Sue," and give him space to do that separately . . . ?

JIM: No, no, I guess I do wish he'd talk to me more about what he's talking to Lynn about. Like, he usually doesn't share a lot with me after one of his appointments.

KARL: So you'd appreciate if Jim decided to share more with you, "Sue"?

JIM: Yeah.

Karl noted that his intent here was "to highlight the pattern of improvements that Jim and Sue had been describing, and to use the content of these improvements to try to invite them to internalize the positive feedback within."

TERRY: Is there a framework of questioning you're following here, like before, or . . . ?

KARL: Yes. I have a general plan: Start simple and go to the more complex. First I ask Jim's internalized "Sue" how it was, coming to the session. Then I try to bring forth the affirming "Sue" as an important part of Jim's inner life. Like, I ask his "Sue" how she's experienced Jim differently, trying to bring forth in him a clearer awareness of how he's contributed to her sense of being loved, so that he can become more grounded in and identify with that more. But he struggles. You can see him in his eyes, working there.

TERRY: You then asked him about Lynn. How do you think he experienced that?

KARL: A bit challenged at first. A shock. He hadn't thought about this much. But maybe it'll open space for him to be more sharing. This can happen in therapy, where there's a drift to sharing outside the relationship, which undermines it. He was a bit defensive, but then said she'd probably want to know what he talks about with Lynn.

TERRY: What's your sense of how Sue might have experienced this?

KARL: I doubt it's something she would've thought to raise. She's probably wondered what's going on, but she wouldn't think to pursue this as an important therapeutic change, a change in their relationship. But I think she'd feel more entitled to pursue it now that I've opened it up.

In fact, Sue was "shocked that he asked that question." But as she said in her IPR interview, "I do wonder. I don't think there's one time when he's come home and told me what he and Lynn have talked about. I used to ask, but he wouldn't say much, so I just learned to accept it. But that was before, when things weren't going well." Jim was also surprised: "What's going on in my mind there is 'Oh, oh, I didn't realize that. Yeah, what do I talk about with Lynn? Sue would appreciate that. . . . ' So Karl's just struck a chord in me. He's just given me something else to think about."

Another important issue that emerged in session 7 and was highlighted by the reflecting team was Sue's anger. This occurred as Karl moved to the internalized-other interview with her and asked, " 'Jim,' what kinds of things have you seen change in Sue that really mean a lot to you?" After a long silence, "Jim" replied, "She hasn't been so—quite as angry all the time—just about anything, everyday things or people or . . . "

Karl then asked how Sue had been instead of angry. "Jim" said that she had been more affectionate and intimate, as well as "letting go her anger." Later in the interview, "Jim" returned to the anger as he was asked what further changes he would value and appreciate in Sue. "For Sue to try harder working on her anger, and not to be so angry with me and with herself." In further discussion, Karl explored the value of Sue's anger, asking whether both spouses could see how it might be a resource for them in identifying areas of unfairness that could be addressed. They struggled with this.

KARL: I was impressed with how eager Sue was to look at her anger. In fact, it was her who raised it through her internalized "Jim." She was enthusiastic about that, instead of reacting defensively and trying to justify it or deny it. I was encouraged by that. I think it's consistent with the shift that she's made in looking at herself.

TERRY: And Jim? Do you think he's as open to exploring it as she is?

KARL: He's open to exploring it, but his way. It's an alien thought to him still—to explore constructive uses of anger and how legitimate it is.

TERRY: What's your sense of the anger?

KARL: Probably [it] has a lot has to do with his domination of her and his involvement with other women. So there's a legitimate basis for her anger, and it's probably been more helpful to him in some of the changes he's made than he's able to acknowledge. I'd like him to recognize that and to affirm her anger as a contribution to his development.

TERRY: But your sense is that he's not at a place where he can begin to do that.

KARL: Maybe begin, but I don't think he's quite there yet, no.

Karl felt it was important to distinguish how much of Sue's anger was coming from her own past history prior to the relationship with Jim. He first invited Jim to become a sleuth in finding out more about Sue's anger, and then to wonder what percentage of it was connected to the past and what percentage to her present experience in the relationship. Both Sue and Jim found this distinction helpful to think about. At the same time, it occurred to Karl to frame Jim as perhaps having a "special sensitivity" to Sue's anger. This came as Jim was attempting to convey how unfair he felt her anger was towards him. Sue had difficulty understanding this.†

> † *Again, this was an excellent point of focus. Perhaps identifying cognitive distortions might also have helped help Jim and Sue to recognize that their reaction to each other's anger was personalized, when it did not need to be.*

SUE: I'm not violent, I'm not abusive, I'm not yelling and screaming, throwing things. I get angry and say things sometimes. But I don't see how my anger is so extreme.

KARL: Do you think maybe he has an unusual sensitivity to anger, because of his own past? He's experienced a lot of anger in ways that he's quite vulnerable to that. And that he has a tenderness, perhaps more than most men. So that you might also consider asking him, "How much of your sensitivity is coming from the present, Jim, and how much is coming from the past?" Maybe he too has a sensitivity that's a "hangover" from some earlier life experiences.

Following this, the couple observed while the reflecting team talked about the impressive changes Sue and Jim had made in their work with Karl, highlighting their willingness to struggle with such difficult issues and to be so open with their feelings. Moved by the team members' affirmations, Sue wept as she said how good it felt to hear them say how far she and Jim had come. Jim responded by taking Sue's hand and offering her his support. As Karl further debriefed the team's comments, the spouses agreed that anger might be an issue they could focus on in their next session.

SESSIONS 8 THROUGH 10

Jim and Sue returned for session 8 reporting that their previous meeting had been quite helpful and that things were going well. The major focus in the interview, however, was not on Sue's anger. Rather, the partners seemed confident and secure enough now in their healing pattern to want to tackle a major difficulty—talking about sensitive issues without falling prey to the complaining/shutting-down pattern. As a result, I (Karl) invited them to discuss this by framing their conversation as an opportunity for Jim to find a way to talk with Sue to explore what kinds of initiatives from him invited her to open up rather than shut down. I offered to "double" for each of them to coach them through (see Lee, 1986); that is, I moved to sit beside either Sue or Jim and prompted each one in ways of talking that would make each more open to hearing what the other had to say. I also invited the spouses to repeat in their own words suggestions I made that fit for them, and to feel free to reject the ones that did not. At one point in their talk, for example, Jim told Sue that he was disappointed with her for not completing her dental assistant apprenticeship, but that he also appreciated her for what she contributed to the relationship. Sue then became tearful, which Jim appeared to ignore.

KARL: *(Prompting Jim)* What's making you sad at the moment, Sue?

JIM: Yeah. Why are you crying?

SUE: *(Long silence)* 'Cause that's all I want, is to be appreciated.

JIM: Well, I try and show you my appreciation. I know I don't—

KARL: *(Prompting Jim)* Are you saying those tears are tears of gratitude because I did appreciate you, a little bit?

JIM: OK. Is that what those tears are about?

SUE: Yeah, I guess so. I just wish I could feel that more.

JIM: Well, I realize that I need to express it verbally to you more. I've always felt that I expressed it to you in my actions, but I see that that tends to go more unnoticed than saying it to you [does]. But I think before we discuss this any more, I'd like to go back and talk about how we can discuss things like this without having a mediator like Karl in the room prompting us. What made today's discussion different?

KARL: *(Prompting Jim)* Or is there something else you wanted to share about your feelings before we go back to that, Sue?

JIM: Right. Is there anything else you wanted to say to me first, or . . . ?

Sue reiterated her need to feel appreciated, which Jim took to mean that he should be positive with her before he expressed his disappointments. Sue struggled to explain that although this might feel good at first, she would still be likely to shut down. Sensing her difficulty, I got up to sit beside Sue and now doubled for her.

KARL: *(Prompting Sue)* Maybe if you can convey to me that we're in this together, Jim. That you're not against me—you're against the difficult situation that we're in. Maybe then it'd be easier for me to stay open and not shut down.

SUE: When you're discussing your disappointments, if you can reassure me that we're in this together, and that it's not me you're against—it's a situation or a problem.

KARL: *(Prompting Sue)* I'd appreciate that if that could happen.

JIM: That's how I've tried to discuss things with you sometimes. But I get a sense that everything I say turns you against me, and that you become opposed to any suggestion I make in order to work together to see our way through something.

KARL: *(Moving over to prompt Jim)* But I'd honestly like to learn how to be able to talk to you so that we can come together against some of our problems that we have.

JIM: Yeah, I'd like to focus on how you and I could learn to discuss and work things through, so that it's just not one against the other.

Because Karl and the couple said that this was another significant session, I (Terry) conducted a third round of research interviews. Briefly, Karl said that his intent in the doubling was to externalize the PIP again and help the spouses to get the better of it by engaging them in the HIP. He noted that he wanted to support Sue in disclosing her experience of Jim's imposing his expectations upon her, and to invite her to feel entitled to talk about how he tended to overpower rather than join forces with her to face things. He also wanted to encourage Jim to express his appreciation of Sue's contributions, and "to affirm him in his efforts to find more tender ways of talking that left Sue feeling safe to respond and not shut down."

Sue, meanwhile, emphasized how safe it had felt to engage in otherwise dangerous dialogue, adding that talking about certain sensitive issues was "no longer something to shiver about." She also highlighted how helpful it was to hear their pattern so clearly identified and described: "Jim having a desire to discuss things, which leads to an expectation. And then his expectation causes me to shut down 'cause I feel like I can't meet it, which then makes me feel bad or worthless. To hear someone else put that cycle into words like that really made me feel good." Jim, however, said he felt frustrated and angry for much of the session. At times it was also uncomfortable and "weird, like I'm in strange, unfamiliar territory, talking about feelings." Jim said that for most of his life he had had to steer clear of emotions and worrying about how other people felt. As a result, he said that part of him experienced their talk as "square, nerdy kind of crap," while another part struggled to acknowledge the importance of emotions and being able to express and talk about them. "Because I've never had to do this, it scares me and makes me feel like I'm in a place where I don't know my way around."

This turned out to be an important disclosure for Jim, as it seemed to open the way to a very significant insight that came to him as we continued our review of the session. This happened as he was explaining how frustrated he was with Sue's "lack of ambition" and his "futile efforts" to convince her of the importance of fulfilling her apprenticeship requirements. Suddenly Jim paused and said that a "tremendous revelation" had just come to him. "Look at me there! I'm trying to get her to buy into my world view. Listen to me, pressuring her to fit into my value system!" As he noted, it was as though he suddenly saw himself expecting Sue to live life the way he felt it should be lived. Jim then said he felt sad as he admitted seeing how he had not been giving Sue the space she needed to create and live her own life, and to find her own meaning in it. Following this, Jim said that he needed to see Sue about his important insight, and suggested that we end our review early so that they could talk.

In the session that followed, I (Karl) explored this breakthrough with the couple and congratulated Jim for recognizing how his expressions of disappointment felt like negative judgments to Sue. I noted that this was a significant revelation, and wondered how Sue had experienced Jim since. She said that the change had brought her considerable relief, and that their relationship had improved accordingly. After some discussion of a car accident that had briefly demoralized Jim, the spouses noted that their sexual relations had been improving and that Sue had been taking far more of the initiative in this area than ever before.

Because it felt as if things were going well, I invited the couple to consider taking a break from therapy. As Sue herself noted, it seemed that their problems had become "more like sandhills than mountains now," and that they could probably manage on their own. We then scheduled a final follow-up session for 5 weeks hence. In this final meeting, Jim and Sue reported that the significant gains they had made were continuing and that they were comfortable with ending the therapy. They added, however, that they would like to leave things open-ended "just in case." I explained that I was starting a sabbatical shortly, but that I would be happy to see them in a year's time if they felt the need.

CONCLUDING COMMENTS

In her final review of her therapy experience, Sue told me (Terry) that it had given her a safe place where she could begin to feel confident in exercising a stronger voice in her relations with Jim. She had a context in which she could express her feelings and experiences in a way that Jim could hear and consider what she said. Sue also noted that it had been helpful to have their relations described in terms of patterns that they were both contributing to and could change. Having things "put into words," however, was especially helpful. "A lot of what was said, we've been trying to deal with or been having problems with for quite a while. But then the way Karl helps put them into words—like in the back of my mind I've known a lot of these things, but not been able to put them into words. But once something's been put into words, you become more aware of it and can face it and deal with it."

Jim felt that the internalized-other interviews had been instrumental in helping him to improve his understanding of Sue's experience. The process awakened in him a concern for others that he had not been aware of before. "The best thing it has done is help me think more about Sue and how she feels. Like, growing up as an addict and drug dealer, I never had time to actually consider other people's feelings. It was all take, take, take. But with this interviewing, it helped me develop those skills. I'm thinking about the other person—about Sue's feelings more often when I go to do something, and Shelly's, too. And in turn that's getting Sue to do things, so we're working together. So I guess that would be my area of growth and why things have changed so much."

Finally, it is important to note that the research process probably added significantly to the therapeutic process. By viewing themselves on videotape and discussing this with a third party (myself), without any pressure to respond to each other or to Karl, Jim and Sue were able to see themselves from an outsider's perspective. This allowed them to disembed themselves somewhat from the emotional dynamics involved, which opened more space for change. A dramatic example of this was Jim's realization, while reviewing the video of session 8, of how his criticisms and expectations were so oppressive for Sue. Thus, it is reasonable to assume that the work in reviewing selected tapes with Sue and Jim also contributed to the therapeutic changes that occurred.

AUTHOR'S REPLY TO EDITOR'S COMMENTS

Dr. Dattilio's comments suggest that he holds a different frame of reference than I (Karl) do for both conceptualizing problems and responding to them. For instance, his emphasis on schemas appears to give priority to intrapsychic rather than interpersonal process, and the use of the Dysfunctional Thought Record suggests that he uses a more directive approach, in contrast to my facilitative approach. Although these may be issues of degree, they are not trivial and would probably yield quite different experiences for clients. I would also not have used the hand-held flags suggested by Dr. Dattilio, as they would have tended to shift too much attention onto surface phenomena rather than continuing deeper experiences. Indeed, my response to Sue's confusion was very different from what Dr. Dattilio's would have been. It was not a problem in the therapy, but an important indicator of a potential domain for further clarifying conversation.

My preference is to minimize my professional status as a directive expert, as it implicitly disqualifies the clients' knowledge and expertise. But I acknowledge that as the therapist I bring something important to the therapeutic process. I do not pretend that I'm not taking significant initiatives. I am very selective in my statements and questions, which are oriented toward what I consider to be preferred directions for the therapeutic conversation. I accept full responsibility for selecting certain distinctions and ways of giving meaning, and for inviting clients to consider these. I also try to respect their freedom to accept or reject what I might see as potentially helpful, and I remain open to changing my direction on the basis of their responses. One important initiative is to ask the clients explicitly whether the therapy is evolving in the direction they prefer, which I did with Jim and Sue. They were also invited through Terry's questions to feel more confident in being able to distinguish and raise their feelings about what was or wasn't happening in therapy. I think it is important for therapists to create space for clients to articulate their experience of therapy, and for therapists to allow this to guide them in collaborative work. A major area of agreement with Dr. Dattilio seems to be our recognizing how important it is for clients to distinguish their own contributions to constructive change so that these patterns will endure. It is more likely that clients can repeat something that "works" if they are aware of what that something is.

ACKNOWLEDGMENT

Lisa Berndt provided helpful feedback on an earlier draft of this chapter.

REFERENCES

Andersen, T. (Ed.). (1991). *The reflecting team: Dialogues and dialogues about the dialogues.* New York: Norton.

Elliott, R. (1986). Interpersonal process recall (IPR) as a psychotherapy process research measure. In L. S. Greenberg & W. M. Pinsof (Eds.), *The psychothera-*

peutic process: A research handbook (pp. 503–527). New York: Guilford Press.

Freedman, J., & Combs, G. (1996). *Narrative therapy.* New York: Norton.

Gergen, K. (1985). The social constructionist movement in modern psychology. *American Psychologist, 40,* 266–275.

Lee, R. (1986). The family therapy trainer as coaching double. *Journal of Group Psychotherapy, Psychodrama and Sociometry, 39,* 52–57.

Maturana, H., & Varela, F. (1987). *The tree of knowledge: Biological roots of human understanding.* Boston: Shambhala.

Roth, S., & Chasin, R. (1994). Entering another's worlds of meaning and imagination: Dramatic enactment and narrative couple therapy. In M. F. Hoyt (Ed.), *Constructive therapies* (Vol. 1, pp. 189–216). New York: Guilford Press.

Tomm, K. (1991). Beginnings of a "HIPs and PIPs" approach to psychiatric assessment. *The Calgary Participator, 1,* 21–24.

White, M. (1993). Deconstruction and therapy. In S. Gilligan & R. Price (Eds.), *Therapeutic conversations* (pp. 22–61). New York: Norton.

White, M., & Epston, D. (1990). *Narrative means to therapeutic ends.* New York: Norton.

Zimmerman, J., & Dickerson, V. (1996). *If problems talked.* New York: Guilford Press.

SUGGESTED READINGS

Gergen, K. (1985). The social constructionist movement in modern psychology. *American Psychologist, 40,* 266–275.

Tomm, K. (1989). Externalizing the problem and internalizing personal agency. *Journal of Strategic and Systemic Therapies, 8*(1), 54–59.

White, M. (1993). Deconstruction and therapy. In S. Gilligan & R. Price (Eds.), *Therapeutic conversations* (pp. 22–61). New York: Norton.

White, M., & Epston, D. (1990). *Narrative means to therapeutic ends.* New York: Norton.

Chapter 14

Internal Family Systems Family Therapy

RICHARD C. SCHWARTZ

The internal family systems (IFS) model has evolved over more than a decade into a comprehensive approach that includes guidelines for working with individuals, couples, and families. The IFS treatment of individuals has been described extensively (Schwartz, 1995; Goulding & Schwartz, 1995), but literature on its application to families is less widely available. This chapter contains the first full-length case report (to my knowledge) of the use of IFS with a family.

THE INTERNAL FAMILY SYSTEMS (IFS) MODEL

The IFS model represents a new synthesis of two existing paradigms: systems thinking and the multiplicity of the mind. It brings concepts and methods from the structural, strategic, narrative, and Bowenian schools of family therapy to the world of subpersonalities. This synthesis was the natural outcome that evolved after I, as a young, fervent family therapist, began hearing from clients about their inner lives. Once I was able to set aside my preconceived notions about therapy and the mind, and really began to listen to what my clients were saying, what I heard repeatedly were descriptions of what they often called their "parts"—conflicted subpersonalities that resided within them. This wasn't a new discovery. Many theorists have described similar inner phenomena, beginning with Freud's "id," "ego," and "superego," and more recently the object relations conceptions of "internal objects." An appreciation of inner entities is also at the core of less mainstream approaches, such as transactional analysis ("ego states") and psychosynthesis ("subpersonalities"); somewhat similar phenomena are now prominent in cognitive-behavioral approaches under the term "schemas." Prior to the development of IFS, however, little attention was given to how these inner entities function together.

Since I was steeped in systems thinking, it was second nature to begin tracking sequences of internal interaction in the same way I had tracked interactions among family members. As I did, I learned that, across people, parts take on common roles and common inner relationships. I also discovered that these inner roles and relationships weren't static and could be modified if the interventions were careful and respectful. I began conceiving of the mind as an inner family and experimenting with techniques familiar to me as a family therapist.

The IFS model, then, views a person as containing an ecology of relatively discrete minds, each of which has valuable qualities and can play a valuable role within. These parts are often forced out of their valuable roles, however, by life experiences that disrupt the harmony of the system. A good analogy is an alcoholic family, in which the children are forced into protective and stereotypic roles by the dynamics of their family. Although one finds common sibling roles across alcoholic families (e.g., the scapegoat, the mascot, the lost child, etc.), one doesn't assume that those roles represent the essence of those children. Every child is unique and, once released from unhealthy roles by intervention, can find interests and talents separate from the demands of the chaotic family. The same process seems to hold true for internal families: Parts are forced into polarized opposition by external circumstances and, once it seems safe, they gladly move into harmonious cooperation.

What are the circumstances that force these parts into distorted and sometimes destructive roles? Trauma is one factor, and the effects of childhood sexual abuse on internal families have been discussed at length (Goulding & Schwartz, 1995). But, more often, a family's values and interactional patterns create internal polarizations within children that escalate over time and spill over into other relationships. Again, this isn't a novel observation; indeed, it is a central tenet of object relations and self psychology. What is novel to IFS is the attempt to understand all levels of human organization—intrapsychic, familial, and cultural—with the same systemic principles, and to intervene at each level with the same techniques.

Are there common roles for parts across people? After working with a large number of clients, I have discovered common patterns. Most clients have parts that try to maintain their effective functioning and safety. That is, they try to control the clients' inner and outer environments by avoiding dependence on others, criticizing their appearance or performance to make them look or act better, and attending to others' needs rather than their own. Because these parts assume protective, managerial roles, I call them the "managers."

People who have been hurt, humiliated, frightened, or shamed will have parts that carry the emotions, memories, and sensations from those experiences. Managers often want to keep those feelings out of consciousness, and consequently try to keep these vulnerable and needy parts locked in inner closets. These incarcerated parts are known as the "exiles." The third and final group of parts clicks into action whenever one of the exiles is upset to the point where it may flood a person with its extreme feelings or make the person vulnerable to being hurt again. When that occurs, this third group tries to put out the flames of feeling as quickly as possible, which earns them the name "firefighters." They tend to be highly impulsive and driven to find distractions that will override or dissociate from an exile's feelings. Bingeing—on drugs, alcohol, food, sex, or work—is a common firefighter activity.

One other key aspect of the IFS model also differentiates it from other approaches. This is the belief that, in addition to these parts, everyone has at his or her core a "Self" that contains crucial leadership qualities, including perspective, confidence, compassion, and tolerance. Working with hundreds of clients for more than a decade—some of whom were severely abused and quite symptomatic—has convinced me that everyone has this competent Self, despite the fact that some people have very little access to it initially. In work with an individual, the goal of IFS is to differentiate this Self from the parts, thereby releasing its resources, and then, in the state of Self, to help parts out of their extreme roles.

APPLYING THE MODEL TO FAMILIES

In work with families, the goals of IFS therapy are quite similar—to elicit the Selves of all family members, and to bring them together to deal with the polarized parts of each member that are involved in the problem. This, in turn, releases family members from their polarized roles in the family.

This belief in the existence of a Self in every family member provides the basis for a collaborative, nonpathologizing family therapy. The role of the therapist is to create a context in which it is safe for clients' Selves to emerge and to interact with one another. Thus, the therapist doesn't have to create competence within family members by, for example, becoming an internalized good object or teaching them the skills of communicating. Instead, in addition to creating a safe, empathic atmosphere, the main roles of the therapist are (1) to point out when polarized parts have taken over and to help family members return to Self-leadership; (2) to help family members create a vision of how they want to relate; (3) to lead discussions regarding the constraints that exist in the family's environment, in the family's structure, or within each family member—constraints that keep the family members from achieving that vision and maintaining Self-leadership; and (4) to collaborate with the family to find ways to release those constraints. This is not to say that there are never times when the therapist makes interpretations or educates. It's just that even during those interventions, the therapist's attitude is one of respect for the abilities of the clients.

The IFS model provides a broad set of principles (balance, harmony, leadership, and development) that guide the therapist's understanding and exploration of family constraints. Also provided is a set of techniques for working with families. These principles and techniques are illustrated in the case below.

FAMILY CASE STUDY

Background

By the time I met with her family, Rebecca, a slight 15-year-old with short dark hair, had been hospitalized four times in the preceding year for anorexia nervosa (she was also bulimic). She was being released from a state hospital, where she'd landed after the family's insurance had been exhausted from the previous hospitalizations in private settings. Two years prior, she had become increasingly concerned about her weight and begun dieting. Eventually her weight dropped to a life-threatening 63 pounds (she was 5 feet 3 inches tall). At this point, the process started of Rebecca's entering a hospital, quickly gaining weight back into the 90s, being released to her family, quickly losing to the 60s again, and being rehospitalized. Now, at almost 90 pounds, she was to come home yet again, and her parents were exhausted, exasperated, and scared.

The first session took place in the hospital just before discharge and included Rebecca and her parents. She had no siblings. The parents were reluctant to try any additional therapy, particularly any therapy that required their involvement. Rebecca was quiet but not unresponsive. She wanted to keep trying, so most of the session consisted of my empathizing with their story and their frustration, while trying to inject some hope that a different approach might work. With unmasked skepticism, they agreed to try some sessions of outpatient family therapy.

During the initial session, I tried to reassure the protective manager parts of the parents, so as to have more access to their Selves. I did this by empathizing with their skepticism and frustration, giving them total control over the decision about continuing, while conveying confidence that their predicament could change and that I was competent to help them change it. I find that this combination of messages often successfully reassures managers.

This first session revealed the following story. Rebecca's father, Bob, a successful dentist, had been divorced from her mother for 6 years. He'd received custody of Rebecca after her mother began having affairs in a flagrant and seemingly rebellious manner. Shortly after the divorce, Bob married Faye, who quickly became very close to Rebecca. Rebecca felt abandoned by her mother and saw Faye as a kind of savior. However, in the following few years their relationship became increasingly strained, to the point where now they fought constantly over Rebecca's eating and other habits. Bob's long hours kept him out of their fray most of the time, but when he was around he tried to play the role of peacemaker, although he usually ended up siding with Faye.

Neither Faye nor Bob could understand Rebecca's eating problems, and both had grown increasingly impatient with her. Unlike some anorexics, Rebecca acknowledged that her weight was too low, but felt unable to control her urge to be thinner and to purge whatever she consumed. She didn't know where the urges came from, but she knew that deep down, she didn't like herself very much.

Introducing the Language of Parts

The tension in the second session was evident from the time the family entered the office. Rebecca had been home for a week and had already regressed into her bingeing and purging behavior. Faye looked furious, and Bob's steely silence betrayed his disgust. Rebecca was quietly weeping. When she did speak, haltingly, she sounded very young. I asked Faye what was happening, and she complained that "a lot of her bulimic behavior is very irritating to me—I find it slovenly, and it bothers me—I have a short fuse when it comes to messiness. I find it extremely irritating."

"So you've been having to struggle with yourself this week," I said. "Would you like some help in that area?"

"No! I don't think it's dysfunctional!" Faye snapped.

"I'm not saying there's anything wrong with it," I said, "but I mean the part of you that gets so activated by Rebecca's behavior. Do you think that if that part wasn't so stirred up, it would be easier for you to help her?"

"Yes," Faye said tentatively. "If I could get help but not have to discombobulate my life any more than it already is, I guess it would be helpful."

As soon as possible, I try to identify the parts of each family member that are connected to the problems the members present. Thus, when Faye talked about her strong reactions, I asked her about whether that part of her got in the way of her relationship with Rebecca. It's usually fairly easy to introduce the language of parts this way—feeding back what clients say about their thoughts or feelings, but construing that as coming from a part of them. This "parts language," in and of itself, is usually very helpful. In this case, for example, it was much easier for Faye to acknowledge that her "irritation" got in the way when it was framed as just a part of her than when I initially asked if she wanted to change her (as in "all of her") thoughts or behavior. I find that clients are more able to reveal feelings and beliefs they're ashamed of when they can speak about a part of them as feeling or thinking it.†

> † *This theory is very similar to the cognitive-behavioral approach, in that it focuses on the internal dialogues of each individual and identifies various schemas, or what Dr. Schwartz refers to as "parts." Dr. Schwartz nicely provides his clients with an avenue to express their various facets; this already suggests in a subtle fashion that these are things that can be changed.*

Also, the parts language helps people feel better about themselves and one another, because if their extremes are contained in small parts of them, there is hope that those parts can change; the implication is that beyond those parts, they have many other resources or feelings. Finally, the language encourages family members to remember that behind the protective parts they often show each other are feelings of caring and love. Thus, simply using this language can change the way family members see themselves, one another, and their problems.† They are not asked to minimize or deny the seriousness of problems or damage done by one another—only to recognize that there is more to one another than those extremes.

> † *The notion of introducing alternative methods of perception is a very important aspect of treatment, and one that is consistent with the basic tenets of the cognitive-behavioral model of family therapy.*

After Faye acknowledged her willingness to work with her angry part, I explained to her, "I don't want you to feel picked on because I focused on that part of you just now. I believe that when families face emotionally charged problems, everyone will at times experience feelings that aren't the way they want to be and are hard to control. My goal is to help each of you have more peace inside, and I know how to help you do that if you're interested. Rebecca will be better able to become healthier in a more peaceful atmosphere, and your life will be easier if you're not so upset by her behavior. So it sounds like you're interested."

Faye said, "Well, particularly to make my own life better, yes."

I turned to Rebecca. "That angry part of Faye seems to trigger a sad, hurt pain in you. Is that right?" She nodded. "Are you interested in finding ways to help those hurt parts of you feel better, so that you won't be so vulnerable to that part of Faye, and maybe won't have such urges to binge and purge?" Rebecca nodded affirmatively again, still sniffling but now making eye contact.

When I ask questions like these, I imply that it is possible for clients to handle their feelings themselves, and that I know how to help them get there. Most teenagers are attracted to the idea that they don't have to be so vulnerable to their parents' parts, and I wasn't surprised that Rebecca perked up when I mentioned this. It was also important for her to hear that Faye was toying with getting more control over her own angry part. Some of the power of family therapy comes from this kind of depolarization process that takes place when each person sees an adversary begin to back down and thinks it may be safe to do the same. This is particularly true if they trust that the therapist can really produce that kind of change, in the others and themselves. For this reason, I frequently say that I can help people change in the ways they want to. There's nothing more healing for a despondent system than a strong injection of hope.

I then asked Bob what parts of him got in the way in this situation, and he replied, "I don't know. Maybe being passive, but I don't think of that as a part of me—just what I do, and I don't necessarily see it as a part of the problem." It was obvious that Bob's managers were not buying into this process, at least not without putting me on notice that I had to deal with them delicately. Faye agreed with Bob, saying, "I think he's more of a peacemaker than part of the problem." Since both parents were lobbying hard to steer me away from Bob, I accommodated them, and the rest of the session was focused on the escalations between Faye and Rebecca.

This initial accommodation to a family's manager parts is often necessary, because many families come into treatment feeling volatile—like a volcano that could erupt, either in the session or at home, if the therapist challenges certain rules, beliefs, or individuals. They also come in afraid of being blamed for the problem and ashamed of having it. In other words, they often "sniff out" the therapist in terms of how much he or she seems to respect their rules and respect them as people, as opposed to blaming them or siding with others. I noted to myself the anxiety connected with my pushing Bob, but decided to do no more with it until the family seemed less distrusting of me.

I asked Faye to elaborate on what her parts told her about the situation. She said, "It's this sort of carelessness about personal property— you know that if you spend money on food, it's going to get trashed. And the lying—that's what I hate the most. I can't trust her, period, end of story."

"So the part of you that gets upset about the food, and the one that's so outraged by what you call Rebecca's 'lying' . . . those parts interfere with the affection you have for her?"

Faye's tone softened considerably as she agreed, "Yeah, it's down there some place, but it's buried under a lot of resentment. I don't like the situation I'm in."

I turned to Rebecca and asked gently about her internal process: "Is there a part of you that agrees with Faye when she gets so upset with you?" Rebecca nodded affirmatively and admitted to getting angry inside also. She tried to push away that angry part, however—"because if I get angry at Faye, she'll get more angry at me, and it will make me feel more sad."

At this point I had enough information to describe a sequence of parts that I saw taking place between stepmother and daughter. When Faye became irritated and disgusted with Rebecca, it triggered Rebecca's own inner critic; this then set off her hurt parts, which in turn released her binge and purge parts, which only further frustrated and infuriated Faye, and the sequence escalated. I made it clear that this was no doubt only a small piece of a larger picture. But it was a place where we could start. Both Faye and Rebecca agreed with this depiction of their interactions as a vicious circle that they had felt powerless to change.† They also agreed that they both wanted to find their way back to the closeness that they used to have and were willing to work on the parts that kept them from achieving it. Faye said, "It seems so simple when you describe it that way." To Rebecca, she said, "I love you, but I also feel a lot of resentment. I know that when I feel those things the love is still there, but I can understand how you wouldn't know that."

> † *It might have been interesting here to explore what images Faye and Rebecca held in their minds regarding what it "looked like" to feel powerless to change. Such images could have led to the thoughts and schemas governing their feelings and subsequently their behaviors. Images are often a strong means for a therapist to get in touch with cognitions and affect that otherwise may not emerge during the cause of treatment.*

Describing this sequence to the family was a bit risky, since it implied that Faye played a role in Rebecca's bingeing and purging. When such a description is couched in the parts language, however, I find that family members usually react in the way Faye did: She was relieved to be able to talk about her complex mixture of feelings without hurting Rebecca. At one point Faye said, "I really want to stress that I don't think it's a matter of affection or love. It's all the other garbage that's been dumped on top of the affection and love that's there. I could draw a picture of it. Love and affection would be down here, and all of this anger and resentment and frustration is piled on top of it like a ton of bricks."†

> † *An alternative that might have been considered here would be to ask Faye just to identify her cognitions as "automatic thoughts" without attaching any affect or behavior to them. In essence, this spewing of random thoughts might have helped her to put things into perspective for herself. This exercise of "cognitive purging" might also have been a subtle way of introducing an alternative to Rebecca's purging behavior, in which she might have been engaging for many of the same reasons why Faye did what she did.*

Gradually it was becoming evident that Faye's and Rebecca's Selves were peeking out from behind their protectors. Faye's voice was very different—less harsh and more caring. Rebecca had stopped crying, and, though she still sounded young, she was taking risks. This is largely the goal of IFS family therapy—to create an atmosphere in which the Selves of family members emerge and interact, rather than the polarized parts that have been dominating their interactions. When this is successful, people often find that the problems they thought were intractable begin to crumble as extreme beliefs and emotions stop obscuring their Selves. Once it's clear that the amount of Self-leadership in the room is increased, I will ask family members to speak with one another directly about their conflicts. Until then, however, I remain fairly central in the sense of talking to each person rather than having them talk to one another, and I try to provide some degree of Self-leadership in my demeanor. I also ask questions designed to elicit their Selves further.

When more Self-leadership is evident (i.e., when family members are calmer and less reactive to one another), I'll ask whether one family member is willing to work with me on his or her parts in the presence of the others. This is not something to take lightly, because it often involves that individual's being vulnerable in front of people who have hurt him or her in the past and may do so again (for warnings and guidelines on this process, see Schwartz, 1995). On the other hand, when this goes smoothly, it generates hope and empathy in the observers, and a feeling in the person who did the work of being accepted and supported by the others. Faye agreed to do this with her angry part, because she didn't know whether she could control it otherwise and because exposing that part wouldn't make her feel so vulnerable. I asked Bob and Rebecca to monitor their reactions as they observed.

After asking Faye to check again to see whether any parts of her were nervous about focusing inside herself in front of her family, and getting the green light, I asked her whether or not she could separate her anger by putting it in a room in her mind. She said she could and saw an image of a dragon, waving its arms menacingly and "doing dragon things." I asked how she felt toward it, and she said, "Kind of amazed. It looks so angry and vicious, with teeth, but it's kind of like watching something in the zoo, so I'm not frightened of it."

I asked Faye to see whether she could find a way to help the dragon calm down. She found that when she approached it carefully, then put her hand out and stroked it like a dog, the dragon stopped raging and sat down. Faye said, "It's really friendly, actually. I'm calm. I stand there. I can assure him." I asked her to ask the dragon what it wanted for her, and she said, "I feel stupid talking to it. It doesn't seem to talk or think much, anyway—it just acts. But it's not so hard to calm down as I thought." Faye told the dragon that when it got upset in the future she would try to be with it in this new way, and the dragon seemed to relax even more.†

†*Once again, the power of corrective self-talk was used here effec-*
tively by Dr. Schwartz. Cognitive-behavioral therapists emphasize the
need to rehearse this self-talk on a regular basis through homework
assignments, in order to facilitate this new technique's becoming a
more permanent part of client's repertoires.

I asked Faye to thank the dragon for letting her help it, and then to
return her attention to the outside world. She came back saying that the
exercise felt weird, but kind of fun, and that she felt like she was 8 or 9
years old. Both Bob and Rebecca also seemed to be in a lighter mood. They
both said that they were familiar with that dragon. Bob said he was glad
to see that Faye could help it calm down. I warned them not to get their
hopes too high; the dragon probably protected hurt parts of Faye that were
still vulnerable, so it might may remain fairly explosive for a while yet.

I was relieved that this exercise had gone well. It's always a bit risky
when someone "goes inside" for the first time with others watching, even
when they're not concerned about the danger. Generally I wait until later
in the therapy before working in this manner, but Faye seemed eager, and
I deliberately didn't ask her about the parts the dragon protected so that
she would not expose any of the vulnerable parts too soon. If Faye had felt
or I had sensed any danger in doing this in front of the others, I would
have asked them to leave. Indeed, midway into the next session, I dismissed
Faye and Bob so that Rebecca would feel safe exploring her own internal
world.

Working Privately with Rebecca's Internal System

The family entered that next session seeming upbeat. Faye's dragon had
had little occasion to get upset, so she didn't have to calm it down often.
However, she said that during mealtimes, when Rebecca became edgy and
seemed anxious to get upstairs, Faye always assumed that she was rushing
off to vomit. Rebecca said defensively that sometimes she was just anxious
to get to her homework, and that she became discouraged when Faye and
Bob accused her even when she was not vomiting. I asked the parents, for
the time being, to trust Rebecca and me to handle her eating problems. I
told them that the best way they could help Rebecca was to keep working
with the parts of themselves that were so worried or angry (just as Faye
did with her dragon), so they could give up trying to coerce Rebecca to
change. Then, as Rebecca felt less concerned about being upset by her
parents' parts, she could work better with me to change her own. Bob and
Faye were clearly ambivalent. But they agreed to try, and then left the room
so Rebecca and I could work with her parts in private.

Rebecca was upset by the preceding conversation, and I asked her what
she was saying to herself about it (this is always a good question for
identifying parts). "Well, I blame myself because I'm so secretive about it,

but when I am doing well and they still think I'm sneaking around, it makes me want to not even try—to give up. It's like I have an excuse—I think I might as well do it if they're going to think I'm guilty anyway. But then I say to myself *I* know I'm doing well and that's all that matters—that I shouldn't be so concerned about their opinion. But I know that I am. It's confusing!"†

> † *At this point, the introduction of a form such as the Dysfunctional Thought Record might have been helpful (see Chapter 1). Because this form provides a structured writing exercise for laying out thoughts and then considering alternatives, Rebecca in this case might have been able to restructure her thinking in a systematic fashion, once she had reviewed it in writing and thought about what she was saying to herself. Cognitive-behavioral therapists often use this as a standard homework assignment to train individuals; eventually, clients can perform this automatically without always writing it down.*

I told Rebecca that I heard several different parts in that statement. One part criticized her for her thoughts and feelings; another told her not to try; and yet another tried to get her to think for herself. I asked whether she would like to help the different parts get along better inside her. She said that she would. I also mentioned that as she talked she seemed very hurt, and asked whether she was aware of a hurt part. She said, "Yes, it's the hardest part to deal with." I asked which of those four parts she would like to begin with. She chose the hurt one. This choice made me nervous, because the hurt part was likely to be an exile that her managers would like to keep us away from. I said that we would eventually work with that hurt part, but first I wanted to know about any fear that she felt when she thought about getting closer to it. She didn't feel any strong reservations, so, with great caution, we proceeded. As Rebecca focused on her hurt, she saw a Raggedy Ann doll slumped in the corner of a room. I asked her to be outside the room looking at it, and she said she wanted to go in and help it. Ultimately in that session, Rebecca was able to hold and comfort the doll. She also found and calmed the part that made her binge, which appeared to her as a frenzied ogre.

After a family member has had a private IFS session, he or she has the option to keep it private or to give some idea of what happened to the rest of the family. Disclosing some details often helps the other family members understand, support, and feel more involved in the work that's being done. It also gives them more confidence that something productive is happening and more hope that their problems can be resolved. On the other hand, when family members' parts are still extreme and threatening, even this amount of exposure can feel dangerous to the client who has done the private work.

Rebecca and I discussed what material she felt comfortable disclosing to her parents, and we had them return to the therapy room. She described to them in a lively way what she did with her doll and the ogre. Her parents listened politely and asked a few questions to clarify what all this meant. Their demeanor was supportive. I told them that I thought the work Rebecca had done was significant, but that she might be feeling more vulnerable as a result of it and might be more volatile during the coming week. When a client first reveals vulnerable parts, it's not uncommon for him or her to feel highly protective for a period afterward. It's good practice to forewarn family members of that possibility following any work with exiles.

Despite this warning, tension was evident when the family returned a week later. Bob's voice dripped with contempt as he described an incident in which Rebecca asked him to help her at the library and "went crazy" when he refused. Rebecca responded assertively, saying that she did not go crazy, but she did get angry because Bob never helped her or did anything with her. She said, "He can't stand it when anyone gets angry, but he never shows that he's upset—he just acts like he doesn't care." Faye jumped in at this point: "That's right. He's not demonstrative in any way, shape, or form, for wonderful things or bad things. That's just the way he is, and we all need to learn to accept it. It's taken me years to figure that out."

I said that for Rebecca it might be easy to mistake Bob's lack of responsiveness for a lack of caring.† Faye said brusquely that the topic of Bob's indifference was nothing new, and she didn't see it as an issue related to Rebecca's problem. Bob said that at his age he was very unlikely to change. He said he thought the problem was that Rebecca was too egocentric, and Faye said she thought Rebecca was just emotionally immature. Rebecca alluded to a recent time when she asked Bob to watch her in a gymnastics meet and he said he had to work, but he came home drunk, so he clearly wasn't working. Faye said, "Maybe he has to release his stress. You do your little number when you're stressed out. Daddy does his."

> †The issue of misattribution receives major emphasis in the cognitive-behavioral approach, which requires couples or family members to become active in gathering more evidence by questioning the other party directly. Instead of making a blind interpretation, Rebecca could have been coached by the therapist to ask Bob directly about his lack of responsiveness. Timing is a crucial factor and should be weighed carefully in such circumstances.

In this session, Rebecca was different. Previously she'd been dominated by her Raggedy Ann part, so she sounded very young and cried frequently. Now she stood up for herself and, in so doing, pointed the spotlight at her father's behavior. This seemed threatening to both parents, and they repeatedly returned the focus to Rebecca's deficits. Faye in particular came immediately to Bob's defense, as if fearing that something awful would happen if he were provoked.†

> † *This might have been a good time to ask Faye, "What's going through your mind right now?", in an attempt to understand her inner dialogue and how she is interpreting the situation. Monitoring cognitions on a regular basis is common in a cognitive-behavioral approach.*

I had to work hard with my own parts to avoid becoming angry with the parents for their denial and scapegoating. From the IFS perspective, people deny or avoid problems because their parts fear facing those problems. The goal of therapy isn't to force people to confront their problems while they are still terrified, but instead to help them feel safe enough to take their problems on. Thus, rather than confronting Faye or Bob at that point, I chose to remind them that I had predicted it would be a difficult week, and asked to meet privately with Rebecca once again.

When Rebecca's parents left, I asked her how she had kept her hurt part, the Raggedy Ann doll, from taking over during those painful exchanges. She said that she had moved it in her mind into a safe, protected back room, and the ogre was holding it. She now realized she had needed to do that during the week, because she had been feeling it more and had been overreacting. She said that the doll believed that her parents didn't care about her, and that she was in touch with those feelings now but not overwhelmed by them. I said that her parents seemed to have parts that reacted negatively to neediness, and that though I hoped they'd be able to change at some point, it wasn't going to be soon. In the meantime, she and I would continue to work on helping her feel less vulnerable to those parts of her parents.

Working with Bob and Rebecca Together

At the next session, I asked to meet with Bob and Rebecca together. This was to provide Rebecca with the opportunity to deal with her father without Faye's protecting him. Clearly Rebecca felt neglected and rejected by her father, and I was curious to see whether I could set up a Self-to-Self interaction between them, centering around those issues. I also wanted a chance to disarm his diffident manager and see whether I could connect with his Self. Bob seemed uneasy; Rebecca seemed scared. I told them that the goal was to improve their relationship.

"Our relationship is fine except that Rebecca expects too much from me," Bob said coldly. "My job causes me a lot of stress, and I don't always have time to attend all of her meets or help with her homework."

I asked Bob what statements he made to himself when Rebecca asked him for something.

"I feel angry because she never understands how busy I am."

Rebecca interrupted in a hurt and defensive voice, "I don't ask you to do anything any more."

I asked her to find the part of her that interrupted this exchange and ask it to step back and not interfere while we talked.

She paused for a moment, and in a stronger voice said, "It stepped back."

I then asked Bob to ask the same of the part of him that got angry with Rebecca.

"I don't understand what you're asking."

I replied that this was just a way to help them talk less emotionally so that they could avoid the painful patterns of the past. I asked what he felt in his body when he became angry with Rebecca.

"I feel a burning in my gut."

I had him focus on his gut and simply ask his anger to step back. He tried it, and his voice softened somewhat.†

> †*This was an excellent example of shifting from an affective point to a behavioral one, in order to help Bob focus on his anger in a more productive fashion. This is one of the beauties of using behavioral techniques, particularly with someone who may experience difficulty with affective expression.*

I then organized a listener–speaker structure between father and daughter that was designed to help them both keep their parts from interfering. In this exercise, each one in turn played the role of speaker while the other just listened. The speaker was to focus inside and then speak for his or her parts about whatever issue was being discussed. The listener was supposed to separate from his or her parts, to try putting himself or herself in the speaker's shoes, and then to repeat back to the speaker what was heard.

In situations where it's difficult for people to maintain Self-leadership, this structure greatly increases the overall sense of safety, as well as the ability of each person to control his or her individual parts. Just to be able to hear and remember what the speaker says, the listener is forced to quiet the parts that are usually so busy preparing a defense that they don't permit real listening. When the speaker senses that he or she is being heard (often for the first time) and not being attacked, his or her protective parts relax. During this exercise I play the role of "parts referee," stopping the action when I detect an extreme statement or reaction, and asking the person to move that particular part and try again with his or her Self in the lead. Gradually both persons find that they don't have to rely on the parts that have been taking over their interactions, and that with Self-leadership they get closer to what they really desire. I also interview the speaker, asking questions designed to bring forth the feelings and intentions that are being protected; I insure that the listener's feedback is complete and respectful as well.

Defensiveness characterized the first several rounds of this exercise, until Bob was finally able to repeat back what Rebecca was saying about feeling hurt because he never had time for her. He said he could understand what she felt and wished he could do more with her, but he felt a tremendous pressure to keep his dental practice thriving. They also discussed how, when Rebecca argued with either parent, the other parent always jumped in to side against her. Bob agreed that he was guilty of that and acknowledged that any kind of conflict in the family upset him a great deal, so he tried to suppress it as quickly as possible. He sided with Faye because he thought parents should support each other, but he could see how this only added to Rebecca's belief that he didn't care about her.

At the end of these exchanges, I asked Bob whether he wanted any help with the parts of him that made him so worried about his work or caused him to fear conflict. He said he would think about it, but clearly he was still uncomfortable with the idea of focusing inside himself, at least in my presence.

At the session's end, both Bob and Rebecca seemed upbeat and playful. I warned them that although they felt good now about having been able to talk, it was likely that their parts would jump back in at some future point, and they could feel terribly disappointed and betrayed if they weren't prepared.†

> † *Dr. Schwartz decided to take a path with Bob that, in my opinion, was ultimately quite effective. Had this not worked, however, an alternative might have been to consider exploring Bob's family of origin; this might have uncovered some of his schemas about dealing with conflict and shed light on how his particular beliefs about his life developed. Focusing on his family of origin might also have taken the emphasis off him, at least temporarily.*

Further Work with Rebecca's Parts

In the next session I met with Rebecca alone. I wanted to continue her internal work and to reassure her parents that we were addressing her eating problems. Rebecca seemed uncharacteristically distant and flat. She said that the closeness with her father had only lasted a few days before he rejected her once again. She was discouraged not only by his change, but also by her own reaction: She felt devastated and returned to the binge–purge pattern, which had abated considerably in the preceding weeks.

I asked her to check with the doll and the ogre, but when she focused inside she said that everything seemed more murky and blurred than before. She could see that the doll had returned to her lonely room and the ogre was again pacing frantically, but these images were hazy and she felt little desire or ability to help those parts inside her. I asked her to find the part that was making things so hazy and making her hopeless and apathetic. She saw a ball that had been deflated by a boy who'd hit it with a bat. Initially she was frightened of the boy, who seemed to have considerable power within her, but upon moving the frightened parts and speaking with the boy, she found that he was trying to protect her from disappointment by discouraging her from trying to improve anything. She told him that she no longer needed that type of protection, because she was learning how to care for the part that got so hurt when she was disappointed (the doll). She asked the boy to let her show him that she could help the doll, and he reluctantly inflated the ball, immediately lifting the inner haze. Quickly she was able to comfort the doll, which by this time was seeming more like a 5-year-old girl, and to return the ogre to his nurturing role.

I then asked her more about what happened internally when Bob or Faye rejected or criticized her. She said that she felt like a loser and attacked herself for not having a perfect body or for not being the perfect gymnast or student. When I asked her to find that perfectionistic part, she saw a woman who looked very sophisticated and perfectly fashionable. Rebecca laughed, saying that the woman resembled Faye.

In the next session, Rebecca told her parents about her parts and what she was doing for them. Faye seemed very interested. She wanted to know what she could do to support this work; she said she could tell it was helping, because Rebecca seemed less moody at home recently. Faye also said that she was thinking about her dragon and seemed better able to contain it—a development that Rebecca confirmed. Bob remained somewhat skeptical but curious. He reiterated that he was unlikely to change much, but was glad that Rebecca didn't seem so hurt by him all the time. Bob and Faye both also noted that she was dashing away from the kitchen table less often, and that they were finding it easier not to worry so much about her eating, as she seemed to be improving. I suggested that because we were making progress, I would work primarily with Rebecca for a few sessions, but we would keep them informed. They liked this idea.

During the next several sessions, Rebecca and I focused on the perfectionistic woman within her. For a long time the woman remained condescending and nasty, saying that Rebecca was basically worthless, so the only way for anyone to pay attention to her was to make her act or look perfect. Ultimately, however, the woman acknowledged that she was trying to get love for the doll (now the little girl) and for an older girl who felt worthless.†

> †*Exploring automatic thoughts such as the ones described above can lead therapists to the underlying schemas that seem to shape clients' feeling or belief of being "worthless." Schemas also exist at different levels; Dr. Schwartz uncovered an example of such a schema here.*

> *According to the cognitive-behavioral theory, the uncovering of schemas is the main road to facilitating change within an individual.*

After she saw that Rebecca was able to help those girls, the perfectionistic woman agreed to "let her hair down" and take on a new role of mentoring the older girl. I had Rebecca ask the older girl to show where in the past she had acquired the feeling of worthlessness. Rebecca saw a series of scenes during the time when her biological mother was constantly distressed and was abandoning her in order to be with a lover. Once this girl felt that Rebecca fully understood and appreciated what had happened to her, she was able to let go of feeling worthless.†

> † *It is important to reach the core of a schema and restructure it, or to do what is commonly known in many models of couple and family therapy as "reframing." Dr. Schwartz did this very nicely in his own style with Rebecca.*

Similarly, the 5-year-old child remembered scenes of her father being drunk and enraged, and her cowering in her bedroom. All this time Rebecca had carried a fear of Bob's temper and the sense that he could shift dramatically, so that she couldn't trust his caring even when he displayed it. As this was revealed to her, Rebecca developed increasing empathy for these parts of her and was able to care for them on a continual basis. Between sessions she spent 10 to 15 minutes each day in focusing on the parts until she found them, and asking how they were doing and what they needed.

During this series of sessions, Rebecca reported that relations between her parents had heated up at home, and that Faye was constantly angry with her again. Things were changing, however: She no longer fought with Faye over picky issues, but instead withdrew to her room and worked with her various parts, or went out with friends. On the other hand, the tension between Bob and Faye seemed to be increasing, with Faye frequently criticizing him and Bob in a constant snit. I regrouped the family for the next session.

Bob and Faye's Withdrawal; Work with Rebecca and Sue

As Rebecca had described, the tension in the room was palpable when the three of them entered. Although Bob and Faye acknowledged Rebecca's continued progress with her eating problems, Faye complained that she seemed distant and aloof. I reassured them that distant aloofness was what teenagers Rebecca's age specialized in. But because it was a sudden shift, I could understand how it would be difficult for Faye. At that point, I decided to inquire more directly about the parents' conflicts. I knew this was risky, but unless these issues were addressed, they would make the work with Rebecca more difficult.

I asked Faye, "How will it be for you if Rebecca continues to distance herself? How will that affect your relationship with Bob?"

She said, "I haven't gotten much from Rebecca except headaches for a while. I can take care of myself. Bob has said many times that he's not changing, and I can live with that."

Bob agreed that he wasn't changing and refused to discuss it any further.

The next three sessions were both frustrating and rewarding. Each week I asked the parents to come in with Rebecca, but each time she arrived alone, saying that her parents were too busy to attend. I spoke on the phone to both Bob and Faye; despite my pleas, both said they were tired of spending so much time and energy on Rebecca. I had no choice but to push ahead with Rebecca individually and see whether I could help her transcend the constraints of living in an emotional war zone.

Rebecca and I continued to work on her parts. She found one that was terrified that if she began to gain weight, she would never stop. It was polarized with the ogre, who was the one who made her binge. Since she had been free from bingeing and purging for several months, the controlling part had begun to trust that Rebecca could regulate her binges, and she had begun to gain weight. She was now approaching 100 pounds. I was frightened that by losing access to her parents, I had jeopardized this delicate improvement.

With the subsequent series of individual sessions, however, Rebecca became stronger and more independent. Predictably, the atmosphere became intolerable at home. Fortunately, she was able to move in with her original mother, Sue, with whom she had had only sporadic contact since her parents' divorce. I spent many sessions with Sue and Rebecca in the listener–speaker format as they explored the wounds from the past that Rebecca's parts had identified. After Sue had left Bob, her life had settled down, and she was quite available emotionally for Rebecca. Indeed, Sue harbored intense guilt about those earlier years and was tremendously relieved at finally being able to apologize to Rebecca. She also wanted Rebecca to know about her predicament at the time—how distant Bob was in the marriage, and how frightened she was by his drinking and temper binges. Although he was never physically violent, these episodes were nonetheless scary.

These sessions had a powerful calming impact on Rebecca's internal system.† Whereas before these sessions Rebecca had to find each part individually, after them her parts seemed to live together more harmoniously—when she looked inside, she would find them together in a peaceful group. Thereafter, my work with Rebecca was pleasant; it involved fine-tuning her inner relationships and trying to arrive at a consensus among her parts about a vision for her future. We gradually increased the intervals between our sessions, and stopped altogether a year and a half after our initial session. Rebecca remained in periodic phone contact with me over the next 4 years. She went off to college, found a boyfriend, maintained her weight, and continued to be free of binge–purge episodes. She reported that Faye and Bob remained married but miserable. Her contacts with them were sometimes upsetting, but at other times OK. She and Sue felt like good friends most of the time.

> † *Rebecca's calmer internal system could be said to reflect the consistency of the newly restructured schema about the dynamics between her and her parents. Dr. Schwartz achieved something here that cognitive-behavioral therapists strive for as a major objective.*

DISCUSSION

This case was not an example of ideal IFS family therapy. Although Rebecca clearly improved, that lasting improvement might not have been possible if Sue hadn't been available. Bob and Faye remained miserable. I failed to create an environment safe enough for Bob and Faye to air their exiled issues (e.g., Bob's drinking). Faye opened herself to me in the second session. In retrospect, I see that I should have maintained that connection by continuing to work with her parts. Bob also showed his Self briefly in the session with him and Rebecca alone. I was so excited and intrigued by Rebecca's internal family that I didn't take advantage of the openings I created with her parents. Thus, when I tried to expand the focus of therapy to include their issues, I did not have enough connection to convince them this could be done safely. My guess is that Bob would have tried to pull out no matter what I had done with him, but that if I had built more trust and rapport with Faye, she would not have allowed Bob to do this (or at least would not have collaborated with him).†

> † *I tend to agree in one sense; yet, in another, it is my impression that Bob's and Faye's individual and joint schemas were rather rigid and would have been very difficult to change. Dr. Schwartz aimed for what was, in my opinion, the most promising target—Rebecca's schemas.*

I highlight this mistake because it's a common one for those conducting IFS family therapy. The techniques illustrated in this case report can bring forth the Selves of people quickly. In 1 hour a week of family therapy, it's difficult to follow up on all of the openings that are created, and the individuals and parts who are neglected will often become even more protective as a result. Also, it's easy to become so enamored of the inner work with the person who opens up first (or most) that other family members and family dynamics are ignored. On the other hand, although this wasn't a problem in this case, the one doing more inner work may be viewed as the "sicker" one. For these reasons, I now keep a closer eye on balancing which family member becomes the focal point and on maintaining connections with others while they aren't immediately focal.

To be completely honest, there's another reason why I lost Bob and Faye: I never totally controlled the judgmental part of me that hated the way they berated Rebecca and complained so often about their precious time. That part never took complete control, but it was frequently in the background, influencing how much I reached out to them. This underscores how important it is for a therapist constantly to monitor and work with his or her parts, particularly when the therapist is experiencing any negative reactions to a family member. I am now better at remembering that arrogant, selfish, and mean behavior comes from parts of people that are protecting them from their pain. This perspective allows me to remain compassionate and to keep offering invitations in the face of hostile rejections.

On the other hand, many valuable IFS techniques for helping families are illustrated in this case. I identify and review some of them here in the order that they were used. These methods would be evident in most IFS family therapy.

1. I tried to deactivate the parents' managers by giving them compassion and control, but also by providing hope that their situation could change and that I was competent to help them do it.

2. I used the parts language to facilitate more open communication; to help family members develop new, nonpathological views of themselves, one another, and the problem; and to create hope for and clear steps toward change.

3. I helped them track the patterns of parts interactions across people, uncovering vicious circles, and then invited each member to focus on his or her own parts rather than trying to coerce change in the others.

4. I elicited the Selves of family members by detecting parts of different family members as these manifested themselves, and then having the members ask their parts to step back and allow their Selves to lead. I also did this by using the listener–speaker framework.

5. I worked with one member's parts privately (Rebecca), or while the others observed (Faye).

6. I warned family members, as things began to change, to prepare for parts' reactions to relapse.

7. I explored and resolved past traumas, both in private sessions with Rebecca and in family sessions with her and Sue.

Aspects of these methods will seem familiar to family therapists from different schools, but they have novel qualities also—qualities shaped by the different view of people offered by the IFS model. Indeed, virtually any family therapy technique can be adapted to fit with this approach, because the IFS model isn't a set of techniques; instead, it's a conceptual package or philosophy.† The techniques described in this chapter represent one way to apply the model.

> †*This statement is certainly consistent with the philosophy of the cognitive-behavioral model, which can lend a flexible "conceptual package" as well to the IFS approach. Hence, Dr. Schwartz presents an excellent model that is compatible and integratable with cognitive-behavioral therapy; the two approaches together may be easily integrated with other modalities as well.*

AUTHOR'S REPLY TO EDITOR'S COMMENTS

As Dr. Dattilio's thoughtful and flattering comments indicate, IFS therapy and cognitive-behavioral therapy have many compatibilities and similarities. In both, the focus is on altering family members' internal systems, and both respect and work with the multiplicity of the mind to do that. Because Dr. Dattilio has already identified several similarities and complementary methods, I focus here on what I perceive to be some differences.

The first difference relates to the way each model views what the IFS model calls "parts" and cognitive-behavioral therapy calls "schemas." My clients find it useful to relate to these inner entities as if they were literally internal family members—that is, full-bodied personalities of different ages, each with a wide range of emotions and thoughts. They enter conversations with these parts and try to show them love and compassion. My understanding of schemas is that they're considered clusters of thoughts and that clients enter less personal relationships with them.

A second difference is in my emphasis on the systemic network of relationships among parts. For example, rather than seeing Faye's dragon as an isolated angry part, I wanted to know about the parts it protected and the parts it was polarized with, and I assumed that for the dragon to change in a lasting way, those other parts would also have to change.

Finally, several times Dr. Dattilio has suggested interventions involving coaching, teaching, or giving assignments. Although I have no doubt that clients benefit from those interventions, I mostly ask questions. This is because I'm trying to release and become partners with the client's Self—the core of leadership that I assume exists within everyone. I'm trying to encourage the client's Self to reorganize the client's internal system and to identify what the client needs to do in the outside world. When clients achieve this kind of Self-leadership, I find that they don't need to be taught or coached because they know what they need to do, and my taking a position of authority sometimes delays the release of their Selves. I'm not sure that cognitive-behavioral theory has a concept that's comparable to what I'm calling the Self.

Having outlined these differences, I want to end by emphasizing that my exchanges with Dr. Dattilio about this chapter and my reading of some of his articles have left me with the impression that far more aspects of our therapy styles are similar than different. I have been disabused of my stereotypes of cognitive-behavioral therapists, because it's clear that he works with affect and imagery as well as cognitions, and is very respectful of his clients. I am grateful for the opportunity to engage in this rich dialogue.

NOTE

1. This case was described briefly in Katherine Fishman's (1995) book, *Behind the One-Way Mirror.*

REFERENCES

Fishman, K. (1995). *Behind the one-way mirror.* New York: Bantam.
Goulding, R., & Schwartz, R. (1995). *Mosaic mind: Empowering the tormented selves of child abuse survivors.* New York: Norton.
Schwartz, R. (1995). *Internal family systems therapy.* New York: Guilford Press.

SUGGESTED READINGS

Breunlin, D., Schwartz, R., & MacKune-Karrer, B. (1992). *Metaframeworks: Transcending the models of family therapy.* San Francisco: Jossey-Bass.
Nichols, M., & Schwartz, R. (1998). *Family therapy: Concepts and methods* (4th ed.). Needham Heights, MA: Allyn & Bacon.
Rowan, J. (1990). *Subpersonalities: The people inside us.* London: Routledge.
Stone, H., & Winkelman, S. (1989). *Embracing each other.* San Rafael, CA: New World Library.

Chapter 15

Feminist Couple Therapy

CHERYL RAMPAGE

THEORETICAL CONSIDERATIONS

Feminism

Unlike other theoretical influences, feminism, as it applies to therapy, has less to do with clinical methodology than with thinking about which belief systems are holding certain problems in place. One may do feminist therapy within a behavioral tradition, or from a psychoanalytic perspective; what is common to both of these is the therapist's consideration of how clients' gender beliefs and gender roles constrain them from solving their problems.

Feminists are interested in how power is distributed and expressed in male–female relationships. The centrality of power draws feminist therapists' attention primarily to heterosexual relationships—especially marriage, as the relationship in which the culturally prescribed power inequities between men and women have their most pernicious effects. These effects are often difficult to change, precisely because the prevailing ideology about marriage is that it is a relation between equals. This ideology itself obscures differences in power that do exist, often by simply attributing the differences to other causes (e.g., he drives the car whenever they're out together simply because he *likes* driving more than she does; she does the bulk of the child care and housework because she *cares* about that sort of thing more than he does [or is better at it]).

Feminism makes therapists sensitive to the gendered uses of power in relationships. Therefore, it leads them to label and challenge the distribution of power in relationships where it is unequal and the inequality is preventing the problem from being solved. This often results in (1) empowering women to claim what they want for themselves in their relationships;

(2) encouraging men first to own and then to cede some of the power that they are used to having, but that may prevent them from having the kind of marriage they want; and (3) using a social analysis to help partners demystify and depathologize the gendered differences between them.

Couples do not come to therapy for assistance with maintaining *in*equality between partners. We live in an age when it is no longer socially acceptable for men to claim that they want to be "king of the castle," or for women to aspire to nothing more than *selfless* devotion to husband and children. Power inequities are thus often obscured by rhetoric and ideology, and yet these inequities continue to exist. The recognition of the disparity between ideology and practice with regard to gender equality compels feminist therapists to investigate how power and responsibility are actually distributed in the small daily routines of married life. These investigations will lead into discussions about such apparent minutiae as who does the laundry, pays the bills, cooks the food, puts the children to bed, and decides when to have sex. A detailed understanding of these transactions is important, because it is in such details that intimidation, coercion, subordination, and oppression are likely to be manifested.

When faced with evidence of gender inequity in therapy, feminists use multiple strategies to address the problem. At times this may involve taking a position of advocacy rather than maintaining neutrality, as when a husband admits that he sometimes screams and throws things when he's angry, but denies that doing so is extremely intimidating to his wife. Advocating on behalf of one client in marital therapy must always be balanced by a strong alliance with the other partner, or in the long run the therapy will fail. Sometimes this alliance is based on nothing more concrete than the therapist's inference about the isolation and powerlessness a man feels, even as he is bullying or intimidating his wife.

Although therapy is not primarily an educational endeavor, there are times when the feminist therapist takes on an instructive role. Given how few role models there are for couples seeking an egalitarian relationship, feminist therapists will often direct couples toward gender-focused readings that will help them conceptualize how their gender arrangements are counterproductive to the marriage they want (see the "Suggested Readings" at the end of this chapter).

For more than 15 years, feminist family therapists have been expostulating on the field's implicit support of sexist ideology (Avis, 1992; Bograd, 1984; Goldner, 1985; Goodrich, 1991; Jacobson, 1983; James & McIntyre, 1983), and suggesting how the field can reform itself to correct this problem (Goodrich, Rampage, Ellman, & Halstead, 1988; Luepnitz, 1988; Rampage, 1995; Walters, Carter, Papp, & Silverstein, 1988). In the project of reforming thinking about female psychology and the development of relationships, the work of the scholars at the Stone Center on Women's Development at Wellesley College (Jordan, Kaplan, Miller, Stiver, & Surrey, 1991) has also been very useful.

The Problem-Centered and Metaframeworks Perspectives

A sophisticated feminist analysis of relationships between men and women is a necessary but not sufficient tool for clinical work with distressed couples. One must also have a clinical framework to guide therapy, organize impressions, develop an assessment, and plan interventions. Like all therapists who have been working in this field for a while, I have learned from many teachers and been influenced by many points of view. My earliest training in family therapy was heavily influenced by the work of Murray Bowen (1978). Later I studied strategic and systemic therapy with faculty members of the Galveston Family Institute. In the past decade, my clinical thinking has been most influenced by colleagues close to home.

The clinical model I use now relies heavily on principles drawn from the "problem-centered" model developed by Bill Pinsof (1995), and the "metaframeworks" perspective developed by Doug Breunlin, Dick Schwartz, and Betty MacKune-Karrer (1992). A detailed description of these approaches is beyond the scope of this chapter, but I have incorporated several salient features of these models into my own work. First, the models are based on a health premise: People are generally believed to be healthy. What brings them to therapy isn't their "pathology," but their inability to solve their problems with the skills and beliefs that they currently hold. The health premise leads us to frame all clinical inquiries from a negative explanation position. In other words, the question isn't "Why are the clients behaving in problematic ways?", but rather "What keeps them from behaving more adaptively?" To answer this question, the therapist engages in a conversation that begins focusing on the problem very much in the present and from a behavioral and systemic perspective. Only if attempts at intervening at this level prove inadequate does the therapist move into more historical and intrapersonal realms. Throughout the process, the therapist is attempting to identify and lift whatever blocks and constraints are preventing the client system from resolving the problem. Clinically simpler problems are generally constrained in fewer ways; more complex and long-standing problems are often constrained in multiple ways and at multiple levels, and they may require much more intervention to be resolved.

For example, two different couples may both seek help for a problem with "communicating." One couple's communication may be constrained only by the partners' reluctance to hurt each other's feelings by complaining. With a little reframing, reassurance, and perhaps some suggestions about how to communicate in nonaccusing ways, such a couple may find the problem alleviated. Another couple presenting with the same complaint about communication may be constrained in multiple ways. She, for example, may be reluctant to voice a complaint because he has a violent temper, because she's afraid for her children's safety, because she doesn't want the neighbors to hear, and because her concerns were ignored in her family of origin (so she has no basis for feeling optimistic about the results of voicing her concerns). He may avoid all affectively stimulating conversation because he doesn't know how to keep his adrenaline in check, because he believes that disagreement is always disrespectful, and because he fears that she will leave him and take his children. When a system is multiply constrained from changing, therapy is likely to require for more time and effort to succeed.

The metaframeworks model suggests several levels of problem analysis, including an analysis of the organization of the system; the recursive problematic sequences; the developmental issues of the system and its members; gender issues; cultural factors that affect the problem; and the internal processes of family members.

Narrative Therapy

A final influence on my clinical work has been the emergence of so-called "narrative" approaches to therapy (Freedman & Combs, 1996; Rampage, 1991; Weingarten, 1991; White & Epston, 1990). Narrative approaches are grounded in social constructionism and based on the premise that what each person regards as true or real is the result of a process of choosing from a number of possible realities or truths. The emphasis in narrative work is on how the stories that people tell (themselves and others) about their own lives become the filter for incorporating and even perceiving new information. Stories brought to therapy are often "problem-saturated" (White & Epston, 1990); that is, clients' problems have permeated every facet of their experience and awareness, rendering nonproblem and solution experiences inaccessible. The goal in narrative therapy is to help clients modify their stories in such a way that their problems are not featured so prominently, and their competence, successes, and pleasures can assume a larger place.

In the following case, the various theoretical perspectives outlined above were interwoven in my thinking as I attempted to assist the spouses in their effort to resolve the issues that prevented them from having the marriage they wished for.

CLINICAL MATERIAL: A MARRIAGE IN TROUBLE

Initial Impressions

It was Peter who made the initial call for therapy. His voice conveyed a mixture of trepidation and exhaustion. He and Liz, his wife of 8 years, had separated 2 days earlier after a particularly rancorous fight. It was neither their first fight nor their first separation, but Peter realized that the marriage had reached the breaking point, and had persuaded Liz to try marital therapy with him.

We spoke briefly, then set up an initial appointment for later in the week. I didn't try to elicit too much information, although Peter seemed to be in the mood to talk. Too much information from one spouse interferes with the rapid formation of an alliance with the couple—a key to positive outcome in marital therapy. From what Peter told me, I anticipated a volatile meeting.

When Peter and Liz walked into my office a few days later, my expectations weren't disappointed. In their mid-30s, both partners were physically attractive. Peter was solid and athletic with sandy hair, while Liz was a brunette and had the long, willowy look of a dancer. Because we met in the middle of their workday, each wore the conventional suit of an urban professional. In spite of some similarities of appearance, however, their demeanors were noticeably at odds. Liz was animated, with an expressive face and a quick smile. She was also, I noted, quick in her movements and her pace of speech. Peter, in contrast, was deliberate to the point of being ponderous. He sat slumped into the corner of the couch; his face looked taut, his jaws clenched. He looked both discouraged and defensive.

I established my intent to ally with them as a couple by opening the session with a general invitation to either of them to begin sharing with me the concerns that brought them to therapy. Not surprisingly, Liz seized upon this opportunity to begin a detailed explanation and analysis of the problem, including her opinion that Peter didn't take any responsibility for their home or their relationship, withheld his feelings from her, and was overinvolved with his family of origin. She added that she had some idea about her own part of the problem and recognized that she tended to be a controlling person—a characteristic she could trace back to her family-of-origin experience. She assured me that she was working on this.

All of this narrative was communicated in a span of less than 2 minutes. Liz would have gone on, but I interrupted her in order to bring Peter into the discussion. As I turned to Peter, he was staring at Liz with a glazed look, as if she were speaking in a foreign tongue. I asked how he would add to or modify Liz's description. He took a long breath, adjusted his glasses, and started, "Well . . . " In the 2-second pause that followed, while Peter struggled to articulate his ideas, Liz jumped back in to explain (to me) what he thought. I waited to see how Peter would respond to this interruption. He made a half-hearted effort to regain the floor, then settled once again into a listening mode. After a minute I interrupted Liz again (trying to calculate how many more times I could do this without impairing our fragile new alliance) and described the sequence that had just happened. I pointed out how Peter's reluctance to fight for floor time and Liz's willingness to speak for him seemed to be interfering with their communication. I suggested that they seemed to process and articulate conversation at different speeds, and that to hear Peter's point of view, Liz would probably have to discipline herself to wait for him to verbalize his own experience instead of jumping in and doing it for him. I also suggested that this particular dilemma probably reflected two gender differences they might do well to keep in mind: (1) In heated discussions, men often talk more slowly than women (Bergman, 1991); and (2) men generally have a smaller affective vocabulary than women, which makes conversations about their feelings more tedious for many men.†

> † *Many therapists have proposed strategies for dealing with such interruptions during the course of couple work, since they can unquestionably be a distraction during the treatment process. For example, Markman, Stanley, and Blumberg (1994) propose that the therapist provide the spouses with a piece of linoleum or another type of floor covering and have each one hold it while he or she speaks. This represents that the individual who is speaking "has the floor" and therefore shouldn't be interrupted. As creative as this sounds, this technique may still fall short of ending interruptions, because impulsive or emotionally charged spouses may not be able to refrain from butting in defensively.*
>
> *As noted on earlier chapters, another strategy that may be helpful in such a case is the "pad and pencil" technique (Dattilio, 1996, in press). This involves providing each of the partners with a pencil and pad of paper. Each spouse is instructed to write down the automatic thoughts that come into his or her mind as the other spouse is speaking. This way both parties can record what they're thinking, and the overt motor activity of writing it down may satisfy their urge to speak out. In this manner, they don't lose what they wanted to say. After each spouse is finished speaking, the therapist is free to ask the other one to read these notes. This allows the spouses to express themselves and eliminates the anxiety that they may have about "not having their say."*

Family Backgrounds

We were less than 10 minutes into the conversation, and I was already engaged in perturbing the couple system, challenging Peter to speak for himself and Liz to stop trying to do it for him. As the session unfolded, the reasons for their difficulties became clearer. Peter described himself as part of a very close family, in which interpersonal differences were minimized to protect the solidarity of the system. Peter felt close to both of his siblings—a brother who lived a short drive from their parents, and a sister who lived next door to them. There was not only little overt conflict, but a high sense of obligation to be there for each other. Although he maintained that he still enjoyed being part of such a close family, Peter had moved across the country when he went to college and had never lived less than 1,000 miles from his hometown since then.

Liz came from a family that was almost the opposite of Peter's: The overall level of conflict was high, and there was a low sense of solidarity. Her parents had divorced when she was 14 years old. Liz had left home to attend college and never returned to live there again. After college she moved several hundred miles from her parents' home. She visited her mother infrequently, never saw her father at all, and spoke to family members only a few times a year.

Peter's description of the marital problem was that Liz "had to have everything her own way." Although she complained of him not taking care of her or the relationship, he said, every time he did initiate something she would criticize it. As an example, he cited Liz's reaction to his driving, which was to do a running commentary on how he was driving at the wrong speed, taking an indirect route, or not paying enough attention in general. Such feedback had, over the years, made him extremely reluctant to initiate anything in the relationship. He was certain that to act would be to fail. Not surprisingly, Liz believed that Peter *purposely* behaved in careless or haphazard ways in order to get her to do more.†

> † *It might have been interesting to probe a bit further into why Liz maintained such beliefs. Perhaps she maintained some cognitive distortions about Peter that were not well founded. This might also have provided the therapist with more of a clue to Liz's thinking style.*

Initial Assessment

As we approached the end of the first session, I was developing a tentative assessment of the problem, drawing on the information the couple told me as well as what I observed. I thought about the marital problem in terms of three dimensions. First, from a feminist perspective, the couple was engaging in some stereotypical and mutually unsatisfying interactions. Liz was overfunctioning both emotionally and in terms of the pragmatics of maintaining their lives together. Peter was emotionally withdrawn and carrying very little responsibility for their daily lives as a couple, in spite of the fact that both of them worked full-time. Second, the gender imbalance was holding in place an organizational problem in the marriage: Although they both subscribed to an egalitarian ideal, the fact that the distribution of labor in the marriage was so unequal kept the relationship skewed and conflictual around issues of balance, harmony, and leadership. Finally, the spouses had described and demonstrated several sequences or patterns in their relationship that created anger and unhappiness. At times these unhappy sequences escalated to such an intolerable level that Peter and Liz would physically separate for a few days, but the separations never seemed to accomplish much more than a temporary reduction of tension. Coming to therapy during the current separation seemed to represent an effort by the couple to disrupt this particular sequence.

Homework

I made two concrete suggestions of tasks the couple could do between the first and second sessions. First, I asked that each of them provide the other with a list of at least 10 specific things the other could do that would increase the first spouse's sense of being cared for in the marriage. Once they exchanged lists, each one was to start doing something on the other's list at least once daily, without commenting on the fact. This is a variation of Richard Stuart's "caring days" exercise that I find very helpful early in marital therapy, as it gets the focus away from the negative and the intellectual, and onto the positive and the behavioral.†

> † This was an excellent suggestion, and in my opinion it was made at about the right time in the treatment process. Such an exercise can also be helpful as a diagnostic aid, in that, should it fail, it will also provide a therapist with additional information about how a couple functions. However, some behaviorists caution against the implementation of quid pro quo exercises too early in the therapeutic process, since it could result in failure. Thus, the decision should be weighed carefully by assessing the partners' readiness for such an exercise.

For their second task, I asked Peter and Liz to spend 15 minutes together at least four times in the coming week. During these 15 minutes, it was to be agreed that neither of them would answer the phone, watch television, or have a computer turned on. I asked that they use these times to talk and listen to each other about whatever was on their minds. I originally developed this task as an intervention to increase marital intimacy; I have come to appreciate its diagnostic significance. The struggle to do the task reveals useful information about a couple's ambivalence regarding intimacy. Few couples successfully complete the task early in therapy (and those that do generally don't require any extensive therapy), but much can be made of how a couple goes about *not* completing it. For example, it's an excellent way to demonstrate the principle of collusion, as generally partners arrange never to be ready to sit down together at the same time.

A Problem Sequence

The second session began with a cautious acknowledgment on both sides that things were a little better. Peter had moved back home, and he had had dinner several times that week with Liz. Liz had "let" Peter drive on a couple of occasions, and she had not been critical of him in doing so. Nevertheless, as Liz was quick to point out, "nothing big" had really changed. Peter hadn't initiated any conversation between them and was still content to spend most evenings engaged in his own solitary pursuits. I blocked Liz from continuing in this vein by asking how it felt to her when Peter *had* made dinner for them a couple of times. She was grudging in her acknowledgment, noting that one evening he had made something he "knew" she didn't care for, and on the other he took so long deciding what to make that they hadn't sat down to dinner until almost 9:00. When Peter spoke up to defend himself, Liz rapidly became very angry; she accused him of being selfish and self-centered and of taking her for granted, and warned that she didn't know how much more she could take.

At one level, this sequence echoed something I had observed in the previous session. When distressed by Peter, Liz tended to escalate rapidly into an angry, accusatory state, to which Peter responded slowly and weakly. His relative lack of reaction only seemed to stir her into a heightened state of intensity. At another level, Peter's lack of response seemed to represent a deeply felt fear on Liz's part that no matter what, Peter would never really be willing to take care of her.

It's important to understand the meaning of repetitive and disturbing sequences in a couple system, and it's imperative to disrupt such sequences in order to limit their corrosive effect on the relationship. With that in mind, I again tried to encourage Peter to speak up for himself, and not to let the pace and intensity of Liz's communication silence him. At the same time, I was careful to validate Liz's longing for some caretaking from her husband and her discouragement about whether it would ever happen. This validation is key; for all the intensity of their longing to be cared for, by the time they reach adulthood most women have completely absorbed the message that their proper role in life is to do for others, and that to want something in return is selfish. Their sense of entitlement, therefore, is often fragile and uncertain. Indeed, I took the intensity of Liz's expression of her distress as a sign of how uncertain she was about the legitimacy of her longing. For a therapist to interrupt a woman's expression of her desire (however poorly expressed), without validating the legitimacy of the longing, is to reinforce her belief that there's something wrong with her for merely wanting it.

Another constraint that interferes with changing the pattern of relational caretaking in marriage is the tendency of women to "hostess" everyone in their lives, especially their husbands. Hostessing involves anticipating and responding to others' needs without the others' ever having to express these needs. Trained from early childhood to value relationships, to be sensitive to the feelings of other people, to subordinate their own needs, and to believe that having a relationship with a man is the *sine qua non* of adult happiness, heterosexual women become expert at hostessing the men in their lives. The trouble with this "gift" is twofold. First, men don't receive the same gender training as women, and so are less adept at subordinating their own desires in deference to others and at recognizing unspoken need. Furthermore, because women are so good at hostessing, men do not appreciate the effort it takes; thus, they either minimize its significance and take it for granted, or assume that women just do this because they want to. The result is that men do not tend to reciprocate the kind of caring that they receive from their wives.

My effort to disrupt this sequence was only partially successful: Liz did cease her attack on Peter, but was quite upset with me. She expressed her fear that I didn't like her, that I found her overwhelming, and that I wasn't willing to listen to her any more than Peter was. The rest of the session was spent trying to repair our alliance, which I took responsibility for having damaged. I acknowledged that it was indeed hard for me to follow and respond to what she was saying when she piled one thing on top of another and spoke about all of it in such pressured tones. At the same time, I let her know that I really did want to hear her. By the end of the session we were all exhausted, but I felt that the alliance had been repaired.

Personal Narratives and Intergenerational Sequences

After that conversation, I began to think that before I tried to make further interventions in their current conflict, I needed to strengthen my alliance with the partners and especially with Liz. There are many techniques therapists can use to accomplish this task. I decided to try to lower the affective intensity of the sessions by redirecting the content from the immediate problem to gathering further information about the families in which Liz and Peter had first learned about being in a relationship. I knew that eventually we would have to return to the present in order to resolve their problem, but I doubted that I could keep the couple in treatment unless I found a way to make the sessions less volatile and strengthened my alliance with each spouse. I also suspected that some of the roots of the marital problem they were experiencing could be traced back to Liz's and Peter's original families. Accordingly, I began the third session by suggesting that we spend a couple of meetings talking about their families of origin. I asked them to tell me the stories of their lives, with particular emphasis on what they had learned in their original families about marital relationships, about being cared for, and about voicing their needs. Both Peter and Liz willingly agreed to this plan and seemed relieved to have a reason not to focus on their current problems for a while.

In the next couple of sessions, each partner told his or her own story while the other spouse and I listened attentively. Not surprisingly, each story reflected themes of not being seen or heard, and of learning that to want something was regarded as either "selfish" or "crazy." Peter's family was religiously conservative; the entire social life of the family revolved around the church community. The structure of the family was rigidly hierarchical, with children and wife all deferring to the wishes of Peter's father. Inducing shame was the principal method of securing cooperation.

Peter had escaped from this environment by winning a prestigious college scholarship. Although he never returned to live in the small town where he grew up, he maintained close contact with his family through telephone calls and frequent visits. In fact, Peter's insistence that he be with his family every Christmas had become a major point of friction between him and Liz. What Peter seemed to have learned from his family was that personal needs must always be suppressed in order to maintain the equilibrium of the system; that happiness consisted of behaving acceptably to the group; and that husbands should be the unchallenged leaders in marital life.†

> † *This was an excellent move, in my opinion—to drop back and focus on family-of-origin issues. The resulting conversation also provided Dr. Rampage with some important information about Peter's schemas, which would later be essential if she were to decide to use some cognitive restructuring techniques.*

Liz's family experience was substantially influenced by her mother's alcoholism, which had reached an acute stage when Liz was a preadolescent. At that point her father had left the marriage and his children, moving to California, from where he made only occasional contact. As the oldest child, Liz was left feeling responsible for her mother as well as for her younger siblings. She was able to continue doing well in school, in spite of the burden she felt. Her younger siblings both left home before finishing high school. Liz worked for a couple of years after high school to save money for college; then she too left home. She put herself through college while working almost full-time. Although she was proud of this accomplishment, she also recollected being almost paralyzed with fear much of the time, feeling that she was only one paycheck or one failing grade away from disaster. She developed several psychosomatic symptoms during this period, including irritable bowel syndrome—a problem that had persisted up to the present.

The most profound lesson that Liz seemed to have drawn from her family experience was that she could never expect anyone really to be there for her. This belief stood next to an equally strong conviction that it was essential to have someone in her life who could stave off her pain and fear of being alone in the world. In her relationship with Peter, she was constantly pulled between longing for the safety and security she had never felt as a child, and skepticism that he could or would provide it.

We were able to use the stories told by Peter and Liz to weave together a description of the marriage that made sense to both of them. They agreed that they had been drawn together, in part, because each saw the other's family as a balance to his or her own: Liz hoped that Peter's close, highly involved family would finally give her a place to "belong," while Peter believed that Liz's capacity to be independent from her family would help him achieve a measure of distance from his own. Nor surprisingly from a family-of-origin perspective, each of their hopes had been disappointed. Far from finding Peter's family a place where she could belong, Liz experienced his family as unwelcoming to her as an outsider. Worse yet, when she and Peter were with his family, he seemed to become remote from her, leaving her feeling even more isolated and anxious than before. For his part, Peter found the interpersonal demands of being a husband even more trying than those of being a member of a rather enmeshed family. He began to use his family involvement as a means of regulating distance between himself and Liz—a pattern that aggravated Liz's reactivity.

Liz and Peter were able to recognize ways in which their personal narratives intersected and, in fact, reinforced their marital discord. They were able to see their mutual participation in some of the more distressing sequences in their marriage, and so to become somewhat less blaming of each other. In addition, I felt that the break from focusing on their immediate problem had helped me to form a stronger and more empathic alliance with each of them.

A Marital Crisis

At this point, approximately 6 weeks into the therapy, a crisis developed. Peter had long since made plans to spend the Christmas holidays with his parents and siblings and their families—a pattern that had begun 3 or 4 years earlier, when Liz refused to accompany him. Now, as the impending visit came closer, Liz became furious and despairing; she feared that he would never change, and that he would always choose his family over her. In sessions, she fell back into the pattern of loudly and angrily attacking Peter for his decision and accusing him of not being honest with her (or with me) about his *real* intentions never to give her what she wanted. She was simultaneously furious at herself for staying in the marriage, defining her doing so as "neurotic" and "dependent."

With the new perspective gained by looking at the intergenerational sequences in their families, Peter was more able to see how anticipating his leaving was triggering another episode of Liz's reacting to his withdrawal by pushing him away. He offered to change his plans, suggesting that they travel together to Paris over the holiday. Liz was not appeased. It was as if the damage had already been done merely by Peter's *intending* to be separate from her for Christmas.

Since crisis destabilizes systems, it also creates the greatest possibility for implementing changes. I worked with Liz on challenging her catastrophic expectations (Pinsof, 1995) that the separation from Peter would necessarily be devastating to her. I also encouraged her to stop seeing herself as a helpless victim in this situation, and instead to focus on taking care of herself by making a plan for Christmas that would protect her from feeling desperate and abandoned. Finally, I urged both partners to collaborate on how they could relate differently to each other through this separation in a way that would strengthen, rather than undermine, their relationship.

We were able to make some headway on each of these issues. Liz decided to use the break from Peter to travel by herself. Since she hated the frigid Midwestern winters and was an amateur archeologist, she planned a trip to the Yucatan to visit a number of Mayan ruins. With some encouragement from me, she was able to ask Peter to take total responsibility for maintaining contact with her during the 10-day period when they would be apart. He was at first reluctant to do so without very specific input from her about how often she wanted him to call her, for fear of not doing it right. I blocked Peter from engaging Liz on this point; I suggested that being in total control of regulating the contact between them gave him an opportunity to demonstrate his willingness to take care of the relationship without direction from Liz, and thereby to disconfirm one of her hypotheses about him that prevented her from feeling good about the marriage. Furthermore, I encouraged Peter to use this opportunity not to practice guessing what *Liz* wanted, but to reflect on and demonstrate what kind of husband *he* wanted to be.†

> †*This was a terrific idea. It not only facilitated the shifting of behavior patterns, but also allowed Liz the opportunity to gather some new data, which she could later use to incorporate into her new schemas about Peter. Firsthand information such as this is excellent for reshaping schemas, since it adds to the veracity of the restructured content.*

The work we had previously done in therapy provided both the encouragement and the conceptual rationale needed for Peter and Liz to try making a change in their relationship through this crisis. Upon returning to therapy after their separate holidays, they reported that their efforts had achieved some success. Peter had arranged for several little gifts to arrive at Liz's hotel during her stay in Mexico. He had called her three times, including at midnight (her time) on Christmas Eve. When she returned home, he unexpectedly met her at the airport. He took great satisfaction in having accomplished the goals of being responsible for reassuring Liz that out of sight would not be out of mind, and of thinking about what kind of husband he wanted to be. Liz reported that she had been surprised and pleased at the flowers and wine in her room, and at Peter's meeting her when she arrived at the airport. The telephone calls, she felt, had been only a partial success, as Peter had shown little interest in what she was doing and had once cut a call short because of some plan with his family.

Organizational and Gender Constraints

The "Christmas crisis," as we came to call it, marked a small shift in the level of optimism Peter and Liz felt about their marriage. In subsequent sessions, we focused on further changes in the marriage—particularly in relation to some organizational features of the relationship, and to the gender constraints that continued to impede the couple's attainment of their goals. Although Peter and Liz both worked full-time in demanding professions, Peter assumed almost no responsibility for the maintenance of their daily lives. He didn't defend this fact as an ideal, but explained that any effort he made to show initiative or leadership in the marriage was opposed by Liz. She asserted that his attempts to show initiative or leadership invariably either were poorly executed or disregarded her needs and preferences. Liz made it clear that she believed Peter's ineptitude in this area demonstrated a lack of caring rather than a lack of competence.

The organizational dilemma contained in this vignette is common among younger married couples. Raised in a generation that takes gender equality as an inarguable right, these couples nonetheless find that the implementation of equality is a challenging task. Both Liz and Peter believed that he should be as responsible for the relationship as she, but they underestimated how much their gender training had directed her toward being responsible for the emotional well-being of the relationship as well as the bulk of their domestic needs. As noted earlier, women learn from early childhood how to read and even anticipate the needs of other people, and they organize their behavior (sometimes to their own detriment) around making their relational partners happy. Because men are trained quite differently, they learn to "tune out" their own emotional reactions (other than anger and disappointment) and to be insensitive to the feelings of others.

These gender role differences create an imbalance in male–female relationships. Because women are usually more emotionally attuned to their interpersonal environment and more expert in a variety of domestic living skills (such as getting wine stains off napkins, finding a reliable babysitter on short notice, and knowing how long chicken can be broiled before it turns into leather), they often find themselves overburdened with the responsibilities of both the emotional well-being of their families *and* the management of countless small tasks required to maintain a family and a home. This was precisely the predicament that Liz found so burdensome.

Changing this imbalance isn't easy. Even when a man expresses his willingness to carry more responsibility (as Peter certainly did), he is unlikely to be as skilled at the requisite tasks as his partner. This creates a dilemma. Should a husband develop his own unique method of doing laundry, even if this means that stains will set and colors will bleed? Should he do the grocery shopping when it suits his schedule, even if it means there's nothing to pack for school lunches once in a while?

There are three constraints that most often make rearranging domestic tasks difficult for couples. First, if a husband is to develop the same level of competence as his wife, he needs to acknowledge his lack of competence, recognize her as the expert and leader in this area, and submit himself to learning from her greater expertise. This situation inverts the "natural" hierarchy of most marriages and forces the husband to acknowledge a limitation. Talking about this in therapy, and inviting the husband to explain why it feels so bad to take advice from his wife, are sometimes helpful simply because the husband can thus let go of some of his nursed resentment. The second constraint that makes this shift difficult is that it does entail an actual loss of freedom for him, since he will be taking on responsibilities that he has not previously had. Third, even women tired of feeling overburdened with responsibility sometimes find it difficult to let it go. They can sabotage their husbands' efforts by being overly critical or by micromanaging. This is particularly true when a woman has derived a significant part of her self-worth from the accomplishment of such tasks, or when she is struggling against (possibly unconscious) gender rules that define the tasks in question as her rightful jobs.

Sometimes it is helpful to contextualize changes couples attempt to make in their gender roles by pointing out that there have been more changes in the expectations we have of ourselves as women and men in the past two decades than there have been in the entire recorded history of humankind. It should therefore not surprise us that these changes have not been smooth and are not yet fully integrated. Like many couples, Liz and Peter found this idea helpful and moderately encouraging.

A Marital Agenda

We began the next phase of our work together by having a conversation about the goals each spouse had for his or her own participation in the marriage. I asked them to speak to each other about what they wanted to contribute to the marriage and what they would like to receive from it. By this time, they were much less reactive to each other, so that direct conversation was not nearly as volatile as it had been. They each developed a set of tasks and responsibilities that they wanted to pursue. There was considerable, but not entire, overlap between their lists. Each partner made suggestions to the other of additional things that might be considered for inclusion on his or her list. In this process, Peter was surprised and pleased that Liz didn't want to add 50 things to his list. She was likewise encouraged to see that Peter had many things on his list that she had not imagined he would think of. They began experimenting with enacting some of these changes in their lives. Over the course of the next few months the therapy served as a vehicle for problem solving centered around their efforts to change the roles that each of them had played in the relationship. There were successes (Peter became a much better cook) and setbacks (it was extremely difficult for Liz to break the habit of interpreting Peter to himself), but all in all, things improved and the couple felt more comfortable.

Efforts to change the distribution of tasks within the marriage were interwoven with efforts to shift the pattern of affective communication. At first, I consistently had to block Liz from interpreting Peter's feelings, and to challenge Peter to take responsibility for naming his own emotional experience. As is often the case, this was not an easy pattern to break. As much as a husband may (rightfully) resent his wife for acting as the authority about his feelings, he may find that neither his emotional vocabulary nor even his awareness of his feelings is sufficient to participate in the kind of relationship she is pressing for. Fortunately, Peter had now been engaged in individual therapy for some time, and through this process he had become much more aware of his own feelings and motivations. Once he felt that Liz was able to listen to him, he began to share more of his emotional life with her. Over time, she gave up her conviction that she knew him better than he knew himself, and became interested in knowing him better by hearing him describe his own experience.†

> †*I would be curious as to how the cognitions of both partners changed as Peter began to reveal more of his emotional self to Liz. This would support the philosophy that affective shifts do influence cognition and behavior; it would also be important to know for facilitating future change with the couple.*

Managing Closeness and Distance

The final stage of our work in the therapy addressed how Liz and Peter handled the fluctuations of closeness and distance in the relationship. Peter's experience in his enmeshed family had left him with considerable ambivalence about being close to Liz. He both craved closeness and believed it to be antithetical to autonomy. He would seek Liz out and then abruptly pull away, leaving her feeling angry and betrayed. Her side of this dynamic was driven by her fear that no one would really want to be close to her. She was often resistant to Peter's efforts to be close, precisely because she expected to be disappointed. When he would withdraw, her worst fears were confirmed.

We worked on helping Peter and Liz to withdraw from each other in a nonhostile, even loving way. Peter began using a "time-out" procedure to get some distance from Liz without rejecting her in a hostile way. Liz agreed that Peter could call a time out from their interaction any time he felt he needed to, provided that he also took responsibility for calling "time in" again. Both Liz and Peter found this procedure a useful tool for regulating the closeness–distance cycles of their relationship, and began to experience greater comfort and satisfaction with the relationship overall.

After approximately 9 months of marital therapy, Liz and Peter felt ready to draw this chapter of their relationship to a close. We ended therapy a week before they embarked on the first of their vacations as a couple that had been mostly planned by Peter. Each spouse felt substantially more optimistic about the marriage, and more appreciative of the role the other partner played in it. Liz felt that she could trust Peter to be as responsible for their lives together as she held herself to be. Peter felt successful as a husband, both as an emotional partner to Liz and as a partner in living.

AUTHOR'S REPLY TO EDITOR'S COMMENTS

Dr. Dattilio's commentary reveals the considerable extent to which my approach to therapy has already been influenced by cognitive-behavioral thinking. There are two bases for this. First, the problem-centered approach has taught me to stay in the present and in the behavioral realm until it is clear that doing so is insufficient to create the desired change. Second, learning about narrative therapy has persuaded me that feelings emerge from beliefs or thoughts. It is extremely difficult to influence feelings directly, but if beliefs change, different feelings often follow. Therefore, I see the cognitive-behavioral emphasis on helping people change their cognitive schemas as highly compatible with my clinical approach.

I was particularly intrigued by the suggestion to have partners write down their reactions to each other's statements as a method of preventing them from constantly interrupting each other to correct, react, or admonish. I like having this kind of easy, practical intervention in my head as I attempt to disrupt a pattern that has been resistant to change.

REFERENCES

Avis, J. M. (1992). Where are all the family therapists?: Abuse and violence within families and family therapy's response. *Journal of Marital and Family Therapy, 18*(3), 225–232.

Bergman, S. (1991). *Men's psychological development: A relational perspective* (Work in Progress No. 48). Wellesley, MA: Stone Center Working Paper Series.

Bograd, M. (1984). Family systems approaches to wife battering: A feminist critique. *American Journal of Orthopsychiatry, 54,* 558–568.

Bowen, M. (1978). *Family therapy in clinical practice.* New York: Jason Aronson.

Breunlin, D. C., Schwartz, R. C., & MacKune-Karrer, B. (1992). *Metaframeworks: Transcending the models of family therapy.* San Francisco: Jossey-Bass.

Dattilio, F. M. (1996). *Cognitive therapy with couples: The initial phase of treatment* [Videotape]. Sarasota, FL: Professional Resource Exchange.

Freedman, J., & Combs, G. (1996). *Narrative therapy: The social construction of preferred realities.* New York: Norton.

Goldner, V. (1985). Feminism and family therapy. *Family Process, 24*(1), 31–48.

Goodrich, T. J. (Ed.). (1991). *Women and power: Perspectives for family therapy.* New York, Norton.

Goodrich, T. J., Rampage, C. R., Ellman, B., & Halstead, K. (1988). *Feminist family therapy: A casebook.* New York: Norton.

Jacobson, N. S. (1983). Beyond empiricism: The politics of marital therapy. *American Journal of Family Therapy, 11,* 11–24.

James, K., & McIntyre, D. (1983). The reproduction of families: The social role of family therapy? *Journal of Marital and Family Therapy, 9*(2), 119–129.

Jordan, J. V., Kaplan, A. G., Miller, J. B., Stiver, I. P., & Surrey. J. L. (1991). *Women's growth in connection: Writings from the Stone Center.* New York: Guilford Press.

Luepnitz, D. (1988). *The family interpreted: Feminist theory in clinical practice.* New York: Basic Books.

Markman, H., Stanley, S., & Blumberg, S. L. (1994). *Fighting for your marriage.* San Francisco: Jossey-Bass.

Pinsof, W. M. (1995). *Integrative problem-centered therapy.* New York: Basic Books.

Rampage, C. (1991). Personal authority and women's self-stories. In T. J. Goodrich (Ed.), *Women and power: Perspectives for family therapy* (pp. 109–122). New York: Norton.

Rampage, C. (1995). Gendered aspects of marital therapy. In N. Jacobson & A. Gurman (Eds.), *Clinical handbook of couple therapy* (pp. 261–273). New York: Guilford Press.

Walters, M., Carter, B., Papp, P., & Silverstein, O. (1988). *The invisible web: Gender patterns in family relationships.* New York: Guilford Press.

Weingarten, K. (1991). The discourses of intimacy: Adding a social constructionist and feminist view. *Family Process, 30,* 285–305.

White, M., & Epston, D. (1990). *Narrative means to therapeutic ends.* New York: Norton.

SUGGESTED READINGS

Carter, B., & Peters, J. (1996). *Love, honor and negotiate: Making your marriage work.* New York: Pocket Books.

Napier, A. (1988). *The fragile bond: In search of an equal, intimate and enduring marriage.* New York: Harper & Row.

Rampage, C. (1995). Gendered aspects of marital therapy. In N. Jacobson & A. Gurman (Eds.), *Clinical handbook of couple therapy* (pp. 261–273). New York: Guilford Press.

Schwartz, P. (1994). *Love between equals: How peer marriage really works.* New York: Free Press.

Weingarten, K. (1991). The discourses of intimacy: Adding a social constructionist and feminist view. *Family Process, 30,* 285–305.

Chapter 16

Narrative Solutions Couple Therapy

JOSEPH B. ERON
THOMAS W. LUND

The approach presented in this chapter has developed out of our 14-year collaboration at the Catskill Family Institute, an interdisciplinary group practice located in New York's Hudson Valley region (see Eron & Lund, 1989, 1993, 1996, in press; Lund & Eron, 1998). Over the years we have studied how therapeutic conversations with people in distress actually work, and we have compared those that reach solutions with those that don't. In the process, we have arrived at general principles for how to conduct helpful conversations that resolve a range of clinical problems appearing at different stages along life's path.

FOUR KEY ASSUMPTIONS

The narrative solutions approach is predicated on four key assumptions about how problems evolve, persist, and can be resolved.

Assumption 1

Assumption 1 is as follows: *People have strong preferences for how they would like to behave, how they would like to see themselves, and how they would like to be seen by others. We refer to this constellation of ideas about self as a person's "preferred view."*

The concept of "preferred view" has appeared in different shapes and forms in the writings of prominent individual and family therapists (e.g., Rogers, 1961; Watzlawick, Weakland, & Fisch, 1974; White & Epston, 1990). In our approach, this concept is basic to understanding how problems evolve, as well as how to plan helpful conversations so that problems can be resolved.

We don't conceive of "preferred view" as a permanent property of a person. Rather, the term refers to a host of possible views or preferences that suit people—that fit with the persons they wish to be. Preferred views change as people move through transitions in life, waxing and waning in importance. For example, young children often prefer to be regarded as good in the eyes of their parents; adolescents as independent and self-sufficient; young adults as successful, autonomous, and capable of intimacy; adults as competent parents and loved partners; and older adults as still useful and deserving of respect. In general, we regard "preferred view" as a narrative concept—a fluid, evolving set of ideas about the self that embraces past, present, and future dimensions of life experience. Preferred views are inferred from the stories people tell about their lives and the ways they describe their experiences.

Assumption 2

Assumption 2 is the following: *Problems emerge when people interpret transitional events in ways that contradict preferred views of self.*

The notion that problems arise during normal times of transition in the life cycle was a major theme in the writings of leading family therapists of the 1970s and 1980s (see, e.g., Weakland, Fisch, Watzlawick, & Bodin, 1974; Haley, 1973, 1980; Carter & McGoldrick, 1980). According to the brief, problem-focused approach developed at the Mental Research Institute (MRI), problems develop innocently from the mishandling of ordinary life difficulties that occur at key transition points in the life cycle (e.g., marriage, birth, leaving home, divorce, remarriage, illness, and death). People can get into problems with the best of intentions; they can also get out of problems without a major overhaul of their personality or family structures.[1]

In the narrative solutions approach, a careful assessment of the mishandling of ordinary life difficulties takes into account shifts in how people think, behave, and interact with others during times of flux. We consider how present patterns of thought and action link up with past stories, and shape how people construct their futures. Events that occur during times of transition are significant to problem development, because they awaken a search for new perspectives. During times of incipient change, people often begin to reconsider how they see themselves and how they should behave.

As people try to negotiate important transitions in life, they not only look inwardly through the lens of history and their own self-narratives, but they also think of themselves in relation to important others. This leads us to our next assumption, which pertains to the persistence of problems within and between people.

Assumption 3

Assumption 3 is this: *Problems intensify and persist as the gaps grow wider among how people prefer to view themselves, how they act, and how they think important others regard them.*

Consider how an event such as job loss triggers the development of a problem in a 48-year-old man. Prior to this event, the man's preferred view of self was congruent with his own behavior and how he imagined others regarded him. For 25 years he fulfilled his wish to be a hard-working, dependable provider and viewed himself as successful in the eyes of his employers, his father (a role model), his wife, and his children. Now downsized and feeling diminished, the man becomes lethargic. He makes half-hearted attempts to prove his usefulness by starting projects around the house, but fails to complete them.

Family members respond to these changes in ways that fit with their own preferences. This is a close-knit family in which being helpful and pitching in are admired. After cheerful pep talks fail to inspire the man to get moving, his wife grows impatient. She chides him to "get off his duff and get a new job," then asks her 20-year-old son to finish the projects his father has started. As the man becomes more convinced that his loved ones see him as useless, his despondency deepens. The more depressed the man acts, the more helpless family members feel, the more critical they become, the worse they feel about themselves, the worse he feels about himself, the more depressed he acts, and so on. Thus, problems intensify and persist as the gaps grow wider among how people prefer to view themselves, how they act, and how they see others perceiving them.[2] The unsettling experience of "disjunction," or contradiction, *within* each person propels more-of-the-same behavior *between* people.[3]

Assumption 4

Assumption 4 is as follows: *Problems are resolved as the gaps narrow among how people wish to be seen, how they act, and how they think important others regard them.*

We believe people are at their best when they think of themselves in preferred ways; act in line with their preferences; and view important others viewing them in these ways. Conversely, people are at their worst when their behavior is "out of sync" with their own preferences, and when they think others regard them in negative ways.

These four assumptions inform how we talk with clients in order to bring out their best and resolve their problems. The therapist follows certain guidelines in promoting "narrative solutions" (see Table 16.1).

CASE EXAMPLE

Thirty-nine-year-old Mary was referred by a friend whom the therapist (Thomas W. Lund) had seen a few years earlier. Over the telephone, she described herself as depressed, having recently separated from her husband of 2 years, Phil. Mary said she had been withdrawing from previously

TABLE 16.1. Guidelines to Helpful Conversations

Step	Effect
1. Discuss clients' preferences, hopes, and intentions.	a. Clients experience the therapist as on their side—as interested in who they are, separate from the problem and its negative effects.
2. Explore the effects of the problem on clients. (How does the problem interfere with clients' acting in line with their preferences, and being seen by others in preferred ways?)	a. Clients talk about the problem openly and with minimal resistance. b. Clients may begin to notice a gap between their preferences and the negative effects of the problem on their lives. c. Clients become motivated to remedy this gap.
3. Connect with clients' preferred views of self. (For example, emphasize our 48-year-old client's propensity to work hard, stay productive, and be there for his family.)	a. Clients begin to see the therapist seeing them in preferred ways. b. Clients become motivated to understand how important others regard them.
4. Highlight contradictions in the storyline by noticing exceptions in the preproblem past, the present, and the future.	a. Clients begin to notice their own strengths and resources. b. Clients may begin to see the current problem more as an exception than the rule.
5. Ask mystery questions. (For example, how did someone with X preferred attributes [hard-working, productive] wind up in Y situation [not working] and being seen by others in Z ways [unproductive, lazy]?) Inquire into the mystery of problem evolution. (How did a problem become such a dominating force in a client's life?)	a. Clients may begin to rethink (or restory) how the problem evolved, with less blame and negativity toward self and others.

(continued)

TABLE 16.1. (*continued*)

Step	Effect
6. Develop an alternative explanation for the evolution of the problem that fits how clients prefer to be seen.	a. Clients may reframe current actions and perceptions in ways more congruent with preferred views of self. b. Clients become inspired to act in ways that confirm their preferences and resolve the presenting problem.
7. Encourage clients to circulate their preferences in conversation with important others.	a. Clients engage in helpful conversations outside the treatment room that support solutions. b. Clients may begin to view important others as viewing them in preferred ways. c. Clients develop less reliance on the therapist as a resource.
8. Review progress, accentuating clients' strengths and resources in resolving the problem. Anticipate future possibilities.	a. Therapy ends with the presenting problem resolved. b. Clients leave with an explanation for the evolution and resolution of the problem that will help them negotiate future predicaments. c. Clients credit themselves, and not the therapist, with the changes that occur.

pleasurable activities, such as her artwork, skiing, and aerobic dancing. She was also calling friends and crying—something that "wasn't like her." Friends advised Mary that she had not fully grieved for the loss of her first husband 5 years earlier. She had to "get over" this loss in order to return to her present husband, a "good man who loved her." These friends suggested that Mary had to learn to work at relationships, and they implied that she was being selfish for leaving her husband. Mary arrived for the first session in a dark business suit. She seemed formal and reserved.

In the first session, the therapist took some of the steps outlined in the "Guidelines to Helpful Conversations" (Table 16.1). First, he expressed interest in Mary's preferences, hopes, and intentions. Second, he was curious about how someone with these preferences would wind up *not* acting in line with them. He wondered with Mary how it was that people she esteemed weren't seeing her positively. We refer to such inquiries as "mystery questions," although it may be more accurate to describe a therapist's general orientation to clients and their problems as a "mystery stance." From the outset of therapy, the problem becomes a glitch or curiosity that fails to represent who people "really" are and demands an explanation.

The First Session: Talking about Preferences

MARY: I'm here because I think I'm depressed—I've lost my passion for life. The only thing I do is work and watch movies. My life is renting movies.

I'm making bad choices with men. Phil's offering me his love and stability—yet I left him.

THERAPIST: Is that what you want?

MARY: Shouldn't I?

THERAPIST: I'm not sure I understand. When you said "Shouldn't I?" . . . .

MARY: Well, he's been good to me. He says he loves me more than anyone could. Shouldn't I be grateful?

THERAPIST: You said something about losing your passion. I've never seen much of a connection between "should" and "grateful" and passion.

MARY: Is that important?

THERAPIST: Is it important to you?

MARY: I think so, but isn't that selfish?

THERAPIST: I'm confused. How did passion get connected to selfishness?

MARY: Phil says I'm selfish.

THERAPIST: Why?

MARY: He's said it at different times.

THERAPIST: Why would he do that?

MARY: I probably am. He says I like things my way and I don't want to work at the relationship.

THERAPIST: Now you're speaking about this relationship with words like "should," "grateful," and "work."

MARY: Aren't relationships supposed to be work? That's what I hear from everyone.

THERAPIST: Does this relationship feel like work?

MARY: Definitely.

THERAPIST: Yet you'd like passion in your relationship with Phil.

MARY: Yes, it's not there. I've really lost my passion for life.

THERAPIST: You care about Phil.

MARY: Yes, I do.

THERAPIST: Is it like you not to talk to someone you care about?

MARY: No.

Mary spoke of her preference for passion, and the therapist learned that she was no longer acting in line with that preference. She felt listless and lethargic, whiling away the hours. Mary said that it wasn't like her to act so withdrawn. She would also prefer to talk intimately with her husband, Phil, although she wasn't doing so at present. The therapist created a climate of mystery around the current problem. He seemed puzzled as to why Mary would be acting out of character. How was it that passion went out of her life and depression took over?

Mary suggested that Phil now regarded her as selfish and ungrateful—views that were disturbing. The therapist notes discrepancies among Mary's preferences, her current behavior, and the imagined views of others. Although Mary wanted to see herself as passionate, energetic, and sensitive to people she cared for, she was now acting depressed and lethargic. She also felt that her husband and friends regarded her as selfish, ungrateful, and uncaring. We assume that these experiences of discrepancy (or disjunction) were fueling the continuation of her depressed behavior (see Figure 16.1).

At this point in the first session, the therapist took additional steps outlined in the "Guidelines to Helpful Conversations" (Table 16.1). He explored how these unsettling views of self (which appeared linked to the presenting problem) evolved over time. How did Mary develop the idea that she was selfish, when she wanted to be passionate, energetic, and connected with people? The therapist looked for contradictions in the storyline—exceptions to the problem in the past and present.[4] Was there a

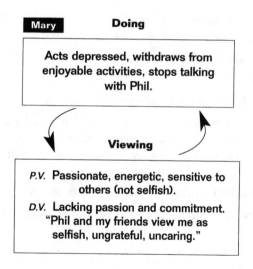

FIGURE 16.1. The evolving problem: I. *Note:* This diagram links current behavior ("Doing") with key views of self and other ("Viewing"). In the "Viewing" box, we highlight preferred views of self and the views of others that contradict the client's preferences at this point. The designation "P.V." is used to refer to preferred views, while "D.V" refers to disjunctive views. The arrows connecting "Viewing" and "Doing" show that the experience of contradiction between how people prefer to be seen and how they see others seeing them is what propels problematic behavior.

time when Mary felt passion without seeing herself as selfish or feeling depressed?†

> † *The therapist was already approaching this situation much in the same fashion that cognitive-behavioral therapists would with respect to attempting to discover Mary's schemas about herself and her relationships. I wonder whether the adjunctive use of certain questionnaires (e.g., the Relationship Belief Inventory; see Chapter 1) might have provided the therapist with additional information on Mary's thinking style, particularly since she appeared to be somewhat sluggish during the course of this first interview.*

The First Session (Continued): Exploring Clues to Problem Evolution

THERAPIST: Do you usually have a passion for life?

MARY: I did.

THERAPIST: When?

MARY: When my [first] husband, Greg, was alive. He died 5 years ago.

THERAPIST: How?

MARY: He was on a business trip and drove off the road. It was unclear whether he had a heart attack or if he fell asleep. I wish I knew.

THERAPIST: It would have been helpful to know?

MARY: I think so.

THERAPIST: Somehow it would have made a difference?

MARY: Well . . . I think so. I always wonder if it was because he was so tired. He had been traveling a number of days and was unsure whether he should continue or not. This leg of the trip was optional. . . . I think he was tired.

THERAPIST: And if he was tired he might have fallen asleep.

MARY: And if he fell asleep, then that's why he died. I feel like I was responsible.

THERAPIST: How were you responsible?

MARY: That's a long story.

THERAPIST: I'm interested.

MARY: Well, he called from Ohio and said he was thinking of coming home, and asked if I missed him. I said that I did, but that I was fine and had a lot of things to do. I didn't want to make him feel guilty and make him end his business trip for me, even though I would have liked him to come home. I guess I should have insisted he come home. He was tired.

THERAPIST: Was he likely to have come home if you had said that you missed him and would have liked him to come home?

MARY: I guess I'll never know. But I think of it often.

THERAPIST: What did other people think?

MARY: *(Her eyes moistened.)* I think they blamed me.

THERAPIST: Who?

MARY: Well, they didn't exactly say it. But I think there were people in his family and some of our friends who thought that I should have somehow provided more of a home—that we shouldn't have both been so independent. I guess they thought that I should have insisted that he come home and spend time with me, rather than doing that last leg of his trip, and maybe he'd still be alive. I just realized that all I'm talking about is Greg and his death. Maybe I need grief counseling. I don't know. I'm depressed . . . I think.

Looking for clues to problem construction, the therapist pursued Mary's story about her first husband's tragic death. Did Mary continue to live her life in line with her preferences, or did problematic views and behavior emerge at this transition point?

The therapist learned that Mary felt responsible for the accident that caused Greg's death. Although she still didn't know the actual cause (heart attack or fatigue), she feared that Greg was tired and fell asleep at the wheel. She knew that she could have urged him to come home when he telephoned from Ohio. Instead, she respected his preference to extend his trip, reassuring him that she'd be fine. Mary recalled that members of Greg's family and some friends frowned upon the couple's independent lifestyle. She felt that they were critical of her for acting so independently and not demanding that Greg come home sooner.

Mary worried that her friends might be right in their belief that "unresolved grief" over Greg's death was the cause of her current depression and withdrawal from Phil. The therapist was interested in an alternative, and more hopeful, possibility. He wondered whether what Mary described as unresolved grief was sadness that she'd stopped living life in line with her preferences. We assume that disjunctive views evolve at critical times of transition. Could Mary have begun to think of herself as selfish, ungrateful, and too independent in the wake of Greg's death? Did she respond to Phil's criticism by submerging her preferences and withdrawing emotionally? The conversation continued in the second session as the therapist pursued this alternative construction of grief.†

> † *I think that the therapist was clearly on the right track in exploring this woman's line of reasoning here. To add to some of his fine inquiry, however, the use of Socratic questioning might have revealed*

> more specifically how Mary came to develop this style of thinking, and, more importantly, to develop the cognitive distortions that were clearly detrimental in her case. I wonder whether she even had much insight into the fact that her thought processes involved a number of distortions, such as "dichotomous thinking," "tunnel vision," and "personalization" (see Chapter 1). Educating Mary about these distortions, even via some bibliotherapy, might have been helpful in beginning to question the validity of her assumptions.

The Second Session: Reconstructing Grief

MARY: I have to realize that Greg is dead, and people say that a relationship like that comes along once in a lifetime, if you're lucky. They say, "Get over it, and get realistic."

THERAPIST: Realistic?

MARY: Yes, they say you have to work at relationships, and if a man loves you and is there for you, you should be grateful.

THERAPIST: Is that what you think?

MARY: I didn't, but maybe Greg was an exception. I mean, maybe I should be happy that I had 10 years of happiness, and [should] accept reality. Maybe that's why I'm depressed. Phil says I'm spoiled—that Greg spoiled me and I'm selfish—that I have to deal with reality.

THERAPIST: I'm very interested in the reality of your life with Greg.

MARY: It's hard to talk about.

THERAPIST: Is it all right for me to ask questions?

MARY: It's OK.

THERAPIST: Did you have what you have described as [a] passion for life?

MARY: For 10 years. It was special.

Initially Mary resisted talking about her life with Greg. She said that friends advised her to get over Greg and be grateful for Phil's love. Phil, too, warned Mary to "deal with reality," suggesting that Greg spoiled her and that Mary's relationship with Greg was the basis of her "selfishness." We can now map how Mary's past and present views of self and other intertwined to support the current problem (see Figure 16.2).

By expressing an interest in Mary's preferences, the therapist assumed a different position from her friends and Phil. When Mary began to view the therapist as perceiving her as capable of passion and commitment, she became more interested in recalling the preferred aspects of her relationship with Greg (an exception to the present problem).†

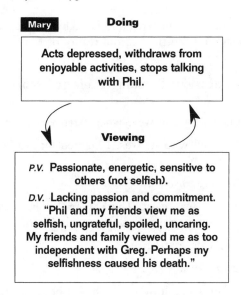

FIGURE 16.2. The evolving problem: II. P.V. = preferred view; D.V. = disjunctive view.

> † *This was a very important move in the establishment of rapport. It also set the stage for what cognitive-behavioral therapists refer to as "collaborative empiricism." The therapist was already indirectly encouraging Mary to challenge the perceptions of her friends by maintaining an objective role, but at the same time he was collaboratively searching for alternatives with Mary.*

THERAPIST: I'd love to hear about what made it special. You glowed when you said that.

MARY: *(Sitting back in her chair and sighing)* I haven't thought about this for years. I try not to think about it. Greg was very nurturing and unselfish. I felt special in his eyes. I looked better through his eyes than I did in my own. When I worked with him in his wood shop, he'd marvel at it. He'd say, "I love it when you work with me." He'd watch me paint and marvel at my work. If I made dinner, he'd act like it was Thanksgiving or something. And, you know, when he made dinner, I would too.

THERAPIST: You appreciated each other. He made you feel good about yourself.

MARY: I felt very special, and I think he did too. Thinking about this is strange. I'm sad, yet I'd like to tell you about it.

The second session ended with Mary's saying it felt good to talk about her relationship with Greg. She said that most of her conversations were about the need to forget about Greg and get on with "reality." In the third session, the conversation returned to the reality of Mary's life with Greg.

The Third Session: Pursuing Preferred Stories (Past)

THERAPIST: You liked who you were when Greg was alive.

MARY: I did, and I liked who he was. I wanted him to be happy, and he wanted me to be happy.

THERAPIST: So you were *un*selfish.

MARY: I guess. But it was easy. That's why I think people think I'm unrealistic. They say you have to work at relationships.

THERAPIST: You didn't do any work.

MARY: It didn't seem like it.

THERAPIST: That sounds like how work should be. Does work have to be unpleasant?

MARY: I guess not.

THERAPIST: I must be selfish myself. I don't seem to want to work too hard. Actually, I don't know a lot of people who do. A lot of people seem to like relationships in which they feel good about who they are and how they are seen by their partners. I'm interested in how hard you had to work with Greg. Did he ever not go along with what you would like?

MARY: Of course. I guess it was easy to negotiate.

THERAPIST: Work wasn't that hard.

MARY: No, it really wasn't.

Instead of "getting over" Greg as her friends suggested, the therapist encouraged Mary to "get with" Greg again. Although Greg was deceased, his positive view of Mary came alive as she reminisced about their life together, and she came alive as she spoke of her experiences with Greg. She recalled passion, happiness, and looking better through her partner's eyes than her own. Through this empowering dialogue, the experience of passion was linked with speaking up about preferences. When Mary talked with Greg about what she wanted, he listened; when she expressed interest in what Greg wanted, he talked.

In this retelling of the story of a happy marriage, Mary became reacquainted with her capacity for intimacy and commitment. She was also inspired to rethink the circumstances surrounding Greg's death. Perhaps when Greg telephoned from Ohio, saying he wanted to extend his business trip, Mary was acting in line with the spirit of their relationship by respecting his wishes. It wouldn't have been like her, like him, or in keeping with their relationship to do otherwise.

This conversation suggested that Mary wasn't *responsible* for Greg's death, but rather that she was *responsive* to him to the very end of their time together. As Mary reconsidered, she herself declared "I wasn't selfish." Once Mary renarrated past events in this manner, she was more motivated to reframe the present and to imagine new possibilities for the future.†

> † *The methods used here were very similar to the methods cognitive-behavioral therapists use in reframing. The only difference is that the therapist might have had Mary examine her thoughts more concretely and weigh them out in a systematic fashion, in order to come to the same conclusion as the therapist has here. The idea behind this would have been to solidify her reframing and to reinforce its permanence.*

The Fourth Session: Preferred Stories (Recent)

In the fourth session, the therapist shifted to the recent past, exploring how the problem evolved in her relationship with Phil. He inquired into exceptions. Was there ever a time when Mary felt Phil regarded her in preferred ways? Did she ever experience passion with Phil? If so, how did passion dry up?

THERAPIST: When did you meet Phil?

MARY: We became friendly about 1 year after Greg died.

THERAPIST: He helped you with your sadness?

MARY: Yes, he was warm, easy to talk to, and I think because he experienced loss in his life, he understood.

THERAPIST: You spent some time thinking of Greg, grieving?

MARY: I did.

THERAPIST: Was anyone else helpful?

MARY: I was in a bereavement group that also helped greatly. I did grieve, and I did feel better for a while. I don't think it's grief I'm feeling. Phil is a caring, kind man. He helped me so much with my sadness about Greg. He's been there for me. Why am I doing this to him?

THERAPIST: You feel that you're not being grateful?

MARY: Yes.

THERAPIST: Do you feel safe with Phil?

MARY: Not really. I feel that he thinks badly of me.

THERAPIST: You don't look better through Phil's eyes than through your own?

MARY: No. I feel like I'm a selfish, disobedient child.

THERAPIST: Do you feel passion?

MARY: No. But how can I expect that? I never had those feelings before Greg. He was special. I'll never get that again, will I?

THERAPIST: But you mentioned that you did feel passion with Phil?

MARY: I did actually, for a while. Phil was very supportive. . . . He was a caring man.

THERAPIST: You felt passion?

MARY: Yes. It seems like it was short-lived.

THERAPIST: When you felt Phil was supportive and caring and felt passion, did he see you as selfish or like a disobedient child?

MARY: No. He saw me as strong and independent.

THERAPIST: Phil saw you like this?

MARY: Yes. He always said how he admired how, even after Greg died, I stayed active physically, I worked hard, I didn't fold. Things were better when I first met Phil than they are now, but I can't do anything I want when I'm with him.†

> † *It might have been interesting to have Mary consider whether or not Phil was engaging in his own cognitive distortions. Mary tended to regard his statements as almost being truth, when in fact these statements might very well be reflecting a distorted view of his own, based on erroneous information. This was something that clearly should have been explored with Mary.*

Early in their relationship, Mary felt that Phil saw her as a strong, independent person. He admired how she continued to stay active physically, and worked at her career. Once upon a time, Mary did feel passion with Phil. Having clarified these exceptions to the current situation, the therapist became curious about what changed in this relationship. How did mutual caring and respect for independence turn to criticism and withdrawal?

THERAPIST: He stops you?

MARY: I feel guilty, like I'm not taking care of him, if I do what I'd like.

THERAPIST: You stopped doing things you would like while you were together.

MARY: Many things—I stopped going to art classes, I stopped skiing, I stopped going to my bereavement group.

THERAPIST: Phil wanted you to?

MARY: He said we didn't spend enough time together—that he wished we spent more time together. He seemed sad when I'd tell him I'd signed up for an art class two nights per week—so I just didn't sign up.

THERAPIST: How was that for you?

MARY: Well, I didn't mind missing art class, but then when it happened with skiing—Phil doesn't ski—and then my group, I started resenting it.

THERAPIST: Were there things you didn't give up?

MARY: Yes. I refused to give up spending an occasional weekend in New York City with friends, "the girls," and conferences. But even then, Phil would ask me to call him morning and night. I felt like I had to report on what I did, and that he would be sad if I said that I had fun—so I stopped calling him.

The therapist inquired into what happened when Mary submerged her preferences. What were the effects of this concealment on Mary, Phil, and the relationship? Were these effects in line with Mary's preferences?[5]

THERAPIST: Phil seemed to want to stop you from doing things you enjoyed.

MARY: He didn't directly say that, but he acted so hurt, so annoyed, that I would want to do anything without him.

THERAPIST: How do you do at giving things up and doing what others want you to do?

MARY: *(Laughing)* Not too good, I guess I get angry.

THERAPIST: Doesn't work so good?

MARY: I get sneaky, then I feel even worse. Like I have no right. I feel even worse. He's been good to me; he loves me.

THERAPIST: You get angry?

MARY: Yes, I rebel by not calling him at times, or not telling him where I am going.

THERAPIST: And you get sneaky?

MARY: Well . . . I met a man from the bereavement group for dinner, and Phil found out.

THERAPIST: How did he react?

MARY: He was really upset—he called me selfish, questioned my commitment to him. I felt guilty.

THERAPIST: Were there other occasions?

MARY: Yeah, actually. I had dinner with a man I met at a conference, and one of my friends got worried—thought I was doing something stupid. I think she told Phil.

THERAPIST: And?

MARY: Same reaction. I was selfish, I don't want to work at the relationship. I *am* selfish—I want to do things I want to do. He is right; my friends are right! I don't want to stop doing what I like to do.

By the fourth session, many of the hoped-for effects of helpful conversations were occurring, setting the stage for change (see Table 16.1). Mary was beginning to notice her own strengths and resources. She could recall times when she acted in line with her preferences and was regarded positively by people she cared for. She was beginning to rethink (or "restory") how the problem evolved, with less blame and negativity toward self and others. She was also beginning to reframe her current situation differently. Perhaps the problem with Phil was that she stopped speaking up about her preferences. After all, she used to do what she wanted to do without feeling depressed, and Phil admired her for being energetic and independent. Maybe she simply needed to become more active again, and let Phil know that she would like his admiration back.

Mary declared at the end of the fourth session, "I *am* selfish." But she said this with a sense of confidence, as if it were OK to be selfish in certain ways. Then, as is often the case between sessions, Mary began to doubt herself again. Wondering whether selfishness is really compatible with caring and commitment, she recalled her first experience with falling in love and having her partner leave.

The Fifth Session: Reconstructing a Past Story

THERAPIST: It's like you to speak up about what you would like?

MARY: Yeah, I guess. Is that selfish? I get mixed up.

THERAPIST: You really don't want to be selfish.

MARY: *(Wrinkling her brow)* I've been thinking about this. I wonder if it's possible to have a relationship while being selfish. I'm lucky I found Greg, but do most men want to be with a woman who is selfish?

THERAPIST: What's been your experience?

MARY: I had very protective parents and only dated one person in high school. I wasn't very experienced when I went off to college. I dated Steven and I was naive, but things seemed wonderful. We were engaged. Of course, right after we both graduated from college, he left suddenly.

THERAPIST: While things seemed wonderful to you?

MARY: Things got to be less than wonderful. I wanted children, but he said he wasn't ready. I guess I wasn't very mature. If I'd given him enough space and time and didn't rush him, maybe he wouldn't have left.

THERAPIST: You sound like you were clear about what you would have liked. How was that immature?

MARY: I don't know. I guess I could have waited to talk about that.

THERAPIST: Could you have?

MARY: Yes, as a matter of fact.

THERAPIST: If you didn't exactly make an ultimatum.

MARY: Oh, no. I did mention it a bit, but I guess that was pretty normal; we were finishing college.

THERAPIST: How did he handle your saying what you would like for your life? Having children?

MARY: Not too well, I guess. He ran off with another woman rather suddenly.

THERAPIST: And *you* weren't mature when you didn't give him more space and time?

MARY: *(Laughing)* You have a funny way of putting things.

THERAPIST: What do you mean?

MARY: Well, you're not really saying it, but by the way you ask questions, it appears rather obvious that if anyone was immature, it was Steven, not me. I just wanted to have kids.

THERAPIST: You weren't interested in anything too unusual there. How did things go after that?

MARY: Actually . . . well . . . I had fun dating a number of men for almost 2 years. My career took off, and I had fun.

Although Mary recounted this story of life with Steven to question the idea of speaking up about preferences, the therapist found contrary evidence. It was only when Mary informed Steven that she wanted to have children that Steven became fearful and left. Often, in the process of reviewing an old story, a new perspective is derived. The therapist helped Mary restory her relationship with Steven in a way that confirmed her preferred views of self. He challenged her assumption that selfishness had anything to do with the "failure" of this relationship. It soon became clear that Mary was capable of intimacy and commitment even at this early time in her adult life. She began to realize that "if anyone was immature, it was Steven." This conversation suggests that Mary was wise to speak up about her preferences, so that she could learn early whether she and Steven were compatible. Mary recalled that after Steven left, her career took off; she also dated and had fun. Thus, a relationship's ending didn't mean an end to passion or commitment.†

> † *This was an excellent example of reframing a schema that had obviously plagued Mary and infiltrated her subsequent relationships. In order to obtain closure on this, I might have suggested that the therapist ask Mary how she would like to reframe this new schema in her mind permanently, now that she had arrived at this new revelation. For example, she might have wanted to practice using the alternative schema ("I was not selfish, but just more mature than Steven at the time, which accounted for the demise of our relationship") instead of the old schema. This might have resulted in more of a permanent change in her thinking about herself, the past, and the present.*

The therapist further explored the wisdom of speaking up about preferences. He went back to Mary's relationship with Greg, inquiring into how the couple managed differences and conflict. This conversation set the stage for Mary to reconsider her present approach to working out differences with Phil.†

> † *From a behavioral standpoint, this might also have been a time to suggest the idea of some assertiveness training in general, since assertiveness appeared to be an important area of deficit with Mary. This could have been addressed in a number of sessions that included role play and practice.*

THERAPIST: Were there ever situations in which you and Greg disagreed— where you had to speak up and tell him how you felt?

MARY: I have to think about that. Well, interestingly, he wanted to pool our finances. I wanted to keep my independence and have separate savings and checking accounts, but then share common expenses.

THERAPIST: How did that go?

MARY: It was rough, but he agreed, and we worked it out very well. It was easy. When he wanted something, I would do it; when I wanted something, he would do it. Even when it was a little bit rough, it wasn't for long.

THERAPIST: Did it ever get into "shoulds" and "obligations"?

MARY: No, never.

THERAPIST: You could speak your mind.

MARY: Yes. With Phil, I feel like a bad child if I don't agree with him. Like I owe it to him, or I'm selfish if I want privacy or if I want to go out with friends.

THERAPIST: How do you negotiate with Phil?

MARY: I don't. I feel guilty and I don't talk.

THERAPIST: And you're sure that Phil doesn't want to hear what you have to say?

The Evolving Problem

At this point, the therapist had a more complete picture of the evolution of the immediate problem from Mary's point of view. The problem began when Phil expressed hurt and resentment about Mary's doing things she liked. Mary suggested that Phil wanted to spend more time with her, but that instead of asserting a preference for intimacy, he criticized her for neglecting him. Acutely sensitive to being perceived as selfish and uncaring (based on her construction of past relationships), Mary stopped doing what she enjoyed.

In the fourth and fifth sessions, the therapist encouraged Mary to compare her current experience with Phil against her past experience with Greg. With Greg, she spoke about her preferences and experienced passion and support. With Phil, she was concealing her preferences and experiencing criticism and shame. Mary recounted with emotion how Phil viewed her as a selfish, disobedient child. Since Mary preferred to regard herself as a mature, independent woman, she felt diminished by Phil's characterizations of her. This experience of disjunction fueled more-of-the-same withdrawn behavior. Mary resolved this discrepancy (1) by withdrawing from many enjoyable activities, and (2) by pursuing some enjoyable activities with people who confirmed her preferences, and then concealing her pleasure from Phil. (See Figure 16.3 for a diagram of the evolving problem from Mary's point of view.)

Through the therapist's purposeful juxtaposition of past and present life stories, Mary noticed that she was not speaking up for a lifestyle of passion, but rather supporting a lifestyle of depression. She was not talking with Phil about who she was, what she wanted, and how she would like him to treat her. Thus, she was not exploring relationship possibilities in sufficient depth to make a decision about the future.

Toward an Alternative Explanation

The stage was now set for Mary to piece together clues to the mystery of problem evolution, and to decide what to do about her current situation. Several mystery questions oriented Mary in her reconstruction of the problem. Why would someone who spoke up about her preferences in her relationships with Steven and Greg (in one case finding clarity, in the other finding passion and commitment) now submerge her preferences? Why would Mary restrict her independence, when it was this same independent spirit that attracted Phil to her in the first place? Why would Mary act sneaky, when sneakiness did not suit her or the relationship? As Mary indicated in the fourth session, sneakiness caused Mary to feel

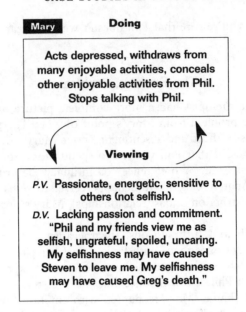

FIGURE 16.3. The evolving problem: III. P.V. = preferred view; D.V. = disjunctive view.

badly about herself and withdraw from Phil; it also brought out the worst in Phil.

Existing negative explanations—that Mary hadn't fully grieved for Greg's death; that she loved once and would never love again; that she made bad choices in men—did not hold up under narrative scrutiny. A more fitting idea was that Mary had simply lost touch with who she was and what she wanted in an intimate partnership. Since Phil was at one time attracted to the independent person Mary preferred to be, it didn't make sense for her to hide this person from Phil. The most compelling explanation for the intrusion of depression into Mary's life was that she submerged her preferences and began acting out of character. It was in the context of this thorough reconstruction of past and present relationships that Mary reconsidered what she needed to do differently to overcome depression.

Mary arrived for the sixth therapy session wearing a brightly colored outfit, and looking more spirited and energetic. She said that she'd telephoned Phil in between sessions and arranged a get-together. Mary went on to describe the ingredients of a helpful conversation they'd had outside the therapy room.

New Conversations, New Solutions

In a problem-dissolving conversation with Phil, Mary spoke up about her preference for intimacy with him. She reassured Phil that she still cared for him, but felt terrible about how he viewed her now. As she did with the therapist in the fourth session, Mary reminisced with Phil about the early times in their relationship. She emphasized how important it was to her that Phil admired her independence, supported her participation in the bereavement group, and encouraged her to pursue what she enjoyed. She said that she wanted to get back to the supportive relationship she and Phil once had.

Mary also told Phil that she was committed to getting beyond depression. To achieve this goal, she had to do the things she felt passionate about doing. She also said that she wanted to spend more time with Phil, but not if he remained critical of her. Mary explained how bad she felt when Phil criticized her for being uncaring and selfish. Feeling criticized caused her to withdraw, feel depressed, and lose feeling for Phil. Finally, Mary conveyed hope for reviving the marriage, if she could once again see herself through Phil's eyes as the person she would like to be.

This new conversation with Phil inspired a change in Mary's depressive symptoms. Although Phil responded in a positive manner, Mary told the therapist that she felt confident about change, regardless of the outcome of their conversation. By committing herself to speaking up about her preferences and reclaiming her previous passion for life, then clarifying what kind of relationship she wanted to have with Phil, Mary set the stage for resolving her depression. She was now looking at the past, present, and future through a nondisjunctive lens. She could envision a future in which she pursued her desire for intimacy and commitment—if not with Phil, then with someone else. She could remember a past in which she lived life according to her preferences and found fulfillment. She could now use the past as a resource in guiding her future actions. She was taking charge of her present circumstances in a way that fit with her preferences and positive intentions.†

> † *This description is quite compatible with the cognitive-behavioral model, which emphasizes the role of cognitive distortions in the development and maintenance of depressive symptoms. The authors' reference to Mary's use of a "nondisjunctive lens" corresponds to the correction of the cognitive distortion of a "mental filter" (see Chapter 1).*

As it turned out, Phil responded warmly to this talk with Mary. He said he would like to attend counseling and reclaim their marriage. Two individual sessions were then held with Phil, followed by two sessions with the couple together.

Talking with Phil Individually

In the seventh and eighth sessions, the therapist explored Phil's preferences, hopes, and intentions, just as he had with Mary. He learned that Phil wanted to be a caring husband who had a close relationship with his wife. Confirming Mary's account, Phil recalled that he was originally attracted to Mary because of her independent spirit. He admired her ability to take charge of her life after Greg died. He loved her creative side, her interest in art, and her commitment to being physically active.

The therapist and Phil then mused over the mystery of why someone who loved his wife for being her own person would be seen by her as critical of her independence. Phil explained that he was under the impression that Mary no longer loved him or wanted to be with him. Since his first wife had left him suddenly and without explanation, Phil was worried about rejection. When he thought he saw history repeating itself, he got panicky. He began interrogating Mary about her pursuits and disparaging the same behavior he'd once admired. (For a completed diagram of the problem cycle at its worst, see Figure 16.4.)

Phil seemed relieved to learn that his own actions were the basis of Mary's withdrawal, not lack of interest on her part. Knowing that Mary wanted to reclaim what they once had gave Phil renewed hope. He felt committed to reassuring Mary that he loved her for being the person she was.

Equipped with an alternative explanation for Mary's withdrawal that confirmed his preferred views of self, Phil decided to change his approach to Mary. He stopped criticizing Mary for doing things separately from him, and instead encouraged her to do what she enjoyed.†

> † *Interestingly, both Mary and Phil appeared to be operating on faulty assumptions based on misinformation. This was clearly a result of their poor communication. The therapist did a nice job of having them consider alternatives. Among the benefits that the cognitive-behavioral approach might have added here were tools or strategies for Mary and Phil to adopt so that they could acquire the skill of questioning the evidence and weighing alternatives automatically. The Dysfunctional Thought Record would have been an excellent structured format to help them accomplish this (see Chapter 1). Its use might also have helped them to acquire the skills permanently and then refer to them spontaneously each time they encountered a situation, such as Phil did in the paragraphs above.*

To Mary's surprise, Phil invited Mary and two of her friends to dinner at his place. An accomplished cook, he prepared a gourmet meal and was pleased that they all enjoyed themselves. Not only did Mary experience Phil as accepting her friends, but she was thrilled to see him enjoying their company.

In the two conjoint sessions (sessions 9 and 10), the couple offered several examples of progress. In a reversal of their recent pattern, Mary discussed how she invited Phil to have dinner at her place. They spent the

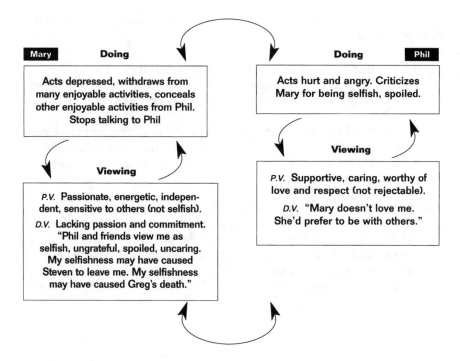

FIGURE 16.4. The problem at its worst. P.V. = preferred view; D.V. = disjunctive view.

evening reminiscing about what had worked in the early days of their relationship and how to reclaim it. Mary also spoke with Phil about how she wanted to remember her relationship with Greg as evidence of her capacity for passion and commitment. Phil listened respectfully as Mary talked about her life with Greg. Instead of being critical of Greg for "spoiling" Mary, he reassured Mary that he could support her independence, just as Greg did. The evening ended with passion. The couple made love, and both partners reported feeling warm, close, and satisfied.

Depression dissolved in the wake of these new conversations with Phil. Mary said she no longer felt depressed. She was acting in line with her preferences, and she saw Phil regarding her in self-confirming ways. She could envision a future without depression—one in which she remained active, energetic, and passionate. If things continued along present lines, she could imagine living together again, although neither she or Phil seemed eager to push for this arrangement. Phil too reported feeling better about himself and the relationship. He said he preferred being supportive to Mary as opposed to being critical, and liked the effects that his support was having on Mary. (The key elements of their narrative solution are summarized in Figure 16.5.)

Therapy ended after the 10th session. Four criteria for concluding therapy had been met:

1. The presenting problem (Mary's depression) was resolved.†
2. Mary and Phil were engaging in helpful conversations that undermined the influence of the presenting problem and supported solutions.
3. Mary and Phil had an explanation for the evolution and resolution of the problem that would help them negotiate future difficulties.
4. The clients credited themselves, and not the therapist, with the changes that occurred.

   † *The authors have not mentioned in the description of this case whether any empirical instruments were used to measure the level of Mary's depression. One possibility might have been to use the Beck Depression Inventory (see Chapter 1), which is a quickly scored measure designed to assess depression in 10–15 minutes. Using such a scale at the onset and throughout the course of treatment might*

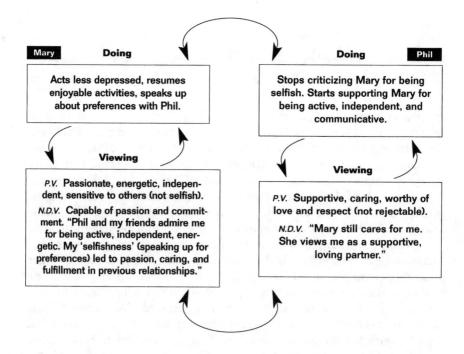

FIGURE 16.5. A narrative solution. *Note:* The designation "N.D.V" is used to refer to nondisjunctive views. The arrows connecting "Viewing" and "Doing" show that the experience of congruence between how people prefer to be seen and how they see others seeing them is what promotes solution-oriented action.

also have helped to reassure both Mary and the therapist that her depression had truly subsided.

An Inoculation Session

Six months later, Mary and Phil called to make another appointment. They wanted to talk over their decision to move back in together. Fearful about returning to old patterns, they hoped to do what they could to prevent this possibility. Mary wondered whether living together would bring out Phil's insecurities again. Would he start watching over and interfering with her independent activities? Phil questioned whether Mary would stop talking with him. Would they lose their newfound passion? When the two of them left the session, they'd accepted that these things might happen, but clarified what they intended to do about it. Mary committed herself to talking openly about her preferences with Phil. Phil said he would discuss his concerns without blaming Mary, and would continue to support her independent pursuits. They left feeling confident that even if old patterns should return, they now had the know-how to engage in helpful conversations to resolve the impasse.

In a telephone follow-up conducted 1 year subsequent to this session, Mary reported that she and Phil had been living together happily for 9 months. Although conflicts had emerged between them, they were able to talk their way through them. Mary was continuing to pursue her interests in art, aerobic dancing, and visiting with friends, free of constraint. She was seeing herself through Phil's eyes as the person she wanted to be, and living without depression.

CONCLUSIONS

The narrative solutions approach integrates ideas across different schools of psychotherapy. In this approach, we therapists may meet with individuals, yet still think about changing interactional patterns. We can alter perspectives with the goal in mind of changing behavior. We can be collaborative, respectful, and nonimpositional in our approach (as in narrative family therapy) and still remain purposeful and planful (as in strategic family therapy). We can talk about problems while still promoting solutions. We can track how problems evolve to obtain clues to how problems can be resolved. We can change present patterns and shift future perspectives by focusing on people's past experiences. We can be brief and practical while embracing the poetic aspects of the human experience (people's reminiscences, hopes, and dreams). We can be empathetic and nonjudgmental in our approach without fearing that we are being idle. When we empathize by connecting with clients' preferred views, we are implementing a key component of an action plan. Solutions begin to develop when clients begin to view others (including us, the therapists) as seeing them in preferred ways.

The decision of whom to see in therapy and when to see them is based on the practical question of what conversations might be most helpful in solving problems. Ideally, conversations between the therapist and one or more family members in the room are only the starting points for productive dialogues between husbands and wives, parents and children, children and their peers, or adults and their friends that take place outside the treatment room. In this case, the therapist chose to meet individually with Mary, although she was reporting marital problems. Imposing couple or family therapy on Mary, when *her* concern was to overcome depression, might have evoked unnecessary resistance. Furthermore, the therapist might have lost the opportunity to understand Mary's preferences, hopes, and intentions in the context of her broad life experiences.

As Mary reconstructed how depression evolved as a problem, she became motivated to talk with her husband differently. This helpful conversation outside the treatment room set the stage for Phil's participation in therapy. If Phil had responded in a critical or uninterested manner to Mary's initiative, couple therapy might not have been pursued. Still, Mary might have benefited from this new conversation with Phil in her quest to overcome depression. A negative response on Phil's part might have led to a decision to pursue a separation or divorce. In such a case, individual sessions might have continued until the presenting problem was resolved and Mary was engaging in helpful conversations with friends and others who supported her preferences.

Change occurs through a process of generative conversations. By maintaining a focus on what conversations are helpful to people, we can decide whom to see, when to see them, and how long therapy should continue. Once people are bringing their own resources to bear on solutions, they are usually not as interested in talking with therapists any longer. In the case we have described, therapy ended because Mary naturally preferred to talk with friends and with Phil, rather than to continue the expensive conversations with her therapist. Therapy didn't end because the therapist artificially imposed time constraints, declaring that solutions must be achieved in 10 sessions or less. Mary and Phil left therapy having experienced the therapist as a valuable resource in fostering helpful conversations between them. Thus, they were more likely to return to therapy for brief interludes (as they did once) to negotiate future impasses.

Brief therapy can incorporate the breadth of the life cycle and still be brief. The narrative solutions approach allows therapists to identify strengths and resources over an expanse of time. Therapists need not restrict their focus to present problems and solutions to achieve rapid change. Brief therapy can help clients develop a coherent storyline that explains how current problems fit into the tapestry of their lives. Not only do clients leave such therapy with symptoms improved or eliminated, but they depart with a blueprint for how to manage life's subsequent challenges.†

> †*It appears that the narrative solutions approach proposed by Drs. Eron and Lund is very compatible with the cognitive-behavioral approach. However, it would be important to use cognitive-behavioral techniques selectively, so as to not infringe on what appears to be at times an indirect posture assumed by therapists in this modality.*

AUTHORS' REPLY TO EDITOR'S COMMENTS

The editor's comments highlight points of similarity and difference between cognitive-behavioral therapy and the narrative solutions approach. Like cognitive-behavioral therapists, we're interested in understanding how patterns of thinking and behavior affect and maintain individual and relationship difficulties. We differ, however, on how to achieve cognitive-behavioral shifts.

In assessing how problems evolve, we inquire with interest into ordinary times of transition that may set the stage for distress, shifting how people think and act. In the case we have described, the therapist explored past occasions when Mary acted in line with preferred views of self and occasions when she felt others, including Phil, saw her in preferred ways. Thus, the therapist was interested in what was right with Mary and Phil and their relationship, as well as in what happened to get them off track.

If the therapist had tried to educate Mary about cognitive distortions (as suggested by the editor on p. 380), Mary might have felt that the therapist thought there was something wrong with her, and that she lacked the resources within her to change her circumstances. Taking a stance that the therapist knew better than Mary about more "functional" styles of thinking would have been less likely to empower Mary to find and enact solutions, and might have invited unnecessary resistance. At this stage in the therapy, the therapist continued a line of inquiry that motivated Mary to rethink how the problem evolved, and to reconsider what to do about her circumstances.

Similarly, the therapist wouldn't have found it helpful to explore possible cognitive distortions on Phil's part (see the editor's suggestion, p. 384). An emphasis on cognitive distortions might have detracted from the more empowering explanation that was emerging for what went wrong in Mary and Phil's relationship. The therapist's purpose at this stage was to invite Mary to recall how Phil viewed her early in their relationship. Notice how Mary recalled that Phil was drawn to her for being strong, independent, and assertive (all preferred attributes). She also remembered that there was passion between them, thus deconstructing the belief that she was incapable of passion or that she could never love again after Greg died. Soon Mary realized that passion occurred when she acted in line with her preferences and viewed Phil as admiring her strengths. Mary arrived at an alternative explanation for the problem—one that carried no implication of deficiencies or cognitive distortions on the part of either person or the relationship. The therapist didn't impose the correct interpretation on or impart it to a client who "lacked insight." Nor did he suggest skills training to a client who "lacked skills."

As the collaborative inquiry between therapist and client continued, Mary reconsidered how she and Phil got off track. She also gathered clues for how to talk with Phil in a way that brought out the best in both of them. It was not necessary to suggest assertiveness training (see the editor's suggestion, p. 388, bottom), because it became evident that Mary possessed the capacity to speak openly about her preferences in her past relationships with Greg and Steven. As the therapist and Mary puzzled over why she stopped "being Mary" with Phil, Mary became motivated to be more assertive. She spoke with Phil about their relationship in a self-affirming, confident, and nonblaming manner, setting in motion positive changes in their relationship. Mary engaged in this assertive conversation without any skills training, because she was able to access an existing resource (assertiveness) once she was properly motivated.

A further concern would be how Mary might have construed the suggestion to pursue assertiveness training from a male therapist. Mary already felt dispirited because she felt Phil now viewed her as flawed. Any implication by the therapist that Mary lacked assertiveness might have resulted in Mary's perceiving the therapist as yet another man who viewed her as deficient. Not only might this have threatened the therapeutic alliance, but it would also have been more likely to perpetuate disjunctive attributions and thus to maintain the problem (e.g., "My husband and therapist both think I am deficient. Maybe I am. I lack passion, commitment, *and* assertiveness; maybe that is why my marriage failed").

In contrast, many of the editor's suggestions are compatible with the narrative solutions approach. For example, the use of a structured questionnaire such as the Relationship Belief Inventory might have been helpful as an adjunct to the therapeutic conversation with Mary (see editor's comments, p. 378). Such a questionnaire might have given the therapist further clues about how Mary was thinking and acting in relation to others, and what needed to happen for her to change. What cognitive-behavioral therapists refer to as "collaborative empiricism" fits with our approach as well (see editor's comments, p. 381). The phrase suggests that a therapist and client are coscientists, exploring what has and has not worked in past and present relationships in an active search for alternatives. We also concur with the idea of solidifying clients' reframings to reinforce their permanence (p. 383).

Based on the shared premise that perspective and behavior are interconnected in the evolution and maintenance of clinical problems, cognitive-behavioral and narrative solutions approaches are indeed integratable. Continued dialogue should serve us and our clients well as we continue to develop more efficient, practical, and empowering ways to be helpful to people.

NOTES

1. Jeffrey Bodgan (1986) has referred to this way of understanding problem evolution as "accidentalism." Steve de Shazer (1985) has used the phrase "damned bad luck." The MRI brief therapy approach contrasted with the structural and systemic family therapies of the 1970s and 1980s, in that symptoms were *not* seen as serving a function to get problems started or keep them going. Furthermore, there was no assumption of negative intention on the part of family members.

2. This "more-of-the-same" cycle of interaction fits within the principles of problem maintenance introduced by the MRI brief therapy group (see Watzlawick et al., 1974). In the MRI approach, the emphasis of assessment and intervention is behavioral. Therapists assess what people *do* about problems to keep them going, and intervene to interrupt problem-maintaining patterns of behavior.

3. The word "disjunction" was used by R. D. Laing and his colleagues to refer to the distress people experience when their view of self is out of sync with their view of others, and with their view of the others' view of them (Laing, Phillipson, & Lee, 1966). We use the word "disjunction" to refer to the gaps among how people *prefer* to be seen, how they act, and how they see others seeing them. Problems evolve as this gap widens, and resolve as this gap narrows.

4. Inquiring into exceptions to the current problem is a practice common to narrative and solution focused therapy. Narrative therapists Michael White and David Epston (1990) use terms such as "preferred stories" and "unique outcomes" to describe this inquiry. Solution-focused therapist Steve de Shazer (1985) uses the term "exceptions." Our aim is to highlight events and experiences in the past, present, and imagined future that confirm how people prefer to see themselves and that contradict current perceptions and actions.

5. This inquiry into the effects of problems resembles what Michael White refers to as an "externalizing conversation" (see White & Epston, 1990). As people recount the negative effects of the problem on their lives and relationships, they often experience the problem as external to them—as separate from who they are or hope to be. They become motivated to act in ways that suit their preferences and undermine the negative influences of the problem.

REFERENCES

Bogdan, J. (1986). Do families really need problems?: Why I am not a functionalist. *Family Therapy Networker, 10*(4), 30–35, 67–69.

Carter, B., & McGoldrick, M. (Eds.). (1980). *The changing family life cycle: A framework for family therapy.* New York: Gardner Press.

de Shazer, S. (1985). *Keys to solutions in brief therapy.* New York: Norton.

Eron, J. B., & Lund, T. W. (1989). From magic to method: Principles of effective reframing. *Family Therapy Networker, 13*(1), 64–68, 81–83.

Eron, J. B., & Lund, T. W. (1993). How problems evolve and dissolve: Integrating narrative and strategic concepts. *Family Process, 32,* 291–309.

Eron, J. B., & Lund, T. W. (1996). *Narrative solutions in brief therapy.* New York: Guilford Press.

Eron, J. B., & Lund, T. W. (in press). Narrative solutions in brief couple therapy. In J. Donovan (Ed.), *Short-term couple therapy*. New York: Guilford Press.

Haley, J. (1973). *Uncommon therapy*. New York: Norton.

Haley, J. (1980). *Leaving home: The therapy of disturbed young people*. New York: McGraw-Hill.

Laing, R. D., Phillipson, H., & Lee, A. R. (1966). *Interpersonal perception: A theory and method of research*. London: Tavistock.

Lund, T. W., & Eron, J. B. (1998). The narrative solutions approach for retelling children's stories: Using preferred views to construct useful conversations. In M. F. Hoyt (Ed.), *The handbook of constructive therapies*. San Francisco: Jossey-Bass.

Rogers, C. R. (1961). *On becoming a person: A therapist's view of psychotherapy*. Boston: Houghton Mifflin.

Watzlawick, P., Weakland, J., & Fisch, R. (1974). *Change: Principles of problem formation and problem resolution*. New York: Norton.

Weakland, J. H., Fisch, R., Watzlawick, P., & Bodin, A. M. (1974). Brief therapy: Focused problem resolution. *Family Process, 12*, 141–168.

White, M., & Epston, D. (1990). *Narrative means to therapeutic ends*. New York: Norton.

SUGGESTED READINGS

Eron, J. B., & Lund, T. W. (1993). How problems evolve and dissolve: Integrating narrative and strategic concepts. *Family Process, 32*, 291–309.

Eron, J. B., & Lund, T. W. (1996). *Narrative solutions in brief therapy*. New York: Guilford Press.

Eron, J. B., & Lund, T. W. (in press). Narrative solutions in brief couple therapy. In J. Donovan (Ed.), *Short-term couple therapy*. New York: Guilford Press.

Lund, T. W., & Eron, J. B. (1998). The narrative solutions approach for retelling children's stories: Using preferred views to construct useful conversations. In M. F. Hoyt (Ed.), *The handbook of constructive therapies*. San Francisco: Jossey-Bass.

White, M., & Epston, D. (1990). *Narrative means to therapeutic ends*. New York: Norton.

Chapter 17

Imago Relationship Therapy

WADE LUQUET
HARVILLE HENDRIX

Imago relationship therapy (IRT; Hendrix, 1988, 1992; Luquet, 1996, Luquet & Hannah, 1998) is a relational model of couple therapy that utilizes behavioral, affective, and cognitive interventions to facilitate understanding and change within a dyad. In addition to helping a couple effect behavioral change, IRT also facilitates in the couple a sense of connected differentiation, and does so through its basic communication skill—the "couple's dialogue." Furthermore, IRT changes the position of the therapist from that of a transferential object in a triad, or of an expert who manipulates thought, behavior, or systems, to that of a facilitator or "coach" who introduces processes that, once learned by the couple, have all of the elements that the couple can utilize in the relationship for further growth, understanding, passion, and behavior change. It is a synthesis and an expansion of various schools, including psychoanalysis, self psychology, behaviorism, systems theory, Western spiritual traditions, and modern physics.

A COUPLE'S POWER STRUGGLES
AS A RUPTURE OF CONNECTION

Inherent in IRT is the concept that a couple in treatment is suffering from a rupture of connection. Each partner is seeking to be understood by the other through a power struggle, but each one is frustrated because the other is also suffering with competing wounds. These wounds often prevent each of them from lowering their defenses enough to appreciate the other's point of view. Seeing the other's world view is what Martin Buber (1958) referred to as appreciating the "otherness of the other"; this term is frequently used in IRT.

In preparing a defense to keep themselves from feeling intrapsychic pain, both individuals go into a necessary self-absorption. Self-absorption is not unlike getting a large splinter stuck in your hand: You tend to focus on the splinter, not on the beauty of the forest that surrounds you. It is from this self-absorbed state, commencing in childhood and solidified over time, that each individual begins to see his or her world as the "right one" and develops a belief that "if only the other would change, things would be better." This is what is referred to in IRT as "symbiosis," or "You and I are one. And I am the one." It is within this symbiotic, self-absorbed state that cognitive distortions (Beck, 1976, 1988) originate. Without fully understanding the other's, or his or her own, motivation or thinking, each partner begins to generate ideas and distortions about the other.

THE COUPLE'S DIALOGUE: A TOOL
FOR REESTABLISHING CONNECTION

The main tool in IRT is a process known as the "couple's dialogue." Prior to any such dialogue, safety must be established. This may take the form of the therapist's asking the members of the couple to center themselves, meditate to calm themselves, or visualize themselves in a safe place. Although this may seem forced and rote initially, this process teaches the partners that they need to create a space in which they can feel safe and be authentic in their relationship. True communication only occurs when the partners can fully understand each other and recognize that they have two very different perspectives on the world that are both seeking validation. It is only when both parties feel fully heard and understood that true behavior changes can take place; otherwise, behavior changes are mainly coerced.

In dialogue, partners are trained to hear each other intentionally, according to a three-part process. First, the receiving partner is asked to "mirror" back what the sending partner said, as accurately as he or she can. When the sending partner feels that the receiving partner has understood the two- to three-sentence "send," the receiver asks, "Is there more?" and intentionally invites the sender to say more about the subject. The receiver is asked to "hold" any comments until it is his or her turn to become the sender. This is no easy task, considering that the receiving partner is being stimulated by what is being said, and naturally wants to respond—often in argument or self-defense. However, both partners quickly learn that if the receiver waits to respond, they both win, because the receiver will more accurately hear the sender. Consequently, the sender is more likely to want to hear the receiver when the partners switch roles, having just experienced a few moments of feeling heard and understood.

When the receiving partner has digested and mirrors back an adequate amount of information to the sender, he or she may be ready to validate what the sender has said. Validation is not agreeing. It is, in essence, a means of acknowledging that the sending partner's world has logic to it from the sending partner's point of view, and that the receiving partner can comprehend how it might make sense. "It makes sense to me that you believe in what you do" and "I can understand how you would see it that way" are validating statements that may be used by the receiving partner. And when this is done, the sending partner typically expresses a sensation of feeling calmer and more clearly understood. He or she is often heard saying, "I don't feel as crazy as I did before being validated." The sender's world finally makes sense to someone. Even if the receiver doesn't agree with it, at least it makes sense.

In the third part of the couple's dialogue, the receiving partner makes an attempt to show empathy for the sending partner. Judith Jordan and her colleagues at the Stone Center (see Jordan, Kaplan, Miller, Stiver, & Surrey, 1991) say that empathy is a two-part process: affective surrender and cognitive structure. In other words, empathy involves (1) momentarily feeling the other person's feelings; and then (2) returning to one's own skin, knowing this is not one's own feeling, but taking a guess at how it might feel for the other. "I imagine that you might be feeling lonely and sad" is a typical empathic statement.

It is through this three-part dialogue process, typically taught to a couple in the first and second sessions of IRT, that connection occurs. The connection, the safety, and the dialogue process invite partners to share more information about themselves. Once empathy is restored, they begin to understand that the sending partner's request for behavior changes is partly a quest for fulfillment of developmental needs not received in childhood, and partly a call for growth on the part of the receiving partner.

CASE EXAMPLE

Background Information

Ron and Amanda came to therapy as a last resort for keeping their marriage together. They'd been married for 10 years and had two children; a 7-year-old boy and a 5-year-old girl. At the time of treatment, Ron was a 35-year-old engineer and Amanda a 33-year-old hospital administrator. They had first met in high school, and later dated in college, so Ron and Amanda had a long history together.

After a romantic 3 years in their early marriage, they had their first child. Although their children were certainly desired, the new additions caused a strain on the relationship. Amanda felt she had to continue her career, because Ron had difficulty staying in one job very long. He was playful and creative; though at times these qualities are desirable in a design engineer, they often caused trouble for him with the other scientists at some of the firms he worked for. Amanda, on the other hand, was driven and interested in succeeding in the sometimes volatile hospital field, where layoffs were frequent and job longevity depended on how much money an administrator could save the facility. They were fortunate in that the hospital had an on-site day care facility, which made Amanda's home-to-work transition easy and affordable.

Amanda said that the problem was twofold: ambition and relatives. She felt that Ron had no desire to succeed in his career—a judgment based on the number of times he'd failed. She thought he had no confidence in himself in spite of her encouragement. She was tired of bailing him out by writing his reports and making sure that he completed assignments on time. She also said that she was at her wits' end with the members of his family. They were always critical of how she did things, and at present she had no desire to be with them. She was also angry at Ron for not speaking up for her when the criticisms began to flow. He had told her numerous times that he would speak to them, but never followed through.

Ron responded that he didn't see Amanda's complaints as "any big deal"; she was blowing things out of proportion. He admitted that he wasn't altogether pleased with his work performance, but felt that he had always landed on his feet in the past. He also didn't want to confront his family with Amanda's complaint. He said to her, "You know how they are. They'll hold it against me. You'll just have to get over it."

Already, in the initial session, both members of this couple had provided clues to their developmental wounding. Ron could never quite do things right, while Amanda was always trying to look good and succeed. In addition, Ron had a critical family of origin. Both Ron's and Amanda's patterns were indicative of a wound in the stage of competence. This wound has its origins at about the age of 4, when a child is attempting to develop skills that will help develop confidence and competence. If these attempts are validated, the child can practice and move on from this stage with a greater sense of his or her ability to accomplish things. However, a child who is shamed or simply not validated may develop the sense either that he or she can do nothing right, or that he or she has to keep trying and become competitive. In the case of Ron and Amanda, these two adaptations to the same wound eventually came together in a love relationship in search of corrective validation for the partners' developmental longing. This process would begin in dialogue.

Session 1: Introducing the Couple's Dialogue

In the first session, Ron and Amanda were introduced to the couple's dialogue. They were first provided with psychoeducational information about the defenses that the brain has developed to protect itself against physical and psychic pain. Some versions of fight, flight, freezing, hiding, and/or submitting are utilized in every threatening couple interaction. These are functions of the reptilian brain, or what we refer to in IRT as the "old brain." Ron and Amanda were told that this is normal and that the brain is only doing what it's designed to do to protect itself. To illustrate this, and to provide the therapist with an idea of their usual means of dealing with frustration, Ron and Amanda were asked to participate in a 3-minute exchange of frustration with each other. The following exchange occurred:

RON: I hate it when we have to attend a function with my family and I feel that I have to attend to all fronts.

AMANDA: What am I supposed to do about it?

RON: I . . . or my family has done all it can to win back your confidence.

AMANDA: Oh, yeah! Right!

RON: That's as far as they get. They've bridged out as much as they're going to. I feel it's time to start reconciling. I'm not saying forgive or to be best buddies. I'm saying respect.

AMANDA: Well, who was it who invited your sister over to talk? It wasn't you!

RON: And I thought you guys worked things out.

AMANDA: Yeah, right. With you stomping all around.

RON: I didn't get involved!

AMANDA: You didn't even want to be there when she's present. You didn't want to be there because you didn't want to see your sister. Why should I make peace with your family and sister if you can't even make peace with them yourself? You've got to deal with your own issues!

RON: I've started to.

AMANDA: And I'm supposed to accept everything after what they did to me?!

RON: I never said you had to accept it.

AMANDA: *(Angrily)* Phew!

RON: I said you have to deal with it. They said they were sorry.

AMANDA: *(Yelling)* They never once said they were sorry! They never told me that. They said they were sorry they hurt you; nothing about me.

RON: *(Long silence)* Well . . .

AMANDA: Your turn.

This short exchange spoke volumes about Ron and Amanda. Because IRT is more concerned with process than with content, the therapist made no attempt to guide the exchange, but did stop the couple to discuss what had just transpired. Both partners recognized that they didn't fully hear each other. They also became aware that they used the old-brain defense mechanisms of fighting and "playing dead" in the exchange. Ron also volunteered that he often submitted at home in an effort to stop the fights.

The next step of the first session was to provide Ron and Amanda an experience of a productive exchange, and this was accomplished through the introduction of the couple's dialogue. The therapist explained to them that it was a three-part process and that they would be guided through each step. For this first dialogue, Ron chose to be the sender, and Amanda chose to listen as the receiver. She was instructed that she would have to hear Ron fully before she would be allowed to respond in the dialogue, so she was guided by the therapist into her "safe place." She chose to calm herself by imagining that she was on a mountain trail in the morning. She was told to return to this place when she felt threatened or if she felt an urgency to respond. She was assured that she would have an opportunity to respond, after she mirrored back what Ron said as the first part of the dialogue process and Ron felt fully heard. The following dialogue transpired:

RON: I want to have the same relationship with my siblings that you have with yours. I feel a sense of conflict as I try to make amends for everyone's feelings but my own. I don't want that sense of conflict.

AMANDA: So if I'm getting this, you said that you would like the same relationship with your siblings as I have with mine. You have a sense of conflict as you try to take care of everyone else's feelings, but your own feelings get neglected.

THERAPIST: Ask him, "Did I get it?"

AMANDA: Did I get it?

RON: Yes, you got all of it.

THERAPIST: Ask, "Is there more?"

AMANDA: Is there more?

RON: I would like to reach a sense of belonging with my siblings that I used to have. I grew up very close to my siblings, and I miss that closeness. I feel like my sister is the type of person I could have a close relationship with.

THERAPIST: (To Amanda) Mirror that. I can see that your old brain wants to respond to that, but hold that and mirror back what was said.

AMANDA: (Giggling) I could feel I wanted to say something, but I didn't act on it. You're right, I could feel that old brain want to respond. OK, I heard you say that you would like a sense of belonging with your siblings. You miss that closeness that you once had with your siblings, and you feel that your sister is the type of person you would like to have a relationship with. Did I get that?

RON: Yes.

THERAPIST: Now for the second part of the dialogue, you want to validate what he said. Validation isn't agreeing, so you don't have to agree with it. Can you see that what he says makes sense to him?

AMANDA: Sure, his feelings are valid even if I don't agree with him.

THERAPIST: That's right. Could you tell him he makes sense?

AMANDA: I can see that. You make sense. I can see that you want to be close to your family.

THERAPIST: Great! Now for the third part, you want to offer him some empathy about this. It's just a guess, and you don't have to be right. Can you guess how he might feel about this?

AMANDA: I can imagine that you might feel conflicted, confused, and divided.

RON: You got it!

Ron and Amanda were at the initial and awkward stage of learning the couple's dialogue. In this first session, they were guided through the process, which allowed them to hear each other from their logical and feeling brains rather than their reactive primitive brains. Instead of the typical emotional distance they experienced after most of their exchanges, Ron and Amanda remained on the "field of play" with each other. After this exchange, Ron spoke a bit more, and Amanda continued to mirror him. When he felt heard, the process was reversed: Amanda had the opportunity to talk, while Ron mirrored, validated, and empathized with her. They were warned that they would not get the process right every time in the next few weeks, but that they should practice the process for about 15 minutes daily.†

> † *The couple's dialogue is a very interesting and effective intervention that allows a couple to slow down and focus more on the feelings and emotions that each partner is experiencing. Since IRT is based on various modalities of treatment, perhaps the use of Socratic questioning by each spouse might enhance the level of insight that each can develop with the other. For example, if the therapist had guided Amanda during this session on how to inquire more directly about the specific thoughts that accompanied Ron's feelings about his conflict with his siblings, she might have developed a clearer sense of why he felt and behaved as he did.*

**Sessions 2 through 4: Practicing Dialogue and Introducing
the Concept of Developmental Wounding**

In the next three sessions, Ron and Amanda had the opportunity to practice
the dialogue process with the therapist present. The therapist also began to
introduce some of the principles of IRT with respect to how couples fall in
love: Each partner in a couple picks just the right person, who, when the
couple enters the power struggle, puts the partner in touch with the places
that most need to be stretched for personal growth. Ron and Amanda were
presented with a developmental lecture and completed several Imago
workup forms during the session.

On one form, they were asked to write down positive and negative
traits of their early childhood caretakers. They were asked to write down
as many traits as they could from as early an age as they could remember:
mean, stern, cold, and so on, or warm, friendly, nurturing, and so forth.
They were also asked to complete the sentence stem "What I wanted and
needed most and did not get from my childhood caretakers was . . . ", and
then were asked to make a column of their childhood frustrations and, next
to these, their behavioral responses to their frustrations. Finally, they were
asked to write down their positive experiences of their childhoods and, in
a second column, how they felt in their positive experiences.

Next, the therapist put this information about their childhoods into a
"formula" about their present relationship. A formula consists of five
sentence stems: "I am trying to get a person who is . . . [negative traits of
caretakers] to always be . . . [positive traits of caretakers], so that I can get
. . . [what I did not get in childhood] and feel . . . [positive feelings from
childhood]. I stop myself from getting this sometimes by . . . [what I did
as a child when I was frustrated]." Ron and Amanda were stunned that
the information from their childhood applied so well to their present
relationship. This exercise dramatically showed them their imagos. (For a
full transcript of the lectures and copies of all forms used in IRT, including
the imago workup, see Luquet, 1996).

From this lecture and workup, they both decided that they had been
wounded in the competence stage. Ron reported that his whole life with
his family was about how he could never do things right. After a while, he
decided not to try, whatever he did would just be criticized anyway.
Amanda also remembered not being able to do things well enough for her
parents. This drove her to keep trying and striving for perfection. Her
problem, she said, was that "I don't know when to stop."†

> † *This sounds similar to some of the early schema work that cognitive
> therapists often do, in order to understand more clearly the basis on
> which individuals generate automatic thoughts about themselves and
> their relationships. Perhaps some aspects of the schema-focused*

> *approach might also have been woven into some of these early sessions with Ron and Amanda, with a particular emphasis on their families of origin. Family-of-origin experiences often set the base for certain beliefs and distortions that develop in individuals and in their relationships. It sounds as though both Ron and Amanda were greatly affected by their respective family experiences.*

The sessions allowed Ron and Amanda to learn about the purpose of marriage and to develop healthy communication skills about the issues that brought them into therapy. They continued to have dialogues in the session:

AMANDA: I don't like that I have to work this weekend. I don't feel like I'm giving to the family the way I want to. There is so much to be done.

RON: So if I'm understanding you clearly, you don't like that you have to work this weekend. You don't feel like you are giving to the family the way you want to, but there's so much to be done. Did I get that? Is there more?

AMANDA: I feel guilty because part of me knows that I should be home and spending time with you and the family. But I feel that I have to go in. And when I am home, there so much to do. I feel that I let you down.

RON: So it feels like you're letting me down, and you feel guilty because you know that you should be home more and doing things with the family. But you don't have to feel . . .

THERAPIST: Whoa, Ron. You're just mirroring. You don't have to take away or fix her feelings. Can you get back to your safe place and listen some more?†

> †*It might have been interesting to return to this issue later on and inquire into why Ron felt as though he might have to "fix things" for Amanda. How did this relate to any of his rescue schemas or distortions about what Amanda really wanted from him?*

AMANDA: And I feel sad and depressed about that.

RON: And you feel sad and depressed about not being home and with us the way you want to. Yeah, I can see that you would feel that way. And I imagine that you do feel sad and depressed.

Amanda leaned a bit toward Ron now. The therapist asked what that was about.

AMANDA: That's the first time you let me have my feelings. Usually you try to tell me that my sad feelings aren't true. You try to tell me that I don't have to feel that way. It's nice to have you let me feel what I am feeling.

RON: I'm so afraid that if I don't counter them, your feelings will be set in stone.

THERAPIST: Amanda, would you be willing to hear Ron about this and mirror him?

AMANDA: Sure. You are saying that you are afraid that if you don't counter what I am saying, my feelings will become set in stone. Did I get that? Is there more?

RON: I do worry so much about your feelings and how fragile they are sometimes. The last thing I ever want is to see you crumble.

AMANDA: So you are saying that you worry a lot about my feelings, and the last thing you want to see is me crumbling because of how I feel. I can see that, and I even appreciate that. I imagine you must feel scared and tense.

THERAPIST: Ron, does that remind you of anything growing up?

RON: Yeah. How my mom was. It was so obvious that she was drunk. I was so filled with rage, but I would kiss her on the cheek because I didn't want her to know that I knew she was drunk. I would smooth that over and pretend it didn't happen.

AMANDA: So worrying about my feelings reminds you of your mother and when she would get drunk. You would try to pretend that it did not happen, and that you did not notice that she was drunk. You would try to smooth things over, even though you were filled with rage and it was so obvious she was drunk. Did I get that? Is there more?

RON: I didn't want to be confrontational, even though I was hurting inside.

AMANDA: So you're saying that you didn't want to be confrontational, even though you were hurting inside. I can see that, and the manner in which you handled things makes sense to me, given the situation. I can imagine that you felt rageful, powerless, scared, and lonely.

RON: You got it.†

> † This unfolded rather nicely as a result of the therapist's subtle initiatives at facilitating dialogue. Perhaps cognitive restructuring can also be used in varying ways in IRT, depending on how smoothly the process described above occurs with each couple. It may be particularly helpful to assign tasks for homework that will solidify partners' understanding of each other's feelings. These may include independent exercises where each partner is asked to challenge some of his or her old beliefs about why the spouse acted in a certain way in the past. In the case described here, the new information gathered in

> this session would have been new evidence for Ron and Amanda to use in restructuring their individual perceptions and beliefs. Such a strategy appears quite compatible with the IRT approach.

Five Processes That Deepen Dialogue

By itself, the couple's dialogue is a powerful communication tool. Imago relationship therapists also employ five additional processes that assist the members of a couple in making greater empathic connection, effecting behavior changes, experiencing daily caring behaviors, dealing with anger, and creating a vision for the relationship. Each of these five processes is taught and facilitated in a session, with practicing of the process assigned for homework. Generally, the couple also practices the process in the next session with the therapist present. When all of the processes are taught and practiced, the couple is taught how to use the appropriate process for the specific situation that may arise. The goal of the therapy is for the couple to acquire skills to utilize when conflict occurs, and to make the relationship a vehicle for personal growth.

Session 5: Imago Process 1—Re-Imaging the Partner

Members of a couple entering therapy typically have a cynical view of each other—a partner-as-enemy point of view. After establishing contact through dialogue, the next step is for each partner to begin to view the other as both an ally and someone who is wounded, rather than as a foe or enemy. The "parent–child dialogue," which was introduced to Ron and Amanda in the fifth session, begins this transformation. In this process, the receiving partner assumes the role of the parent, and the sending partner assumes the role of himself or herself as a young child. The receiving partner asks the question, "I am your mother/father. What was it like to live with me?" The sending partner then speaks to that partner as if the partner were the parent. This process typically reveals some deep pain to the receiving partner, which helps him or her to begin understanding the other's vulnerabilities and wounds. To go further, the therapist may introduce the "holding" process, in which the receiving partner is asked to hold the sending partner in his or her lap in a hug position. The sending partner then tells the receiving partner about the frustrations in his or her childhood. The receiver mirrors back the frustration in an empathic setting.

By this time, Ron and Amanda were well on their way to learning the importance of hearing each other. They'd learned that if each listened long enough to the other, the other's ways of doing things and reactions in power struggles would begin to make sense, given the additional information. The couple's dialogue process provided each of them as the sender with a sense of feeling understood and of centeredness. At the same time, it brought about a cognitive restructuring in each of them as the receiving partner, as the images of why the partner did what he or she did were affected. In the first few sessions, in short, the partners began the process of "re-imaging" each other.

In fifth session, Ron and Amanda deepened this re-imaging process through the parent–child dialogue. This exercise aided them in seeing and experiencing each other's vulnerable side, and it gave the partners a chance to express their childhood wounds in a nurturing environment. To many, this process might appear regressive. Yet the aim of this type of dialogue is for the wounds to resurface, to be articulated, to begin to be healed through understanding and empathy, and to reveal to both partners what some of the underlying motivations for their behavior really are. When partners are able to see what is motivating their behavior, they can make more genuine and lasting changes.

The parent–child dialogue began with the therapist's setting the tone for what was to evolve. The receiving partner was asked to go to his or her safe place, and to listen as if he or she were a parent, but this time to listen with an open and nurturing heart. The partners were then given questions to ask each other. In this case, Ron chose to talk to his mother.

THERAPIST: Amanda, ask Ron this question: "I am your mother. What was it like to live with me?"

AMANDA: I am your mother. What was it like to live with me?

RON: It was evilness. I was always trying to stay away from you. I didn't want you to tell me what to do. I wanted to stay away from you when you were drunk. I'd hide downstairs, or in my room, or outside. But then I wanted attention from you for the things I was able to do well. And I wanted you to notice. You never realized that I was trying to stay away from you when you'd come after me. You never got into your own world. And although you let me set up my own world, I wanted you to notice that I was doing good things. It was not until I was 23 years old that you noticed that I was important. But by then it was too late, because I don't have a lot of sympathy for you. I don't have a lot of feelings about what concerns you, other than you are alive. I don't have much consideration for the things that are important to you, because if things were ever important to me, you didn't care about them. I know that sounds callous, but I'm sorry.

THERAPIST: And it makes me feel . . . ?

RON: It makes me feel sad, because you could have been someone I looked up to, but instead you are someone I look over. I do love you very much, but you have to understand that as you get older and need me, I can't help but treat you like you treated me. It is not because I feel vengeful. I don't have it in me because I don't know how to take care of you.

THERAPIST: Amanda, ask this question: "I am your mother. What did you need from me that you did not get?"

AMANDA: Ron, I am your mother. What did you need from me that you did not get?

RON: I needed for you to say, "Hey that's really neat," or "Hey, don't do that." Two extremes that were never there. I needed you to help me with my homework, but you never did. I needed for you to tell me not to get involved with drinking and drugs, but you just said, "Well, you'll grow out of it." And that made it OK to you. I needed to know that you loved me. I needed to know that I was someone special. I needed to know that I was better than average . . . or worse than average. I feel that I got cheated out of something special. I know it did not have to happen this way. I don't have many memories of my childhood, because things were so bad I didn't pay attention, either. I think I was really good at being a kid, but now I don't know how to capture that spirit again.

At this point, Ron and Amanda were asked to disengage from the role play in order to process the material that had just surfaced.

THERAPIST: Amanda, what did you see?

AMANDA: A lot of pain. It was so visible. It is not like Ron to be so open.

RON: Wow!

THERAPIST: Were you surprised?

RON: Yeah, I didn't think I would come up with that much. I thought I might keep it on the surface or say, "You didn't do that bad," or "I'm an OK person, so I guess you did your job right." But that stuff came from way down. I didn't expect that to happen.

AMANDA: It makes sense to me now why he doesn't speak up for me with his family. I still don't like it, but it makes sense to me why he hasn't talked to them about how they hurt me.†

> †*It would have been interesting to see how Amanda eventually incorporated this new material into her existing schema about Ron and his behavior. From a cognitive-behavioral perspective, this is the point where the true restructuring process begins.*

For homework, Ron and Amanda were assigned the task to switch roles, with Amanda talking to one of her parents. This exercise helped both partners to restart their "empathic engines," which had been turned off over the past few years. To listen to each other's pain, they had to become less self-absorbed and more focused on each other. Ron and Amanda were beginning to understand the foundation of the IRT concept of appreciating the "otherness of the other." Interestingly, many of the presenting problems they'd arrived with now seemed less important to them, even though nothing had been done thus far toward making actual behavior changes.†

> †*This is an interesting statement, since to some theorists, such as some who espouse humanistic or emotionally focused approaches to therapy, such a transaction would be sufficient for behavioral change to occur in and of itself.*

Sessions 6 and 7: Imago Processes 2 and 3— Re-Romanticizing and Re-Visioning the Relationship

Couple researcher John Gottman (1979) reports that long-term stable marriages have one thing in common: There are five positive behaviors for every negative behavior. Partners in distressed couples have to learn how to please each other intentionally. The "re-romanticizing" process teaches partners to flood each other with caring behaviors. In the sixth session, each partner is asked to come up with a list of behaviors that would make him or her feel loved and cared for. The couple is then asked to engage in a dialogue about the lists, and each partner is told to begin giving the other partner one caring behavior from the other's list each day. The couple is also told about the importance of regular surprises for both partners, and about daily "belly laughs" as a way of maintaining safety. The more they experience pleasure with each other, the more they will experience safety, passion, and thus connection.

Much of the business motivation literature currently available says that "if you can dream it, you can build it." In the "re-visioning" session, the partners are asked to design their dream relationship. They are given the task of creating what they both consider to be the ultimate in marriage and to write it down in the present tense. Typical aspects of a dream relationship include the following: "We take walks together," "We talk using dialogue," "We respect each other's work," "We have a pleasurable sex life," and "We are financially secure." The partners are given the task to review their dream relationship each month and to develop goals to attain this relationship. Through this process, the relationship becomes intentional as the couple makes an effort to make the dream come true.

For Ron and Amanda, the sixth session started with a short presentation about the importance of pleasure and caring behaviors in relationships. The therapist especially emphasized that a caring behavior needs to be pleasurable to the person receiving the caring gesture rather than the person providing it. To give football tickets to a person who does not really like football is not a gesture of caring. Too often, however, couples live under the false assumption that each partner should know what makes the other happy. This assumption has produced many unhappy birthdays and anniversaries. So it is important for each partner to generate a list of behaviors for the other partner to perform, instead of simply letting the other partner guess.

Ron and Amanda began composing their lists in the session and discussed several items in dialogue. This session was a good opportunity for the two of them to learn how to use dialogue for positive conversations; good news needs to be heard and validated as much as bad news does.

THERAPIST: Amanda, would you be willing to tell Ron one of your caring behaviors—a behavior that, if he did it, would make you feel loved and cared about/

AMANDA: I really love when you bring a towel to the shower for me when I forget.

RON: So you really love when I bring you a nice clean fluffy towel when you forget it when you take a shower.

AMANDA: Yeah. Sometimes I forget it on purpose, so that you can bring it and we can spend some time together.

RON: Oh, so sometimes you forget it on purpose, so I will bring it to you and we can spend some time together. Well, I can understand that. And imagine that you feel special, cared about, and loved.

THERAPIST: Great. Ron, do you have one?

RON: Not as good as that, but I really like it on Saturday morning, when I wake up and have a crick in my neck, you bring me a nice cup of hot coffee and rub my neck.

AMANDA: So you really like it on Saturday morning when I bring you a cup of coffee and spend some time rubbing your neck. Did I get that? Well, I can understand that, and I imagine that you feel cared for and nurtured.

RON: Yep.

Ron and Amanda laughed as they shared several more of the caring behaviors on their lists. They were instructed to keep adding to the lists and to put them someplace where they could both see them easily. This gave each of them ample opportunities to begin the assignment of performing one caring behavior a day for the other partner. Each was also instructed to begin giving the other partner a surprise once a month, that the partner would enjoy, as a way of increasing pleasant anticipation in the relationship. Finally, in this session, they were asked to participate in some activities led by the therapist that would elicit a "belly laugh." Although they initially found this hard to imagine, Ron and Amanda participated in a game called "suck and blow," in which they passed a credit card back and forth between themselves by mouth. This elicited howls of laughter from them, and they seemed to enjoy it thoroughly. Since shared laughter is one of the things many unhappy couples lack, they were instructed to try to elicit and participate in a "belly laugh" with each other once each day.

In the next session, Ron and Amanda worked on their dream relationship. Again, this seemed unrealistic to them at first, but they were told about the importance of defining what kind of relationship they would like to have eventually. Working on separate worksheets, Ron and Amanda wrote down the qualities they would each like to have in their relationship. They were instructed to start each item with "We," so that it could be a shared goal, and to write it in the present tense, as if they already had it. The document they were about to write together was not unlike a business plan; businesses that write down their yearly goals are more likely to achieve them.

Ron and Amanda each compiled an extensive list, and then came together in dialogue to discuss the lists. They took one item on each list at a time and decided together whether that was something they wanted in their dream relationship. Those goals that seemed heated and caused tension were not included; they would be discussed in future sessions in the form of behavior change requests. Here are some items from Ron and Amanda's joint dream relationship list:

> We have fun together.
> We talk using the couple's dialogue.
> We eat out once a week.
> We are financially secure.
> We support each other at family events.
> We have an enjoyable sex life.
> We kiss at stoplights.
> We have fun traveling.†

> †*I think that it would also have been important for the partners to assess how realistic their expectations for their dream relationship actually were. Unrealistic expectations are among the primary causes for marital tension and stress (Baucom & Epstein, 1990).*

Sessions 8 and 9: Imago Process 4—Behavior Change Requests

At this point in IRT, the members of a couple are developing an understanding of each other and have developed ways of increasing passion and safety in the relationship. They now need a method of requesting behavior changes without the use of criticism, devaluation, or coercion. In the eighth session, the couple is introduced to the idea that a frustration is a desire stated negatively: "I hate it when you're late" becomes "My desire is for you to be on time." The couple is then taught to take a desire and turn it into a specific "behavior change request" that is positive, achievable, and measurable. For example, "My desire is for you to be on time" becomes "Twice this week, I would like for you to be home within 5 minutes of the time you said you were going to be." The receiver is instructed that he or she does not have to fulfill the request. Rather, if the receiver chooses to, the request is fulfilled as a gift—a way of showing concern for the developmental wound that "being late" may be triggering. Because a behavior change request is made without criticism and in the dialogue process, connection is maintained and the power struggle is avoided.

The behavior change request also facilitates mutual growth. The thing one person requests of the other is usually the most difficult thing for the other person to give. This is because the frustration of one partner usually coincides with a social self-expression that was not fully developed in the other partner. The request "I would like for you to listen to how I feel for 15 minutes three time a week, using dialogue" is typically given to the partner who needs to develop his or her feeling abilities. "I would like for you to make a list of five chores you can complete on the weekend" is typically given to the partner whose growth lies in developing the ability to accomplish a task. Through behavior change requests, partners call each other into mutual wholeness.

Readers have probably noticed by now that Ron and Amanda had not yet dealt directly with changing specific problems. In IRT, to change a problem, a couple has to understand it fully. Ron and Amanda were learning that their frustrations weren't what they thought they were when they first came to therapy. They had progressed from "He said/She said" to "What can we learn from this frustration?" In the eighth session, they began the process of turning their frustrations into desires and then into specific behavior change requests. It was important for them to know that this session was not about changing each other, but about educating each other in what they needed to do over a period of time to use the relationship for growth and to reclaim lost parts of their selves.

To help them with this, they were each given a form with a series of sentence stems. They were asked to think of a few frustrations and write them down on a separate sheet of paper. If they were to read those frustrations as they were, an argument would probably ensue, so they were each asked to pick one and bring it through the series of sentence stems so they could engage in dialogue about the frustration and begin to educate each other about the changes needed for relationship and individual growth. As an example, here is how one of Ron's behavior change requests was developed through this process. (Ron's responses to the sentence stems are in italics.)

I get frustrated when . . . *you never let us see a stupid movie.*
Then I feel . . . *inhibited.*
And I react by . . . *giving in and seeing something more intellectual or dramatic.*
My hidden fear is . . . *that by insisting we see a stupid movie, I will appear immature.*
My desire is . . . *that I would like to take you to a really stupid movie that we don't have to think about.*

To obtain my desire, I would like to request from you . . . [make three requests]:

1. *Once this week, I would like to take you to a really dumb movie.*
2. *Once this month, I would like for you to pick out a really dumb movie and take me to it.*
3. *For the next 2 months, when we are making movie choices, I would like you to be open-minded by including two dumb movies on our list of possible selections.*

Although this example may seem simple, Ron's request centered exactly on an area of growth for Amanda. She was brought up in a critical home in which work was important. Consequently, it was difficult for Amanda to let down, have fun, and waste some money on a dumb movie. It would take a stretch on her part to participate in this request; yet, to do so, she would begin to reclaim some of her liveliness that she lost (probably as a result of losing trust in her instincts). If she exercised this part, like an atrophied muscle, she might be able to reclaim at least part of it.

Amanda also had a request for Ron in this session. Because this session was about each partner's educating the other on what each needed regarding behavior changes, she presented it by reading from her sheet and while Ron mirrored her back.

AMANDA: I hate when we go to your parents and I don't feel taken care of by you.

RON: So I'm hearing that you really don't like it when we go to my parents and you don't feel that I'm taking care of or support you.

AMANDA: That's right. And I feel vulnerable.

RON: And you feel vulnerable.

AMANDA: And I react by getting quiet while we're there and feeling distant from you for a few days.

RON: So when this happens, you get quiet and feel distant from me for a few days.

AMANDA: And my hidden fear is that I will have to fend for myself.

RON: And you're afraid that you'll have to fend for yourself.

THERAPIST: Amanda, does this remind you of anything growing up?

AMANDA: Yes—when my dad would badger me about not doing my chores right, and my mom would just watch. I did not feel taken care of, and I would get quiet and withdrawn.

RON: So when your dad would badger you the way he does, and your mom would look on without helping you, you felt vulnerable and you would get quiet and distant.

THERAPIST: And your desire is?

AMANDA: My desire is that I feel supported by you, and you speak up when you see me being attacked or feeling vulnerable.

RON: So you would like for me to support you and speak up when I see you being attacked by my family.

At this point Amanda made three requests of Ron, which he mirrored back to her:

1. Once this month when we are at your parent's house, I would like for you to say to your parents, "Do not bring Amanda into this conversation," when you see me feeling uncomfortable with how they are treating me.
2. Twice this month, I would like for us to have a dialogue before and after our visit to their house about my uneasiness about being there.
3. Once this month when we visit your parents, I would like for you to approach me and say, "How are you feeling? I am willing to listen to you now," and to listen to me using dialogue.

Again, these requests were made to someone who had difficulty in feeling and in motivating himself to accomplish things. These requests from Amanda not only would meet her needs, but would restart the feeling and doing parts of Ron.

Ron and Amanda were assigned the task of filling out more behavior change request forms and having dialogues about at least two of them. They brought their completed forms back with them the next session, where they were checked to make sure they called for positive, measurable, and "do-able" behaviors. This was very important, because couples in general tend to be vague about what they want (e.g., "I want you to be nicer"), rather than specific ("Twice this week, when you come home, I would like you to come to me, hug me around my waist for 15 seconds, and ask me, 'How was your day?' "). A specific request allows the receiver of the behavior to feel taken care of in the way he or she needs to be taken care of. At the same time, it allows the sender of the behavior to reclaim his or her lost parts through the performance of the details of the request.

Session 10: Imago Process 5– Resolving Rage through the Container

The "container" is a seven-step process used to express anger safely. It is the most complicated and least often used of the imago processes, and is only introduced after the couple fully understands the IRT concepts of safety and dialogue. The container begins with the sending partner's making a request for an appointment to express anger. Though making an appointment may seem odd at first, a couple learns that this step gives the receiving partner the opportunity to find a safe and centered space for fully hearing the sending partner's anger. The sending partner then sends one sentence to let the receiving partner know what he or she is angry about, and this is mirrored. Then for the next 10 minutes, the sending partner "explodes" his or her anger, with the receiving partner listening attentively. The receiver is taught to do this in the session and to realize that if he or she waits through the anger, this will provide the opportunity to hear the sender's hurt that lies beneath. It is at this point, sometimes referred to as an "implosion," that the empathic connection occurs and we typically see the anger turn into passion. This is followed by a moment of rest and recovery.

The process then moves into the behavior change request step in which the sending partner makes three requests for changes that would have a positive effect on the frustration. These requests are mirrored back by the receiving partner. The process ends with the couple's participating in a few minutes of high-energy fun or a "belly laugh." This is a way of maintaining the connection through fun, caring behaviors and of increasing the passion begun in this session.

It should be noted that containers unfold in many ways with couples. Some are very loud, dramatic, and powerfully moving, while others are quiet and rather uneventful. Whatever the outcome, the idea is to give couples a safe and structured way to deal with anger and rage. Couples often report benefits from containers no matter what form they take.

Ron and Amanda came to the 10th session having spent 2 weeks working on frustrations and behavior change requests. It was important for the therapist to start this session by checking on their homework and dialogue. They reported that they had completed several of the behavior change request forms and had talked about them. They said that what would have typically been a heated conversation turned out to be fairly rational because of the structure of the forms and dialogue. They now each had several behaviors that they could attempt to change, written out for them in a positive and practical format.

THERAPIST: Can you see how the request taps into your adaptations?

RON: Yeah. It goes against your psyche. You don't really want to do them, but you can see why it's important.

THERAPIST: Did you get that if you do the behaviors, your partner gets [her] need met, and you grow into those lost parts of yourself?

RON: Oh, yeah!

AMANDA: It makes sense.

THERAPIST: So you are learning that nature is not concerned with your comfort. Nature is concerned with your growth.

It was important to let Ron and Amanda know that this work isn't easy. Reclaiming parts of yourself using behaviors you don't typically use is like going to physical therapy; it requires a stretch.

This session focused on how to handle rage in a relationship. As stated earlier, in IRT this is done, rather oddly, by appointment. This enables the couple to create a safe space for the anger to unfold, and to experience a productive rather than a reactive transaction. The seven-step container process was used to guide the couple through anger to empathy and passion. Ron and Amanda had made the appointment and had decided to do the container work in the session. The session started with the second step of sending the trigger sentence:

THERAPIST: Ron, can you send in [no more than] two sentences what this is going to be about?

RON: I'm angry about your bringing work home with you.

THERAPIST: Amanda, could you mirror that?

AMANDA: So you're angry about me bringing work home.

THERAPIST: Good. Now, Ron, I'd like you to build up your anger about this. Amanda, I want you to get ultra-safe and prepare yourself to provide a safe place for Ron to express his anger. The only thing you're allowed to say during this is "Tell me more" or "Say that louder." There are three rules to this: no hitting each other, no property damage, and no leaving until all of the steps are completed. Listen long enough, and you'll find the prize underneath. When you're ready, tell him that you're ready to hear him.

AMANDA: OK. I'm ready to hear you now.

Now came the third step—exploding anger.

RON: I hate your boss. I hate what that company has done to you—what it has done to your spirit, your body, your mind. I want you to change your job as soon as possible, if that's what you want.

AMANDA: Tell me more.

RON: In the past 2 years since you've been there, I've seen your smile get smaller. I've seen—and I don't mean this as a cut to you—your waist size get bigger. I've seen you get more and more unhappy, and all we ever talk about is your job and how much we hate your boss. You have to either get rid of the job or get rid of your boss.

AMANDA: Tell me more.

RON: I hate your boss.

THERAPIST: Say that louder.

RON: I hate your boss!

THERAPIST: Louder.

RON: *(Loudly)* I hate your boss! I hate what your boss has done to you and how happy you used to be. I can't stand when I come home after a long day myself and find that this guy has had another fit and has taken his unhappiness out on my wife

AMANDA: Say it louder.

RON: I hate that this guy and this job [are] making us so sad. Things have got to change. I'm so unhappy because the whole time I've been thinking that it's me, and it's not. You and I are unhappy together, and the cause of the unhappiness is not totally me.

THERAPIST: And it reminds me of when I was a kid.

RON: It reminds me of when I was a kid, and my father would go away every other weekend with his job and leave me in the evil clutches of my mother. This wasn't something that I could change, and it made my mom more and more unhappy when he'd go away, so nothing would get done. Then he'd come back and he would be mad. He could have changed his job arrangement, but he never did. He never did and he still hasn't. He's doing it today. My sister is still living at home taking care of my mother, because my father won't change his job. I don't want us to fall into a trap like that.

THERAPIST: I needed my mother's smile.

RON: I did need my mother's smile and my father's presence. Then maybe she would not have drunk so much and she would not have ignored me. *(Ron's eyes filled with tears.)*

THERAPIST: Stay with the feeling.

RON: My mom hurt me bad. She hurt me bad by being hurt herself. And a lot of things could have been different. She never spoke up about how much she hated it. She couldn't change that, and he couldn't change that. We aren't them. I want to see our lives change for the better.

THERAPIST: Amanda, would you be willing to hold Ron for a few minutes?

The fourth step, holding and implosion of feelings, followed naturally. Amanda held Ron as he quietly sobbed. She was obviously quite touched by his show of emotion as she softly stroked his face. He talked quietly to her about how he hurt and how he wanted a better life for the two of them. After a few minutes, Ron sat up and wiped his tears. He took a few moments to pull himself together and thanked Amanda for listening to him. This was the fifth step—the moment of rest and recovery.

In the sixth step, Ron made three behavior change requests of Amanda, and she mirrored each one. Ron's requests were as follows:

1. Four times this week when you come home, I would like for us to talk about work for a maximum of 20 minutes; then I would like us to talk about other subjects or do something active, like walking together or going to the library.
2. Within the next 2 weeks, I would like for you to make one call to the university to get financial aid information and an application to the graduate school.
3. I would like you to ride the exercise bike for 20 minutes three times a week; then I would like to ride it also for 20 minutes three times a week.

Amanda said that she thought she could comply with these requests, and she made a commitment to contact the university within the next 2 weeks for information.

The seventh and last step of the container process is designed to help the partners regain some of the energy they have expended in this highly emotional process, and to allow them to experience pleasure with each other. Ron and Amanda asked to participate in an activity that would produce a sustained 15-second "belly laugh." As they had done in a previous session, they chose to pull out a credit card and play "suck and blow." The session ended with Ron and Amanda in a loving embrace.

Sessions 11 through 15: Learning to Use All of the Processes in a Fluid Manner

Ron and Amanda returned for five more sessions. At this point, they had learned the couple's dialogue and the five imago processes. These last five sessions were spent helping the couple learn to use the processes in what is referred to as a "seamless flow."

Ron and Amanda became quite proficient in the processes. As with all couples who learn and utilize IRT, theirs was not a "happily ever after" story. There were many more power struggles, and many times when they didn't use the dialogue to resolve the struggle. Yet, when things calmed down a bit, they seemed to come back to the processes they'd learned in the earlier sessions.

Follow-Up

A 6-month follow-up found the couple moving forward, with Amanda registered for graduate school, talking less about work, and going to an occasional "dumb movie." Ron was standing up to his family more, and found himself being more supportive of Amanda and talking more on a feeling level with her in dialogue. They both acknowledged that they had a long way to go, but felt safe and connected enough to proceed with the marriage—something they hadn't been quite as sure about 9 months earlier.

CONCLUSION

IRT teaches couples connected differentiation, primarily through the couple's dialogue. When one person fully understands another in the dialogue process, it defines not only the sender but the receiver of the message. This is what Jordan et al. (1991) refer to as finding "self-in-relation." In IRT, the self is defined in relationship by partners' seeing that each other's world makes sense. There is no push for agreement between partners; rather, the push is for partners to understand that if each one listens long enough, he or she will see that the other's way of seeing things, shaped by adaptations from childhood, has validity to that partner. When partners are understood, they feel safer. When they feel safer, they let their guard down. And when the guard is lowered, they are more available to make behavior changes that are significant and long-lasting.

AUTHORS' REPLY TO EDITOR'S COMMENTS

It's refreshing to see the cooperative spirit that Dr. Dattilio brings to his comments interspersed throughout this chapter. There is a sense of wanting to add to rather than detract from a model that, though in its infancy, has many strong adherents. They are certainly comments to take seriously as IRT expands its therapist base and extends and evolves its theory.

Specifically, the suggestion on page 410 that an exercise be added to help a couple challenge old beliefs may be very useful. Perhaps after the partners experiences through dialogue that they have distorted beliefs about each other, an exercise could be formulated that would help increase their curiosity about each other's true nature. An example would be a few rounds of "Let me tell you who I really am. I am . . . " with the sending partner being listened to in the couple's dialogue.

On page 408, Dr. Dattilio's comment about the imago workup's helping the partners understand the basis of their automatic thoughts about themselves and each other is quite accurate. Part of the reason the imago workup is so effective at doing this is that it catches the couple off guard: The partners write about their parents, and find out that what they've written applies to each other. We have witnessed people being very shaken by this information in workshops when they realize they have married a composite of their parents.

On page 414, Dr. Dattilio finds interest in the statement that "many of the presenting problems they'd arrived with now seemed less important to them, even though nothing had been done thus far toward making actual behavior changes." He says that according to some proponents of humanistic and emotionally focused approaches, "such a transaction would be sufficient for behavioral change to occur in and of itself." And it is true that these emotional transactions, where empathy is evident, do bring about behavior change. Yet we have found that empathy isn't enough. Deeper behavior change requires a stretching of the limits of the self. We have found that this occurs best in the form of a specific, positive, measurable, and "do-able" behavior change request. When empathy is present, these deeper behavior changes feel less coercive to the partners granting the changes.

One comment we have some reservations about is that on page 407, where Dr. Dattilio suggests that Socratic questioning might have been a useful modality to attempt with Ron and Amanda. Questions often take people out of their feelings and into their logic. This is useful if that's the therapist's intent, and cognitive-behavioral therapy seems to utilize behaviors and thoughts for much of its work. IRT makes use of sentence stems and a type of questioning that allows the sending partner to stay in his or her affect while the receiving partner gains additional information. For example, in the dialogue given just prior to Dr. Dattilio's comment, the therapist might have instructed the receiving partner to pose a question (e.g., "Can you tell me more about wanting to have a relationship with your siblings?") or send a sentence stem (e.g., "If I had a relationship with my siblings, I would feel . . . " or "Having a relationship with my siblings would . . . "). This means of inquiry would have allowed the couple to stay in an affective mode while at the same time discovering additional information.

In sum, cognitive-behavioral techniques are certainly valuable to IRT. Many such techniques have already been incorporated in the imago processes, and we would do well to investigate how additional techniques might enhance our model. It is possible that cognitive-behavioral techniques that can be couched safely in the dialogue process may help partners to take the time to understand each other in deeper and more authentic ways.

REFERENCES

Baucom, D. H., & Epstein, N. (1990). *Cognitive-behavioral marital therapy.* New York: Brunner/Mazel.

Beck, A. T. (1976). *Cognitive therapy and the emotional disorders.* New York: Signet.

Beck, A. T. (1988). *Love is never enough.* New York: Harper.

Buber, M. (1958). *I and thou.* New York: Scribner's.

Gottman, J. (1979). *Marital interaction: Experimental investigations.* New York: Academic Press.

Hendrix, H. (1988). *Getting the love you want: A guide for couples.* New York: Henry Holt.

Hendrix, H. (1992). *Keeping the love you find: A guide for singles.* New York: Pocket Books.

Jordan, J. V., Kaplan, A. G., Miller, J. B., Stiber, I. P., & Surrey, J. L. (1991). *Women's growth in connection: Writings from the Stone Center.* New York: Guilford Press.

Kuhn, T. S. (1970). *The structure of scientific revolutions* (2nd ed.). Chicago: University of Chicago Press.

Luquet, W. J. (1996). *Short-term couples therapy: The imago model in action.* New York: Brunner/Mazel.

Luquet, W. J., & Hannah, M. T. (Eds.). (1998). *Healing in the relational paradigm: The imago relationship therapy casebook.* New York: Brunner/Mazel.
Swimme, B., & Berry, T. (1992). *The universe story.* New York: HarperCollins.

SUGGESTED READINGS

Hannah, M. T., Luquet, W. J., & McCormack, J. (1997). Compass as a measure of efficacy of couples therapy. *American Journal of Family Therapy, 25*(1), 76–90.
Hannah, M. T., & Luquet, W. J. (1997). Brief imago therapy and changes in personal and relationship distress: Preliminary findings. *Journal of Imago Relationship Therapy, 2*(2), 55–65.
Hendrix, H. (1988). *Getting the love you want: A guide for couples.* New York: Henry Holt.
Hendrix, H. (1992). *Keeping the love you find: A guide for singles.* New York: Pocket Books.
Jordan, J. V., Kaplan, A. G., Miller, J. B., Stiber, I. P., & Surrey, J. L. (1991). *Women's growth in connection: Writings from the Stone Center.* New York: Guilford Press.
Luquet, W. J. (1996). *Short-term couples therapy: The imago model in action.* New York: Brunner/Mazel.
Luquet, W. J. (1996). To what end, couples therapy? *Journal of Couples Therapy, 6*(1–2), 13–30.
Luquet, W. J., with commentary from others. (1996). Case study: Don and Bonnie, a rigid/diffuse couple. *Journal of Imago Relationship Therapy, 1*(2), 67–77.
Luquet, W. J., & Hannah, M. T. (1996). The efficacy of short-term imago therapy: Preliminary findings. *Journal of Imago Relationship Therapy, 1*(1), 67–75.
Swimme, B., & Berry, T. (1992). *The universe story.* New York: HarperCollins.
Wilder, K. (1996). *A brief history of everything.* Boston: Shambhala.

Chapter 18

Psychoanalytic Couple Therapy

FRED M. SANDER

"No." That was my initial reaction to the invitation to contribute a chapter on psychoanalytic couple therapy to this volume on how cognitive-behavioral approaches can be integrated with others. These disciplines are, despite occasional attempts at integration (Seagraves, 1982; Wachtel, 1977), basically antithetical. I was prepared to decline the invitation. To do so, however, would have contributed to the increasing isolation and insularity of psychoanalysis, which until recently played a central role in establishing and defining the nature of psychotherapy. Whereas the Copernican and Darwinian revolutions challenged our convictions of being at the center of the universe and of being descended from God rather than from apes, respectively, the Freudian revolution challenged our illusion of free will by showing that we are all too often controlled by unconscious forces. Another revolution is now upon us: The computer-driven information revolution, part of our rapidly changing ecosystem, is once again changing how we define ourselves. As computers increasingly take on human characteristics, will our identities, epiphenomena of our computer-like brains, increasingly mirror this rapidly changing technological world (Turkle, 1995)?

Not to engage in this (r)evolution would have threatened the survival, in a Darwinian sense, of the psychoanalytic perspective. It would also have run counter to the "fundamental rule" of psychoanalysis. Freud encouraged his patients to "say whatever came to mind." Silence, whether in the clinical situation or in the scientific arena, interferes with the discovery of new truths—be they insights into the unconscious mind or into the complex patterns and determinations of human behavior.†

†*I tend to agree with Dr. Sander that the psychoanalytic and cognitive-behavioral approaches are antithetical in many ways. However, there are some areas that lend themselves to rapprochement, and I hope that these will begin to emerge within the context of this chapter.*

Although some scientists, like many artists, initially flourish in isolation, communication of their work is critical if it's to be tested, confirmed, refuted, and refined. A work of art, a scientific paper, a person's way of experiencing the world—all are ultimately communicated to and interpreted by an audience, a witness. Artists, scientists, patients, and therapists, in communicating with those around them, facilitate the discovery of new truths. It is in that space between artist and audience, scientists and their peers, patients and therapists, or authors and their readers that new "co-constructions" (to borrow a term from postmodernism) evolve. I can imagine you, the reader, either nodding in agreement at this point, or questioning the emphasis thus far on words and speech. "What about nonverbal communication?" you may ask.

In the consulting room, a husband stares out the window as his wife berates him for never talking with her. Does the therapist ask the husband to put into words the possible meaning of his behavior and how he feels when criticized? Or ask his wife how she feels as he avoids her? What memories do these behaviors stir in them? Should the therapist assign a task of having each speak and listen without being interrupted, preferably using the boundary-setting personal pronoun "I" rather than the boundary-invasive and blaming "you"?

How can we begin to address and understand the current bewildering array of theories and practices reflected by the varied chapters in this book? Because human behavior is so multiply determined, there are multiple ways of defining and treating it. Like a Rorschach blot, our behavior and emotions are defined by each of us with *Rashomon*-like idiosyncrasy. In addition, each era defines mental illness and its treatment differently. I am reminded of Henri Ellenberger's observation about the emergence of psychoanalysis: "Curing the sick is not enough; one must cure them with methods accepted by the community" (1970, p. 57).

When Ellenberger wrote those words, he probably didn't imagine the "methods" introduced by the pharmacological and managed care revolutions we're now experiencing. These revolutions, driven by an economic system that seeks to maximize profits, encourage the briefest possible treatment. In such a context, mental illnesses or problems are best defined narrowly and treated narrowly. Furthermore, with this narrower focus we are more able to "document" results. Labor-intensive listening to patients isn't encouraged in this climate, even though such time spent has been shown to reduce absenteeism at work and unnecessary visits to the doctor.

The couple I'll be discussing later in this chapter presented with a conflict over whether to have a third child. The wife threatened divorce if her husband denied her a third child. How does one assess outcome in a case such as this? The couple, after they've had or haven't had a third child, divorces or doesn't. What constitutes a positive result? From whose point of view? How do we evaluate the spouses' decision, whatever it may be, and its impact upon their children and their children's children? Follow-up studies of narrow behavioral sequences rarely go beyond a few months or a year. The more precisely defined the variables, the more measurable—but also the more trivial the findings.

Ironically, the psychoanalytic revolution, "the talking cure," began 100 years ago with the briefest of treatments, hypnosis (Sander, 1974). But Freud, finding his initial successes to be short-lived, began to explore his patients' unconscious conflicts, which he found to be rooted in childhood sexual and aggressive impulses. He found that these conflicts, and the associated feelings of shame and guilt, contributed to adult character structure and to the inhibitions, symptoms, depressive affects, and anxieties his patients suffered from. By the end of his life, Freud's view of the complexity of the mind and the persistence of sexual and aggressive conflicts led him somewhat pessimistically (or more realistically?) to see psychoanalysis as interminable (Freud, 1937/1964). Managed care would have a problem with that, as human as it is. Then again, can care *be* "managed"? As I was writing this chapter, one managed care company declined the marital treatment of a husband, the insured patient, who had recently revealed an extramarital affair to his wife. "We don't cover personality disorders," they said, even after I reported that over the weekend the "patient's" wife had had an acute asthmatic attack from which she almost died!

THE CORE OF PSYCHOANALYTIC THEORY

Before turning to the case, I would like to outline briefly what I consider the essence of psychoanalytic theory and practice. I won't be able to do justice to the numerous schools of psychoanalysis or the many subtle controversies that have evolved over the past 100 years. The emphasis here is on what I consider to be *core* concepts applicable to the treatment of couples. Mainstream psychoanalysis has rarely applied these elemental insights to couple and family treatment. I believe that the recent decline of psychoanalysis is partly attributable to this insularity and neglect of family treatment. Freud questioned at an early stage how psychoanalytic treatment, which he compared to a surgical procedure, could succeed "in the presence of all the members of the patient's family, who would stick their noses into the field of the operation and exclaim aloud at every incision" (1917/1963, p. 459). Though he was exquisitely aware of the family's impact on an individual's behavior (Sander, 1978, 1979), the exclusive emphasis on treating the individual was, in part, in synchrony with our Western emphasis upon the fullest development of an individual's autonomy and potential. In a letter to Karl Abraham, Freud (Abraham & Freud, 1965) commented that, in his experience, analysis almost universally resulted in divorce.†

> †*This is indeed an interesting statement. It's not surprising that unilateral change in a relationship would tend to cause major friction or eventually even the fracturing of a relationship. Perhaps this was something that troubled Freud as a family man.*

The theories, technique, and aims of psychoanalysis, especially since the days of the surgical metaphor, have changed dramatically (Sandler & Dreher, 1996). Nonetheless, despite the universal and comprehensive applicability of psychoanalysis, it has continued to limit itself to one-to-one treatment. This is so despite the limited number of analyzable individuals and the unlimited potential of extending psychoanalytic insights to a broader range of therapeutic modalities, including couple, family, and group therapy.

Psychoanalytic theory is at bottom an account of how each child's complex imaginative inner life interacting with the environment becomes intrapsychically structured, and later is played out in his or her family and work life. The fact that each person's internal conflicts are enacted with important others whose conflicts are so often complementary and shared is the key to applying analytic theory to couple therapy (Sander, 1989). It is this "mutuality" that drives what systems theorists call "reciprocal determinism." With some recent exceptions (Dicks, 1967/1993; Scharff & Scharff, 1992; Slipp, 1984), psychoanalytic theorists and practitioners have focused more upon the inner conflicts that emerge in individual treatment, especially in transferences to the analyst. The analytically oriented couple therapist attempts to address those transferences that are already enacted within the couple and also expressed toward the therapist. What are some of these core conflicts that so readily translate into rigidly patterned marital and family interaction?

The Central Role of Childhood
and the Unconscious in Psychoanalytic Theory

From its beginnings, psychoanalysis has emphasized that in addition to genetic predisposition, early childhood conflicts and experiences are critical. The contending forces of childhood conflicts, generated by the interaction of inner drives and external experience, are repressed because of the pain associated with them. Nonetheless, these repressed impulses linked to memories of early relationships have a way of influencing the present.

A couple with one child aged 10 consulted me after 15 years of marriage when the wife insisted upon a separation. What triggered the need to separate now after so many unhappy years of marriage? The immediate precipitant was the husband's going to meet a woman he'd first met on the Internet. When I asked about the wife's history, I learned of her father's sudden death at 43, when she was 10. While wanting a separation, she was also insisting that her 43-year-old husband see their child regularly. She had no conscious feelings or memories of the events surrounding her father's death. It did seem that she was unconsciously identified with her about-to-be-abandoned child and was reliving the death of her father. She was attempting to undo that loss by seeing to it that her child, while she and her husband were separated, was still able to see her father. She was also set on being abandoned again by losing her husband this time. On the other hand, the husband's wish to continue their unhappy marriage seemed partly influenced by an identification with his own unhappily married parents, who were staying married to the bitter end.

What are the core developmental anxieties of childhood that contribute to such life histories? In Freud's (1926/1959) monograph "Inhibitions, Symptoms and Anxiety," he stated that these anxieties involve the calamities of childhood: loss of the love object, loss of the love of the object, castration, punishment by our consciences, and/or not living up to our ideals.

As toddlers, we must all give up the secure place on our parents' laps and develop a separate sense of identity. Not only must we learn to separate from our first love objects, but we must also learn that the love of those adults is conditional upon our conforming to their demands. These universal developmental crises lead to the ambivalences linked to what analytic theory has called the oral and anal stages of psychosexual development. Particularly relevant is René Spitz's (1957) view that the child's first saying "no" is a critical development milestone. The child thereby indicates his or her emerging separateness, and at the same time discovers the ability to turn the tables on those who've been saying "no" to him or her. We see derivatives of these conflicts in the seemingly petty conflicts of everyday adult life. Arguments over lateness or minor differences in points of view can express feelings of abandonment or not being of "one mind." Arguments over socks not put away, dinner not served on time, or dishes not washed often reverberate with childhood experiences of once having been expected to conform to the dictates of elders.

After the deprivations and humiliations of early childhood, we must all come to terms with the reality of gender differences. The discovery of anatomical differences stirs new aggressions in boys and girls. Boys, fearing being called "sissies" and already trying to escape identification with their mothers, may run from girls—miniature versions of their mothers—or gang up with the other boys to torment them. They may also, fearing competition with their fathers, prefer to remain identified with their mothers, thereby leaving the arena of competition with their fathers in order to be loved by them.

Girls biologically, and until recently culturally, have tended to repress overt competitiveness and aggression. They struggle with their own ambivalence toward the opposite sex; they imagine one day that they may grow up to be like their fathers, or have babies like their mothers, or outshine their mothers in their careers. Both boys and girls must work out the unique blending of their constitutional bisexual potentialities.

Feelings about gender differences are further compounded, in both boys and girls, by the growing awareness that their parents share an intimacy that excludes them. Feelings of inferiority based on comparisons with their very large parents contribute to intense aggressive and competitive feelings toward one or both parents. By identifying in varying degrees with each parent as well as with other significant adults, they metabolize some of this aggression. They imagine that they will realize their ambitious fantasies when they become adults.

Children must also deal with guilt feelings and anxiety that their aggressive strivings stir up. These guilt feelings may be especially magnified if their aggressive and sexual fantasies appear to be realized. For example, when a child is preferred or imagines being preferred by one parent over the other parent or over a sibling, the stage is set for heightened feelings of guilt, especially if a preference is reinforced by the other parent's unconscious collusion. These feelings may be manifested as low self-esteem, heightened vulnerability, anxiety about success, or behavior designed to elicit punishment. All of these childhood conflicts contribute to the formation of adult personality; in varying ways, they are repeated or transformed in everyday adult life.

These repetitions manifest themselves in the multiple "transferences" we make to the important others in our lives. We do unto others what was done—or what we imagine was done—to us. We try to avoid losses while paradoxically behaving in ways that bring losses about. We try to dominate, or allow ourselves to be dominated; we stop at nothing to achieve success, or, just as often, avoid success lest we be punished for bettering our parental models. These conflicts and behaviors, intrapsychic or interpersonal, come to the attention of the individual therapist when they reach a level of unacceptable pain within the patient, or to the couple/family therapist when they result in interpersonal conflicts. In traditional analytic treatment, these transferences and related countertransferences are experienced, interpreted, and (ideally) worked through. In couple and family therapy, transferences among family members are more in focus than transferences to the therapist, though these can be present and dealt with also.

Psychoanalytic Goals and Technique

The highly condensed summary above of core psychoanalytic concepts emphasizes the guilt-ridden, largely unconscious conflicts of childhood that are repeated in the ubiquitous "transferences" of adult life. When patients gain understanding and insight into these neurotic patterns, they can become freer to experience themselves and others in their lives more realistically. Simply put, if the aggression and related guilt rooted in childhood can thereby be reduced, there is a greater likelihood that pleasurable experiences can begin to outnumber painful ones. Change through emotional insight and understanding is the generally accepted goal of psychoanalytic treatment.

As mentioned earlier, psychoanalytic theory and practice began 100 years ago with the directive intervention of hypnosis. Over time, however, the hallmark of treatment became its nondirectiveness. Analytically trained therapists avoid direct interventions such as guidance, suggestion, and advice, seeing them as gratifying regressive wishes to be parented. Although psychoanalytic therapy isn't without its quietly gratifying aspect (De Jonghe, Rijnierse, & Janssen, 1992), the goal is to interpret and work through regressive transference wishes. Because these regressive wishes are often acted out between family members in the clinician's office, it's usually necessary to intervene more actively in couple/family therapy than in one-to-one therapy. Couples inevitably ask me to take sides, to judge, or to suggest quick solutions to their conflicts. Such resistances to self-awareness must be addressed tactfully and interpreted, as details of their defensive patterns and life histories become better known. *What makes the treatment analytic is the predominance of interpretive over directive interventions.*

Psychoanalytically oriented couple therapy is best conducted in at least once-weekly sessions. For practical reasons, I have found it hard to follow Graller's (1981) recommendation of twice-weekly sessions. Regularity of sessions over time permits a degree of continuity and depth that facilitates the exploration of unconscious motivations.

Some Technical Matters

1. *Must both members of a couple be present at each session?* Personally, I suggest all of us discuss whether to start sessions before both partners have arrived, or whether to meet if one of them cannot attend. Such a discussion tends to reveal how the partners negotiate and how they perceive themselves in relation to the therapeutic process. For example, the husband in a somewhat competitive couple I treated worried that his wife would resent time he might spend alone with me. Was this an accurate reading of his wife or a projection of his own feeling? In this exploration I encourage husband and wife to participate actively in being responsible for decisions, while we create a space to discuss their conflicts and their differences of opinion about the decisions. If possible, I prefer to start sessions on time and to meet with one partner if the other is late or unable to attend. Occasionally individual therapy and couple therapy are combined (Sander & Feldman, 1993).

2. *What of confidential communication?* I indicate that I do not keep partners' secrets about their current lives. Occasionally one partner shares a secret with me—for example, some homosexual experimentation in adolescence—which I don't tell the other. If an extramarital affair is revealed, usually it's out of a wish to tell the partner, and I try to work out the appropriate time for the revelation of the "secret" (which often isn't a secret).

3. *What about the financial responsibility for sessions?* Although I make every effort to reschedule when both members of a couple know in advance that they cannot make it to an appointment, I generally charge for missed sessions, as in analytically oriented individual treatment.Many couples challenge this policy, which addresses our mutual responsibilities. To increase understanding, I explore their feelings about this policy, their personal expectations, and the partners' conflicts with each other and with me.

CASE EXAMPLE
Background and Early Sessions

Larry and Louise are professionals in their early 40s; when first referred, they had a daughter aged 6 and a son aged 3. Their marriage of 10 years, following 5 years, of courtship was deteriorating. Whereas many couples complain in the initial consultation about a "communication" problem, Louise was clear in her insistence on wanting a third child, and Larry was absolutely opposed to the idea. Louise was prepared to divorce Larry if she didn't get her "reasonable" wish. Larry felt that to comply would be yet another capitulation to her demands; she had been granted her wish for a larger engagement ring and, more recently, a larger apartment. On a more mundane level, Larry complained that Louise shopped for more groceries than they needed. He felt that she was both controlling and out of control in her perennial optimism that everything financial would work out, while she felt that he was too controlling in his fearful, pessimistic worrying. He was drawing the line and saying "no" this time, citing his sense that they were already living beyond their means.

As is so often the case with couples in conflict, each partner saw the problem as being in the other—an obvious indication for couple therapy. Sexual relations had stopped months ago, and they were alternately angry with and withdrawn from one another. Neither had any capacity, at this juncture, for seeing the other's point of view. The stubborn compulsive and narcissistic features in each partner were the only hints of DSM-IV psychiatric diagnoses (namely, the applicable personality disorders). I mention this only to underscore the inadequacy of individual diagnoses in capturing relational dynamics.

Although there is also a glaring paucity of relational diagnostic descriptions, nevertheless this couple's interaction fit fairly well into a dynamically oriented nosology of relational patterns developed by Sheila Sharpe (1997). Her categories, based on psychoanalytic developmental psychology, include the "symbiotic merger," the "push–pull oppositional," the "gender competitive," and the "triangular Oedipal" styles. This particular couple manifestly presented with a power struggle characteristic of an oppositional pattern. However, such a description was only the starting point. In order to understand and treat their problems, both the couple and I would have to explore the sources, defensive nature, and less conscious meanings of their particular conflict. I recommended this course of treatment to them.

I also inform the members of a couple at the start that it's helpful to me—and, I hope, to them—to know something of their earlier lives in order to begin to understand how they came to their current difficulties. This history taking, together with the exploration of the presenting complaint, usually takes about three sessions. Often I tell them this when they call for the first appointment.†

> † This is consistent with the cognitive-behavioral approach, which is often misunderstood as not being concerned with a couple's history. In fact, when developing a conceptualization of individual and joint schemas in a relationship, a cognitive-behavioral therapist will often delve into the partners' families of origin for a better understanding of how they arrived at their current beliefs and styles of thinking and interaction.

Initially, Louise was pleased to have persuaded a resistant Larry to come for a consultation. Soon, however, Louise herself expressed irritation with my treatment plan. She saw the explorative analytic approach as interfering with her pressing wish to become pregnant. Larry, on the other hand, so initially reluctant to submit to any kind of therapy, began to enjoy and benefit from coming to the sessions. He wanted to talk about their conflicts.

How do we understand this reversal in their early reactions to me and the therapy? In part we have to look at their individual histories. Louise, the middle of three children, had a rather positive view of her family. Her parents were reasonably affluent, and she felt that most of her needs—certainly those for material things—were met. An aspect of her past life that was less than ideal, she stated, was her father's tendency to "always get his own way." On weekends, if he wanted to play tennis, it was tennis they played regardless of anyone else's wishes. She resented his authoritarian approach.

Larry was the only child of less affluent parents. His father was rarely home; he worked two jobs, hoping, as he would often say, "to become a millionaire." His parents lived modestly and sacrificed a great deal for Larry. For example, they gave him their master bedroom when he was a teenager. Although he was always well provided for, he felt it was at the expense of pleasures, such as vacations, to his parents.

I was initially impressed with how little personal or family pathology appeared to exist in either of them. This seemed to be explained in part by the fact that each of them felt well cared for by their mothers, who were homemakers when they were children. Nonetheless, we began to explore those characteristics of their respective family structures that could be contributing to their present difficulty. Louise's optimistic wish to replicate her relatively happy family with its three children clashed with Larry's pessimistic fear that a third child would plunge them into the painful poverty of his youth, so strongly connected in his mind with his father's overworking.

As therapy progressed, several important issues and dynamics surfaced. One was their commitment to their children. Larry's professional responsibilities as a management consultant gave him more flexibility than Louise had as a pediatrician. Consequently, Larry functioned more often as the hands-on parent. This fitted his conscious wish to be more present for his children than his own father had been for him. He did feel, though, that at this point in his life he didn't want the responsibility of an additional child. Larry said that if they had more economic security and Louise would be willing to be home more often, he would consider a third child. However, this would be difficult, given Louise's demanding profession. (Larry had left the private sector, where he was unhappy, for a lower-paying governmental job that he enjoyed.)

In the fourth session, Louise complained that Larry rarely showed affection to her. He responded by saying, after all, "he was not a crazy man with a rifle"—a comment that presaged his acknowledgment, several sessions later, that he was controlling a great deal of anger. Moreover, this need to control his anger exhibited itself in treatment through his wanting their communication with me to be almost contractual. In keeping with this, he angrily accused me of not sticking to "the contract" of giving them my evaluation and treatment plan after the third session, as I had promised in the first session. It had seemed evident to me—and, I thought, to them—that conjoint therapy was the only possible setting within which to explore some of their latent conflicts. I then did spell out how I saw the work ahead, repeating the initial features of their families as noted above.

Insights and Explorations

In the sixth session, Louise reported that Larry had been "a most unhappy camper" during their attendance at her college reunion. The heat, the long hours of travel, and the inadequate housing made him sulk most of the weekend, ruining it for her. He felt he had again sacrificed and given in to her wish to go to the reunion.

In the very next session, another problem arose: Larry's constant feeling of disappointing Louise. She was angry that Larry hadn't reminded her about his upcoming annual weekend away with a male friend. She was also still angry at Larry for sulking about her reunion the week before. I asked whether his failure to remind her of his plans was his way of getting even with her for the previous weekend. He agreed that this was possible, and added that his general anger was also related to feeling that he repeatedly disappointed her. Both these sessions were evidence to them that they were in a cyclical or reciprocal power struggle.†

> †*In the interest of maintaining an analytic frame, perhaps the therapist could have questioned Larry in a more Socratic manner, in order to uncover his schema or belief system that caused him to think in this fashion. For example, was this notion of repeatedly disappointing his wife due to Larry's perception of Louise's expectations of him? Perhaps using the "downward arrow" technique (see Chapter 1) might have caused this information to surface more readily, without requiring the therapist to be too directive. That is, the therapist could have asked Larry to state what his initial fear would be in disappointing his wife. This would then have been followed by asking, "If so, then what would that mean to you?" successively, until the core of his fear was uncovered.*

More significant insights seemed to come in the next session. After Larry's weekend with his friend, Louise felt that "Prozac must have been put into his cereal," because Larry had realized several things: (1) Talking and finding time to talk with each other were important. (2) Louise should have at least the same amount of time off as Larry had had over the past weekend, or should have had her wish to go as a family to the reunion. (3) They could improve their lives if he could understand his misplaced anger.

He gave, as an example for exploration, his continued anger at her siblings for what he felt was opposition to their marriage. Larry's mention of Louise's siblings led me to ask about his feelings about being an only child. He remembered that his parents had talked about having a second child when he was about 6. In fact, he recalled quite vividly being told that if they went ahead, he would have to share his tiny bedroom with a sibling. He remembered shouting, "No, no!" At this point, I noted that his older child was now the age he was when his parents had brought up the possibility of another sibling. The parallel wasn't lost on him. When I asked where a third child would sleep, they indicated that it would require the division of one of their three bedrooms. To that idea, Larry let out a resounding "No!" In the same session, he reiterated his commitment to being home with the children more than his father had been. He said that some of his anger at his wife, who was away from home more than he was, seemed meant for his father for spending so many hours away from home. This clear example of insight into the displacement of his feelings was followed by his reporting that he'd confided to a friend how well he thought the marital therapy was going.

Insightful sessions like this are the exception, but they do come periodically if unpredictably in the open-ended, exploratory analytic approach. I don't know why I chose to ask about Larry's being an only child when he mentioned Louise's siblings. I may have preconsciously recalled that, as an only child at 8, I had asked my parents for a sibling. I mention this to emphasize the relatively unfocused and intersubjective nature of analytic therapy: It permits the emergence of those childhood memories and conflicts that in turn shed light on current problems. Since the conflicts that create interpersonal difficulties are universal and multidetermined, as long as the therapist is broadly attuned to the couple, he or she can address and interpret a number of—if not all—the determinants. I emphasize "not all" because people rarely fully resolve all the multifaceted conflicts of childhood. However, as a therapist provides enough evidence of the patterns linking past and present behavior and needs, a more positive unfolding of a marriage should become possible.†

> † This sounds very similar to the type of collaborative empiricism that cognitive-behavioral therapy involves. It appears that a bit more emphasis may be placed on the therapist's and the couple's combined exploration in cognitive-behavioral therapy. It is through this discovery that the therapist attempts to explain the maladaptive pattern of conflict to the couple and to develop a strategy for change.

Larry and Louise continued to open up and work on their problem. After this particular insightful session, they both began to acknowledge that there was an emptiness in their relationship, because their children and jobs held a higher priority for both of them. When I asked about the 8 or 9 years before they'd had children, they reported seeing each other only on weekends during 5 years of courtship, when she was in medical school and he was already working. There was little feeling of romance or sense of needing or missing each other during those years; even then, their work came first. And so they are at present—busy professionals, committed to their children, but with a limited sense of attachment to each other. From the beginning, they had feared relying on each other to satisfy their needs for affection and intimacy. This lack of trust, as was pointed out to them, made it difficult for each of them to compromise, because compromise meant loss of control to the other. In fact, they both said that a divorce would hurt their children more than it would hurt them.

Evidence of their pseudoindependence exhibited itself prior to my 1-month summer vacation. They showed little reaction to my impending departure. Upon my return, however, they reported having had a "generally good summer," although they didn't get along well during the first couple of weeks after I left. Things improved as my return neared. Louise also reported that she had felt intense anger toward me and Larry, because her wish for a third child had remained unsatisfied. Three months of therapy had achieved nothing, she said.† Larry, on the other hand, was all smiles when I saw them in the waiting room. I wondered aloud in our session whether Larry seemed pleased to see me again because the exploratory nature of the therapy had reinforced his wish not to have a third child, and because he experienced me upon my return as a more present male than his father had been.

> † *At this point, unless it would have been too much of an intrusion, the therapist could have inquired directly into Louise's automatic thoughts about why she thought that nothing had been achieved in 3 months of therapy. This might have encouraged her to reveal some of her expectations about the process of treatment. Perhaps questioning her in more detail would have revealed that she was maintaining distortions about therapy. It would also have been important to determine whether her statement was an attempt at manipulation on her part.*

As we explored the differences in their reactions to me and to the therapy, Louise said that she saw me as a reincarnation of her arbitrary father. We were doing the therapy "my way" rather than gratifying her wish. She had hoped that my authority would by now have brought Larry around to her way of seeing things. Larry responded to her complaints and disappointment by noting that she seemed to have become like her father in insisting on doing things her way. Unconsciously confirming this observation, she insisted once again that her wish for a third child required "no reason."

At this point, in order to break the blaming cycle, I asked Louise what her childhood fantasies had been about the family she might have one day.† She reported that she had always imagined having five or more children. Unable to even hear this, Larry said that if he were to have to prove his love for her by complying with her wishes, it would be "like cutting off my right arm." At this point, I did not suggest my sense that components of their struggle were masculine strivings on her part, reflected in her partial identification with her father, and complementary fears of femininity in him, equating compliance with losing his right arm. Such deeper interpretations require appropriate timing.

> † *This seems to have been an excellent move, particularly with regard to the use of imagery or fantasy material in determining her level of expectation and how this might be contributing to her conflict with Larry. Perhaps these fantasies were totally unrealistic and needed to be discussed.*

In the next few months, their defenses generally loosened and they became willing to discuss not only each other's obstinacy, but their own wishes and anxieties. In this context, I mentioned that their dreams might be of interest. Larry indicated that he dreamed regularly, while Louise said she rarely remembered dreams; she added that she didn't need to dream, as she was already living a "nightmare" in not having her "dream" for another baby fulfilled.

Larry's Dream

Two sessions later, somewhat compliantly, Larry related a brief dream. A child was giving him and another person a pair of shoes. He wanted casuals rather than wingtips, but he was given the wingtips, and he was very unhappy. The context for this dream was a shopping trip earlier that week to buy shoes for their children. Their daughter was unhappy because it turned out her old pair still fit. When Larry asked me what I thought the dream meant, I interpreted his wishes for dependence by noting what seemed to be his identification with his deprived daughter—his wanting to be indulged rather than to be in the role of responsible parent. I suggested that this might be contributing to his opposition to a third child: "Would a part of you rather be the child?" He acknowledged a wish to be taken care of—a wish already expressed when one of our sessions fell on his birthday and he hoped, half seriously, that I would provide an appropriate treat. He again added that if they were wealthier and Louise were able to be home with the kids—thereby gratifying his and vicariously his children's needs for dependence—he would have no problem with a third child.

Some Tasks or Assignments

In the introduction, I have indicated that the analytic approach is mostly an interpretive one. Nonetheless, I occasionally give an assignment that may serve as a stimulus for further work. For example, early in the treatment with Larry and Louise, I saw a *New York Times* editorial on the intransigence of the Israeli–Palestinian conflict. It focused on a Babylonian Talmudic dictum about the virtues of compromise that goes like this: "Where there is complete truth, there is no peace. And where there is peace, there is no complete truth." I gave a copy of the editorial to Larry at a session Louise couldn't attend and asked him to share it with her. At the next session, when I asked about their reactions to the piece, I learned that Larry had left it on her desk without bringing it to her attention. She hadn't read it, and they hadn't discussed it. I thought this showed how disengaged they were from each other, as well as from me, at this early stage of the treatment.

From time to time, I will ask a couple to see a play or movie that reflects some aspect of their situation. Sometimes people are more able to gain insight into something in themselves if it's seen as external to them, on stage or screen. A number of months after the first assignment, I had seen a performance of Shakespeare's *The Winter's Tale,* a play about an autocratic tyrant who virtually destroys his family because of his psychotic irrationality. I asked Larry and Louise to see the play. My purpose was both to get them to spend more time together as a couple, and to give them an indirect stimulus to look at themselves.†

> †*This was an excellent behavioral exercise; it is also used quite frequently by cognitive-behavioral therapists. A structured homework assignment such as this may serve as a diagnostic indicator, as well as a strategy for improving a relationship. For example, adding the assignment of keeping track of the expectations that the partners each secretly held prior to the event, and later comparing this to their respective reactions after the event, may be helpful in determining levels of expectation and attribution—two things that are essential in understanding relationship discord. This assignment is also a nice suggestion for having the partners spend more time together and assessing how this affects their relationship.*

Ostensibly, the conflict between the autocratic king and submissive queen in the play was an exaggeration of Larry and Louise's manifest relationship—an autocratic wife and a submissive husband. Indeed, when they came to the next session, they reported having had a pleasant evening together; they thought the production excellent; they saw the parallel I had made; and they acknowledged that each of them was dictatorial at times. Larry added another twist that dealt with his identification with the king, whose wife was pregnant with their second child. Like the king, Larry also didn't want another child! The assignment thus offered another opportunity for a shared insight—a way they could bridge the distance between them.

Further Developments

Larry's wish to be more indulged as a child, and Louise's child-like insistence on having her way, left this couple in a continuing though less intense stalemate. Although we worked intensely on this, there was no simple compromise here. As the saying goes, "You can't be a little pregnant." However, they began getting along better in other ways. For example, after about 5 months, they were in the midst of one of their extended arguments when they again felt at the "breaking point"; however, the tension was defused when Larry put his arm around Louise and they cuddled. Clearly, Larry didn't feel that he was "losing his right arm" by making peace. And Louise could accept his comforting her. Not surprisingly, when they were able to give and receive solace, they also resumed a condom-protected sexual life. They seemed ready for more intimacy.

About this time, 6 months into the treatment, I asked to meet their children. Their daughter was described as having mild separation anxiety when she was dropped off at school. In addition, I wanted to get a feel for how they interacted as a family. Louise brought them to the session, and when they arrived, they rushed to greet their father with warm embraces. Their daughter drew colorful and happy pictures, while their son played ball with his father. When I asked Larry and Louise to return to the waiting room during the latter half of the session, the children accepted this separation with ease. During some doll play, I asked their daughter how many children she would like to have when she grew up. She smiled and interestingly answered that she would like triplets. Then, with a gleeful smile, she changed that to "One child!" It was as if she were expressing some aspect of her parents' conflict, not to mention her own wish to have been an only child.

Some months later, Larry and Louise began having unprotected sex. This, however, didn't mean that their conflicts were resolved. Larry continued to feel that he was capitulating, but was unprepared to have his family break up over this issue. His generally contained anger did erupt after Father's Day, when he felt especially neglected. Louise had served breakfast in bed for him, but later that morning a neighbor whom they hadn't seen in years came unannounced for support with a family crisis. Louise invited her in, despite Larry's hinting that they had other obligations that day. In the session he let loose a machine-gun-like barrage of anger, which made me think of his earlier disclaimer that he was not a "crazy man with a rifle." He felt that at least on Father's Day, he deserved complete, uninterrupted attention. I was struck by his seemingly disproportionate anger, especially after he had been served breakfast in bed. We began to address how much of his anger over "sacrificing" all the other days of the year was released on this day, which was ostensibly set aside for him. The idea that the neighbor in distress might have unconsciously represented the arrival of a third child did not occur to me until I was writing this chapter.†

> † Once again, it sounds as though Larry's anger came as a result of the violation of his expectation about the day's events. Could these automatic thoughts not have been addressed more directly by inquiring of Larry what went through his mind just prior to his exploding at his wife? Perhaps he was misperceiving the situation or had developed unrealistic expectations about how things would unfold during the course of the day. Cognitive-behavioral techniques may be useful for such inquiries.

I suggested to Larry that behind his sacrificing for others was a wish that, as in the earlier dream, he be the recipient of such generosity. I reminded him of his identification with his parents' way of sacrificing for him. I pointed out that he might also have felt guilty that he benefited as a result of his parents' sacrifices. Moreover, I wondered to myself whether he felt guiltily responsible for having vetoed a sibling in his family of origin (Arlow, 1972). Perhaps out of such guilt, he was now, in identification with his parents, ambivalently permitting Louise and his children to be the beneficiary of his sacrifices.

Beyond their sacrificing for him, I hadn't obtained a fuller picture of Larry's parents' marriage. He reported that in the context of his parents' stoical existence, his mother nonetheless did express wishes for more pleasure and material things; however, his father would inevitably veto these wishes, saying that they couldn't afford them. Larry thus developed a further insight into his identification with his father's withholding, while at the same time showing periodically that he could be a better, more accommodating husband than his father had been.

At the end of a year of approximately 40 sessions, their marriage had improved, but Larry came to feel that there was little likelihood of any further change. Though Louise would occasionally express wishes for more intimacy, their relationship was still relatively distant. She would suggest that they go for dinner after the sessions before returning home to their children. In keeping with his wish to be more present and available than his father, he would opt to be with the children, but he did begin to go for dinner with Louise without feeling coerced. At this point, we began to discuss the possibility of terminating treatment.†

> † *As a cognitive-behavioral therapist, I would be curious to inquire of Louise whether her general schema of the situation had changed any, and if so, how. What had she done, or what had occurred, to result in any actual change in her behaviors? Did she view the situation differently? Was she thinking about or cognitively processing the situation with Larry any differently than previously?*

Types of Termination in Couple Therapy

1. A planned termination involves both the couple's and my satisfaction that we have sufficiently resolved the initial conflict and the couple appears ready to move on without therapy.

2. Sometimes after a period of 6 to 12 months, the individuals in the couple begin to appreciate the contribution of their individual conflicts and ask for a referral for individual therapy. They may agree to continue to work further in couple therapy on their problems while simultaneously engaging in individual treatment.

3. Couple therapy sometimes ends with the abrupt acting out of some conflicts that the partners can't deal with. They sometimes terminate by phone. To avert such an ending, I ask the couple to return for a couple of sessions to try to talk about the conflict the partners are having, either with each other or with me. Often this is a valuable chance to focus on a core

conflict. Sometimes talking about this impasse may allow the treatment to continue.†

> † *A popular behavioral technique is to institute a contract at the very beginning of treatment in which both partners agree that regardless of what occurs, they will not end treatment abruptly, but will at least permit a follow-up session over the telephone. This may also be a method of securing their commitment prior to the start of therapy. I sometimes find that such a contract will eliminate couples that are prone to end treatment abruptly when it does not seem to be going in the direction they desire.*

4. It's not uncommon for a couple to reach a plateau after 6 to 12 months. The partners will then begin to discuss termination, though we all have a sense that further work may be helpful. Over the past 15 years, I have found that some such couples benefit from a couples group, for reasons I describe below.

I recommended the option of a couples group to Larry and Louise. Their relationship had improved, but the core oppositional problem and emotional distance persisted. I thought that their seeing other couples who were more in touch with problems of closeness and distance might help them to see this as an area to work on; too seldom did they recognize it as a problem in their shared defense of distancing. We had also come no closer to a fuller understanding of Louise's insistence on a third child, other than that she wanted a girl. She had cried when their son was born. To have given birth to another girl would have given symbolic birth to herself as the younger sister she was in her family of origin, rather than to her younger brother. She could appreciate this, but only intellectually. How the birth of her brother had affected her would probably be accessible only in a more intensive individual analytic therapy, in which she had no interest. In fact, whenever Louise saw me individually, she felt uncomfortable in the dependent patient role; she greatly preferred her role as "the doctor" to her own young patients. Almost all couples to whom I recommend this shift oppose it vigorously. Larry and Louise were no exception, but finally they agreed to give it a try.

Psychoanalytic Couples Group Therapy

Increasingly, Louise and Larry came to realize how their conflicts dovetailed and contributed to their impasse. Their relationship improved, but they were no closer to a satisfactory resolution about whether or not to have another child. They weren't inclined to pursue individual treatment and felt there was little to gain from continuing in couple treatment.†

† *A cognitive-behavioral strategy to use here might have been a very gentle exploration of some of the myths or false understandings that Larry and Louise held about continuing further in treatment, particularly in a group setting. They might have harbored some reservations about being exposed to a group milieu, which would be prone to confront them more heavily.*

As I have mentioned above, over the years I have found that couples stuck at this plateau, such as the one in the case of Larry and Louise, benefit from a couples group. I've been running such couples groups for 15 years. In a general way, these groups of three or four couples provide the members with a holding environment that includes the support of others who often empathize with them. Marriage is such a private institution that couples know little about what goes on in other families. In the group they come to feel that they aren't alone in their suffering, and they learn firsthand how others handle similar conflicts.

In the first meeting of the group that Larry and Louise attended, one woman talked of how her wish for a child 20 years previously had led her to have one out of wedlock. This empathic response to Louise's pressing wish for a child was balanced by other group members' puzzlement regarding her willingness to jeopardize the family's integrity over this one pressing issue.

There is another benefit of couples group therapy. As I have indicated, marital partners suffer from shared complementary "transferential" views of each other. In a couples group, each member experiences each of the others from the other's own psychological perspective. These independent views usually differ from the spouses' views and provide another way for all members to see that, just as in courtship, love can be blind to the complexity of the loved one. Spouses' perceptions have their own blind spots. This offers another opportunity of seeing one's partner and one's own conflicts from a wider perspective. The support of the group as a "good family," combined with newer perspectives, leads to diminished aggression and an opportunity to explore conflicts at every developmental level. Because different developmental conflicts are variably manifested in each couple, latent conflicts in one couple may be catalyzed by their manifest expression in another.

As it turned out, the group focused in its first session on Larry and Louise's problem. Larry did most of the talking, almost as if he were the only child in the group. Toward the end of the meeting, Louise questioned whether Larry really had to leave early to visit a hospitalized family member; she also insisted that I get new chairs, as hers was uncomfortable. The group immediately picked up on her authoritarian stance toward Larry and me, and on Larry's quickness to be compliant (to say "yes" to his wife's insistence that he stay until the end of the session). The group thus confronted them at the start with their characteristic styles, which continue to be a source of conflict for them.

Of course, at the group level, one meaning of Louise and Larry's conflict over a third child resonated with the group members' discomfort in shifting from the familiar conjoint setting to the enlarged, "multisibling" couples group.

CONCLUSION

Although psychoanalysis has been central to our 20th-century under-standing of the human mind, it has been, with its individualistic focus, reluctant to address couple or family treatment. In this chapter I have outlined how core psychoanalytic concepts, such as the often unconscious developmental conflicts of childhood, can be applied to couple therapy. In describing my work with a couple over whether to have another child, I have tried to show how such a manifest conflict is multidetermined and deeply embedded in character traits. The interpretation and working through of such deeper conflicts usually require longer-term treatment than our emerging managed care culture seems to favor.†

> †*Psychoanalytic therapy has a rich texture to offer in work with couples in conflict. Perhaps one of the ways to make this "individualistic focus" more adaptable with couples is to consider integrating it with some of the cognitive-behavioral principles I have mentioned in my comments throughout the chapter. At the same time, respect should be maintained for the analytic frame with careful compromise.*

AUTHOR'S REPLY TO EDITOR'S COMMENTS

It's a puzzlement. Dr. Dattilio and I apparently agree, "for the most part," that the psychoanalytic and cognitive-behavioral approaches are antithetical. None-theless, we surprisingly seem to agree on a number of fundamentals. His comments, in fact, are quite respectful of the analytic model and raise no major issues of disagreement. Especially germane are our views of behavior and cognition as having histories learned largely in past relationships, and as having their usually reciprocal, often fantasy-driven influences in current relationships. After reading his largely positive comments, I began to wonder whether I was more of a behaviorist and/or he more analytic than I thought!

So why are these approaches seen as so antithetical? Let me emphasize the differing role of the therapist, as I see it, in these two approaches. As I have noted in the text of my chapter, the main characteristics distinguishing psychoanalytic treatment from other treatment types are these: (1) Uncon-scious factors play an important role in human behavior; and (2) the uncov-ering of these unconscious wishes and conflicts requires the establishment of an atmosphere of listening and interpretation in an open-ended setting, rather than active direction, counseling, or the more active questioning Dr. Dattilio suggests a number of times during my case presentation.

I respond specifically to two of his comments. Dr. Dattilio suggests in regard to Larry's explosion on Father's Day (p. 442) that I could have asked what might have been going on in his mind just prior to his exploding. "Perhaps," Dr. Dattilio wonders, "he was misperceiving the situation or had developed unrealistic expectations about how things would unfold during the day." In general, I would see such a question as especially valuable in an early stage of treatment. At this stage, however, not only had Larry actually stated his expectation of "uninterrupted attention" on Father's Day; I knew enough of his story to interpret that the explosion took place in the context of his identification with his parents' long-standing and long-suffering sacrifices most days of the year. This contributed to his entitled expectation of a payoff on Father's Day. As psychoanalytic treatment deepens over time, one aims for the realization that such explosions come from deeper layers of the recent and distant past.

As to the exploration of their myths that might have been interfering with furthering the treatment (p. 445), Dr. Dattilio is here interestingly more analytic than I. I had come to feel that analysis of Larry and Louise's joint distancing defenses would not work in the diluted once-weekly sessions. They were too entrenched in their shared emotional independence and unmotivated for individual treatment. At this point I bypassed their resistance and intervened *very actively* by suggesting a couples group, where I thought their exposure to others dealing more directly with dependence-related conflicts might get them to see their distancing more clearly. I suppose Dr. Dattilio's being here more psychoanalytic than I illustrates that as therapists gain more experience they become less ideologically pure.

Of course, the clinical reality of seeing a couple requires a more active stance than that in more traditional individual analytic therapy. I have nonetheless tried to show that the interpretive analytic approach can be utilized with certain cases. Freud (1940/1964), toward the end of his life, warned that "however much the analyst may be tempted to become a teacher, model and ideal for other people and to create men in his own image, he should not forget that it is not his task in the analytic relationship." In the same paragraph, I should mention, he added that "the amount of influence which he may legitimately allow himself will be determined by the degree of developmental inhibition present in the patient. Some neurotics have remained so infantile that in analysis too, they can only be treated as children" (p. 175). Our current emphasis upon brief treatments puts a premium on active interventions, which may reinforce the dependent position of the patients. Although there is a place for such active interventions, I believe that they should follow a careful assessment of the clinical situation and should not be applied universally.

The achievement of greater emotional maturity is a slow process, usually requiring the working through of painful unconscious childhood conflicts centering around separation, dominance–submission, and competition. The short-term treatments in current vogue are, in my opinion, a denial and cultural repression of what the Freudian revolution is all about (cf. Jacoby, 1976).

REFERENCES

Abraham, H. C., & Freud, E. L. (1965). *A psycho-analytic dialogue: The letters of Sigmund Freud and Karl Abraham (1907–1926).* New York: Basic Books.
Arlow, J. (1972). The only child. *Psychoanalytic Quarterly, 41,* 507–536.
De Jonghe, F., Rijnierse, P., & Janssen, R. (1992). The role of support in psycho-analysis. *Journal of the American Psychoanalytic Association, 40*(2), 475–499.
Dicks, H. V. (1993). *Marital tensions.* New York: Basic Books. (Original work published 1967)
Ellenberger, H. (1970). *The discovery of the unconscious.* New York: Basic Books.
Freud, S. (1959). Inhibitions, symptoms and anxiety. In J. Strachey (Ed. and Trans.), *The standard edition of the complete psychological works of Sigmund Freud* (Vol. 20, pp. 75–175). London: Hogarth Press. (Original work published 1926)
Freud, S. (1963). Introductory lectures on psychoanalysis: Part III, Lecture 28. Analytic therapy. In J. Strachey (Ed. and Trans.), *The standard edition of the complete psychological works of Sigmund Freud* (Vol. 16, pp. 448–463). London: Hogarth Press. (Original work published 1917)
Freud, S. (1964). Analysis terminable and interminable. In J. Strachey (Ed. and Trans.), *The standard edition of the complete psychological works of Sigmund Freud* (Vol. 23, pp. 216–253). London: Hogarth Press. (Original work published 1937)
Graller, J. (1981). Adjunctive marital therapy: A possible solution to the split-transference problem. *Annual of Psychoanalysis, 9,* 175–187.
Jacoby, R. (1976). *Social amnesia: A critique of conformist psychology.* Boston: Beacon Press.
Sander, F. M. (1974). Freud's "A case of successful treatment by hypnotism: An uncommon therapy." *Family Process, 13,* 461–468.
Sander, F. M. (1978). Marriage and the family in Freud's writings. *Journal of the American Academy of Psychoanalysis, 6,* 157–174.
Sander, F. M. (1979). *Individual and family therapy: Towards an integration.* New York: Jason Aronson.
Sander, F. M. (1989). Marital conflict and psychoanalytic therapy. In R. Liebert & J. Oldham (Eds.), *The middle years: New psychoanalytic perspectives* (pp. 160–176). New Haven, CT: Yale University Press.
Sander, F. M., & Feldman, L. B. (1993). Integrating individual, marital, and family therapy. In J. Oldham, M. B. Riba, & A. Tasman (Eds.), *American Psychiatric Press review of psychiatry* (Vol. 12). Washington DC: American Psychiatric Press.
Sandler, J., & Dreher, A. U. (1996). *What do psychoanalysts want?: The problem of aims in psychoanalytic therapy.* London: Routledge.
Scharff, D. E., & Scharff, J. S. (1992). *Object relations couples therapy.* Northvale, NJ: Jason Aronson.
Seagraves, R. (1982). *Marital therapy: A combined psychodynamic behavioral approach.* New York: Plenum Press.

Sharpe, S. A. (1997). Countertransference and diagnosis in couples therapy. In M. Solomon & J. Siegel (Eds.), *Countertransference and couples therapy.* New York: Norton.

Slipp, S. (1984). *Object relations: A dynamic bridge between individual and family treatment.* New York: Jason Aronson.

Spitz, R. (1957). *No and yes: On the genesis of human communication.* New York: International Universities Press.

Turkle, S. (1995). *Life on the screen: Identity in the age of the Internet.* New York: Simon & Schuster.

Wachtel, P. (1977). *Psychoanalysis and behavioral therapy.* New York: Basic Books.

SUGGESTED READINGS

Dicks, H. V. (1993). *Marital tensions.* London: Karnac Books. (Original work published 1967)

Sander, F. M. (1978). Marriage and the family in Freud's writings. *Journal of the American Academy of Psychoanalysis, 6,* 157–174.

Sander, F. M. (1979). *Individual and family therapy: Towards an integration.* New York: Jason Aronson.

Sander, F. M. (1989). Marital conflict and psychoanalytic therapy. In R. Liebert & J. Oldham (Eds.), *The middle years: New psychoanalytic perspectives* (pp. 160–176). New Haven, CT: Yale University Press.

Sander, F. M., & Feldman, L. B. (1993). Integrating individual, marital, and family therapy. In J. Oldham, M. B. Riba, & A. Tasman (Eds.), *American Psychiatric Press review of psychiatry* (Vol. 12). Washington, DC: American Psychiatric Press.

Chapter 19

Emotionally Focused Couple Therapy

SUSAN JOHNSON

Emotionally focused therapy (EFT) for couples, although still a relatively new approach to changing distressed relationships, is now one of the few couple therapies that has demonstrated clinical effectiveness (Dunn & Schwebel, 1995; Alexander, Holtzworth-Munroe, & Jameson, 1994); it generates large treatment effects (Johnson, Hunsley, Greenberg, & Schlindler, 1997) that persist over time (Gordon-Walker & Manion, 1997). EFT has been successfully used with many different kinds of couples, including those in which individual partners suffer from significant problems, such as extreme family stress (Gordon-Walker, Johnson, Manion, & Cloutier, 1996), depression (Dessualles, 1991), and posttraumatic stress disorder (Johnson & Williams-Keeler, in press). EFT is a short-term, structured approach (Johnson, in press-a) that focuses on changing negative interaction patterns and building secure emotional bonds. The interventions used in this approach have been clearly specified (Johnson, 1996; Greenberg & Johnson, 1988), as have the stages of treatment and a couple's journey through the change process. The EFT perspective on relationship distress focuses particularly on emotional responses and rigid, self-reinforcing patterns of interaction; empirical research on the nature of this distress (Gottman, 1994) particularly stresses the crucial significance of these two elements. This research also stresses the crucial importance of emotional engagement in relationship satisfaction and stability (Gottman & Levenson, 1986). In addition, there is research addressing the question of who is best suited to this kind of intervention (Johnson & Talitman, 1997), so that therapists can match clients to treatment. Key change processes and events have been identified as well (Johnson & Greenberg, 1988).

EFT fits with the present *Zeitgeist* in the couple and family field, in that it is a collaborative model and is nonpathologizing in its orientation. It is also a constructionist approach, focusing on the process of how individual partners actively organize and create their ongoing experience and schemas about the identity of self and other in the context of their interactional dance. Partners are viewed as being "stuck" in certain ways of regulating, processing, and organizing their emotional responses to each other, which then constrict the interactions between them and prevent the development of a secure bond. In turn, constricted interactional patterns then evoke and maintain absorbing states of negative affect.

THE DISTINCTIVE ELEMENTS
OF EMOTIONALLY FOCUSED THERAPY

How EFT differs from many other approaches is that it gives priority to emotion as a determinant of attachment behavior and as a positive force for change in couple therapy, rather than seeing emotion as something to be overcome and replaced with rationality. In attachment relationships, emotion tends to override other cues; it primes and organizes key attachment responses, such as requesting and offering comfort and affection, which define the bond between partners (Johnson & Greenberg, 1994). Emotion not only organizes attachment behavior, but communicates with others, pulling for particular responses and so organizing interactions. When vulnerability is expressed, for example, it tends to disarm and pull for a compassionate response. Emotion is the music of the attachment dance; changing the music rapidly reorganizes the partners' interactional positions and so the dance. For example, when a previously hostile partner touches and expresses his or her fear and desperation, a whole new dance of confiding and compassion may begin. EFT is also based on a specific theoretical approach to intimate relationships. Attachment theory (Bowlby, 1969, 1988; Hazan & Shaver, 1987) is used as a guide to partners' needs and as an overall metaframework from which to view and reframe partners' responses to each other (Johnson, 1996).

The goal of EFT is to help couples expand the emotional responses that prime their interactions and to structure interactions that facilitate secure bonding and emotional engagement. The EFT therapist makes the following assumptions:

• The couple therapist needs to focus on both self and system, on intrapsychic and interpersonal realities, and on how each reflects and generates the other. Reciprocally determining affective states and interactional patterns are viewed as priming and maintaining relationship distress.

So one partner's anger may prime the other's avoidance. This avoidance then heightens the first partner's insecurity, which is then expressed as anger.

• Emotion is a primary link between self and system; it primes key responses to intimate others, orients people to their basic needs, and colors the meaning of their interactions by priming key schemas about the nature of self and other. When expressed, emotion pulls for specific responses from partners, and so plays a major role in organizing interactions around key dimensions such as affiliation and dominance. The EFT therapist focuses upon either the most poignant emotion that arises in the therapy process, or the emotion that is most salient in terms of attachment needs and the organization/reorganization of interactions. Fear is addressed extensively in EFT, primarily because fear especially constrains information processing and interactional responses. When partners are preoccupied with regulating fear and protecting themselves from threat, they are often unable to see and respond to relationship cues. In fact, couples often talk of their relationship problems and hurts in life-and-death terms. A wife might say to her husband, for instance, "You watch me drown. You turn away and watch me drown."

• Emotion is particularly relevant and central in attachment contexts, where basic security and safe connection with irreplaceable others is at stake. Attachment needs for secure relationships with accessible and responsive others are viewed as adaptive and natural (Bowlby, 1988), rather than in any way being signs of immaturity or dysfunction. Secure attachment and independence are seen as two sides of the same coin rather than as dichotomous; as Minuchin and Nichols (1993) point out, to be fully connected is to be more fully oneself. Attachment is viewed as an inherent survival mechanism that gives rise to a particular sequence of behaviors when the security of a bond is threatened. These behaviors are protest and anger, designed to elicit a response from the attachment figure; clinging and seeking; depression and despair; and, finally, detachment. Insecure attachment is associated with problems with emotional regulation. Partners are often either in alarm or numb and disengaged. Insecurity influences the processing of attachment information and colors others as untrustworthy and/or the self as unlovable, making it more difficult to maintain emotional engagement, especially when engagement is most needed by the partner or the self (Simpson, Rholes, & Nelligan, 1992). Attachment theory gives the EFT therapist a powerful focus, a clear sense of direction, and a compelling perspective from which to frame and reframe partners' responses.

• Attachment needs and desires and most emotional responses are essentially healthy and adaptive; it is the way these desires and responses are enacted in a context of perceived danger that becomes problematic. Therefore, needs for contact infused by fears of loss are expressed as coercive demands. The EFT client who would get up every morning, march to his wife's side of the bed, and aggressively shout "Kiss me!" is an example. Needless to say, he did not get kissed. The EFT therapist assumes not only that people have very good reasons for being the way they are, but that people are greater than their problems, possessing an inherent capacity for growth and health.

• For significant and lasting change to occur in complex interactional systems, the therapist needs to help the couple construct new corrective emotional experiences, which subsequently will organize new relationship events. The assumption is that insight, skill building, or negotiation will be less than effective. As Einstein commented, "Knowledge is experience. Anything else is just information." Therefore, the EFT therapist continually moves between helping partners reprocess and reorganize emotional responses (so that reactive anger expands into helplessness or desperation) and using these reprocessed responses to expand interactions in the direction of increased connection (e.g., "So can you turn to your spouse, please, and help her to see how desperate you are?").

The two main therapeutic tasks in EFT are, first, eliciting and expanding core emotional experiences that prime partners' interactional positions; and, second, restructuring interactions. A positive therapeutic alliance is a prerequisite for effective intervention. This alliance is collaborative and is an essential part of EFT. It's characterized by empathic attunement on the part of the therapist, as well as a willingness to let the clients teach him or her about the nature of their experience and how it creates and reflects their interactional dance. The interventions used to address the first task are taken from experiential individual therapy, as first formulated by Rogers (1951) and developed by Greenberg and colleagues (Greenberg, Rice, & Elliott, 1993), and the restructuring of interactions involves the directive, task-oriented interventions typically found in systemic therapies (Minuchin & Fishman, 1981). Specific interventions, and the times they are most appropriately used, are outlined in detail elsewhere (Johnson, 1996) and are illustrated in the case description that follows.

The EFT therapist focuses on "three P's": (1) on the present context; (2) on intrapsychic and interpersonal process patterns—that is, how people construct their emotional experience and interactional cycles in the present; and (3) on primary affect. "Primary affect" concerns here-and-now direct responses, rather than secondary reactive responses—for example, the hurt and fear that precede the expression of anger, or the helpless despair that underlies numb withdrawal. These primary responses are often unattended to, undifferentiated, or disowned, and only the secondary responses are expressed as part of the cycle of distress. The therapist reflects and validates these secondary responses, in order to join with partners and describe the cycle, but then expands these responses to access primary affect. The therapist stays close to the affective responses and interactional steps that define the relationship, and avoids becoming caught in content issues and pragmatic problems.

The nine steps of change in EFT are as follows: (1) assessment; (2) identifying the destructive interactional cycle that maintains attachment insecurity and marital distress; (3) discovering the unacknowledged feelings underlying interactional positions; (4) reframing the problem in terms of the cycle and unmet attachment needs; (5) promoting the owning of needs and of new, expanded aspects of self and experience; (6) promoting acceptance of these aspects of self and experience by the other; (7) facilitating the expression of needs and wants, and creating safe emotional engagement; (8) fostering collaboration in regard to problematic issues; and (9) consolidating new positions and new cycles of attachment behavior. Steps 1–4 constitute cycle deescalation, and steps 5–7 involve changing interactional positions. Steps 8–9 are concerned with the integration and consolidation of positive change.

Below, I present a case study. Included are lengthy excerpts from the first session (steps 1 and 2) and fourth session (step 3). Also included are the specific change events occurring in steps 5–7—namely, withdrawer reengagement (session 8) and blamer softening (session 10). These are associated with successful treatment (Johnson & Greenberg, 1988).

CASE EXAMPLE: BETWEEN THE HAMMER AND THE ANVIL

Nancy and Will were a professional couple in their late 40s, married for 4 years. Both partners had been married before, and Will had two sons in college. Will was a senior administrator, and Nancy had a successful career in management consulting. Will had initiated therapy following a particularly painful fight after which Nancy had gone to stay with her aunt for 4 days. Will had been divorced for 3 years before he met Nancy at a tennis club. Nancy had been married very young and had been divorced for 13 years before meeting Will. During this time, she'd had many relationships, but had focused mostly on her career. Will had seen me for three sessions of therapy during the dissolution of his first marriage.

Session 1

In the first session, Will asked whether I remembered him, and I replied that I did. The spouses then immediately launched into presenting their problem.

WILL: Perhaps I should tell you why we're here.

NANCY: *(Interrupting)* We're here because I don't have confidence in Will. He's always looking at other women.

WILL: She believes I'm always flirting *(passing his hand over his face and looking weary)*.

NANCY: I'm not stupid or crazy. We went out to a supper party last Saturday, and he smiled at the woman sitting beside him all evening.

WILL: I can't even remember what she looked like.

NANCY: *(Very coldly)* Really? Amazing.

SUE J: This is what happens at home? These are the kind of conflicts that happen?

WILL: All the time. It never stops. I'm on trial constantly. I can't win, no matter what.

SUE J: So if this is what's happening at home, how would it unfold? What would happen next?

WILL: I either keep trying to defend myself, or I just give up and I withdraw. There's lots of distance.

SUE J: How do you see it, Nancy? Often partners experience things differently.

NANCY: I try to be calm, but he always denies everything, like he is now, so I get angrier and angrier, and then he just leaves. I don't want to live like this. *(She leaned forward toward Will.)* You never do anything, do you *(scathing voice tone)*, so innocent always. So I'm angry at nothing, is that it? Poor you, poor you.

SUE J: Nancy, that is happening here too, isn't it? You're getting angrier and angrier. *(Nancy nodded.)* It's upsetting for you to hear Will talk to me about this and draw a picture of himself as innocent. I think that's the word you used, isn't it? You're protesting that he doesn't seem innocent to you, and you don't want to be painted as the villain. Is that correct?

I moved to contain the escalating cycle of complaining, contempt, and defense by reflection, and to begin to build an alliance with this lady, who was already enraged 2 minutes into the session.

NANCY: Yes. The way Will puts it, I'm out of my mind.

SUE J: Perhaps you could help me understand how this problem looks to you. Perhaps you could help me understand what happens from your point of view when you have these discussions at home.†

> † *This was an excellent direction to proceed in at this early stage of the therapy process—to begin to investigate Nancy's perception of the situation. However, it's not clear to me whether Dr. Johnson had a reason for using vague phrasing such as "what happens from your point of view," or whether this is her general style of questioning. I would be curious how a change in her questioning might have elicited*

> *more of Nancy's exact thoughts—for example, asking Nancy, "What thoughts or images go through your mind when you have these discussions at home?" In this manner Dr. Johnson might have obtained more insight into Nancy's true perceptions or belief system, as opposed to simply a behavioral description of what Will did, as seen in her subsequent lines of responses. Also, would such a question have inhibited the type of emotional response that Dr. Johnson was seeking from Nancy?*

NANCY: Oh! He is very good at not listening. He'll walk away. He'll even pick up the newspaper *(Will started to interrupt, but she cut him off)*. Yes, yes, you do. On Sunday morning, you picked up the newspaper like I wasn't even talking.

SUE J: And then what do you do?

WILL: *(Interrupting)* She gets outrageous. She even hit me once. I can't stand there and listen to all this stuff. I'm about as far from being a philanderer as you can ever get. I never cheated on anyone in my life. She's so suspicious. I don't understand her. She seems to see me as some kind of predator. She never says anything good about me. I smoke too much, I don't play the right sports, I don't play tennis well enough, and it's like—her image of me is that I'm always looking to make it with some other woman.

SUE J: *(Turning to Nancy)* Is that right? Is that right, Nancy, that you never see anything good about Will?

NANCY: *(More slowly)* No, no. Part of me sees that he's honest; part of me doubts him.

SUE J: Oh, so part of you believes him, but part of you is—what word did you use? "Suspicious," is that OK? *(Nancy nodded.)* Part of you is watching and expecting he'll hurt you. Is that it? *(She nodded again.)* Can you tell me about the part that believes him, that he's honest? When does that part come up?

I wanted to know how rigid their perceptions of each other were and how global this pattern of conflict in their relationship was. Did they have any close time away from this cycle, and how did the cycle evolve over time?

NANCY: Well, sometimes things are going well, and I start to think it's OK. But it never lasts for long. Like at the beginning of our marriage, we had about 4 or 5 months that were really good, but it never lasts for long. In the beginning of our relationship, I thought that he was solid, reliable.

I then directed the session into a brief history of this relationship and the partners' former relationships. The most salient points in the emerging picture were as follows: Will had grown up as a loner—the introverted child in a family with two precocious, extroverted older brothers. His parents separated when he was 8, and he stayed with his father and grandmother, while his two older brothers went with the mother. He wasn't able to remember being close to anyone growing up. He'd married young, and the marriage dissolved into a distant friendship after a few years. Nancy was the oldest girl in a stable family, where she had been "replaced" by her younger brother. She challenged me to compare her distress at her mother's transfer of attention to her rival brother to her present situation with Will, commenting that she had heard this analysis from Will and from a previous individual therapist, and it wasn't helpful. Nancy had also married young to an older man, who had systematically deceived her and had many affairs. Nancy and Will had married after a short courtship. The presenting problems had emerged after the first year and had grown steadily worse, to the point where Nancy scanned Will's mail and checked up on his presence at his office.

When I inquired about the positive part of the present relationship, the couple painted a picture of a very limited, occasional companionship. Nancy was turning more and more to her female friends, and physical affection and lovemaking were now very infrequent. The "attack/accuse–withdraw/defend" cycle seemed to exemplify the patterns that are identified in Gottman's (1994) research as the "apocalypse" for marriage.

The reactivity of emotional responses and the rigidity of the cycle, particularly the heat of Nancy's hostility, made this couple quite difficult to intervene with. I often interrupted and defused this hostility with reflection and reframing, focusing on Nancy's experience rather than Will's "crimes." I also reminded myself that she had good reason for her insecurity, which was constantly reinforced by Will's distance. This helped me empathically attune to her and honor her experience. Seeking the hidden rationality in seemingly extreme or irrational behavior is an active part of EFT.

At the end of the first session, I formulated the problematic interactional cycle (step 2 of EFT) and highlighted the attachment issues in that cycle, particularly the issue of the lack of trust. We seemed to have formed a basic collaborative alliance and a contract for therapy. I suggested that both Bill and Nancy wanted to work on their marriage and were, in their own ways, fighting for the relationship. They were both framed as hurting and needing things to change, so that jealousy was not the hub of their interaction and they could achieve some closeness and security with each other. An expectation was set that therapy would take from 12 to 15 sessions.

The cycle was formulated in terms of Will's protecting himself by staying distant and avoiding Nancy's anger, and Nancy's being vigilant and fighting to avoid being betrayed again. As she became more insecure and distrustful, Will then felt more helpless and distanced himself further. As he distanced, she felt betrayed and became more enraged. Both were framed as victims of the cycle, which I continually framed as a common problem that the partners needed to help each other with. I also described the creation of the cycle in a nonblaming manner; I stressed that Nancy had very good reasons to doubt a man's commitment to her because of her experience in her past marriage, and that Will had a natural gentleness that led him to withdraw rather than to stand his ground. I then heightened the statements they had made to each other in the session—that for both of them this was the closest relationship they ever had, and one neither of them wanted to let go of.

In the following session, my goals were to move the spouses into formulating and expressing the emotions underlying their interactional positions (step 3 of EFT), and to help them begin to expand their constricted emotional experience and interactional responses. The cycle of interactions continued to be framed as the problem, and the couple adopted this frame (step 4 of EFT). My aim here was to deescalate this cycle and create a secure base in the session, in order to evoke new emotional responses and new steps in the interaction. The typical sequence is that the more passive, withdrawn partner is encouraged to take the lead in progressing through steps 5 to 7 of therapy.

The first few therapy sessions with this couple were a roller coaster. They would begin to talk of the cycle and begin to be less reactive; then an incident would occur that would prime the cycle again. For example, Nancy found a picture of Will's ex-wife in his briefcase. This kind of priming would also occur in the session, and Nancy would call Will names and derail the process of therapy. I framed these cues as alarms that suddenly called attention to the lack of safety inside the relationship. I would then refocus the session on the trust and safety between Nancy and Will, rather than on discussing the "facts" of some incident that included a third person. I also emphasized how afraid they both were at this point; in particular, I framed Nancy as trying to prove to Will that he couldn't hurt her with impunity and therefore render her helpless. By session 4, both partners were able to begin to express the feelings implicit in their attacking and withdrawing positions, as in the excerpt below.

Session 4

SUE J: Nancy, you're saying that it's so hard for you to trust Will. There's a part of you on guard all the time, looking for evidence that he's about to betray you. *(Nancy nodded.)* It would feel very precarious to let down that guard and believe that Will wanted to be with you, even to take care of you, yes? Even maybe take care of you.

NANCY: I'll be vulnerable! *(She leaned back in her chair and braced herself.)*

SUE J: Yes, and you're a fighter, right? And that part of you that stays on guard, the part that says "Never again," doesn't want to let you be vulnerable. You were a young girl once, looking to your husband, your first husband, hoping for all the caring you felt deprived of in your family. And he betrayed you, and some part of you said, "Never again. I'll never let anyone hurt me like that again." Is that it?

NANCY: Yes *(pause)*. I swore I'd never let that happen, I'd never be hurt like that again *(pause)*. I had to learn to fight. No one was ever there for me, no one.

SUE J: Ah! So it would be a leap of faith for you to see Will as someone who's trying to learn how to be close and may hurt your feelings sometimes, but as someone who won't deliberately betray you. That would be a leap of faith, and it would mean being willing to be vulnerable with Will.†

> † *A very definite schema was emerging here with Nancy—that seemed to tap into some family-of-origin issues. In fact, later on in this case study, a similar type of schema obviously emerged with Will. In order to obtain a more definite picture of the individual struggles both of these spouses brought to this relationship, perhaps a more in-depth focus on their respective families of origin might have helped each of them see how such schemas or belief systems developed. I would also think that focusing on schemas from their families of origin would have allowed each spouse to identify with some of the emotional elements that caused so much difficulty for the other. In my opinion, this notion of focusing on schemas would have been particularly important in with Nancy, who had just revealed a fear of vulnerability that seemed crucial to her sense of preservation in this relationship.*

NANCY: I told myself, "Never again," but some part of me knows he's a good man. But then he keeps things so superficial, he's so closed, he's so . . .

SUE J: You can't see him, is that it? Yes? How can you trust a stranger? The alarm goes off, does it, when he is hard to reach?

NANCY: Right, and I get angry, and I'm between the anvil and the hammer. *(Her voice became very clipped, very matter of fact.)* If I trust, I'll be scared and be disappointed again. If I prove he's a cheat, a liar, I'll be alone, but . . .

SUE J: But not shattered. [This was Nancy's word for her feelings when she watched Will "flirt."] Between the anvil and the hammer, caught between the hope that Will will be there and the dreadful fear that he won't be. That must feel kind of helpless, doesn't it?

NANCY: *(Long pause, voice much softer)* Yes, and I don't *like* feeling helpless, and then something happens.

SUE J: Something happens when you pick up even a hint that Will could turn to someone else, and at last you're out from being between the anvil and the hammer. You're fighting, enraged, and that feels better maybe, and no one will ever hurt you again? Hmm?

NANCY: *(Voice flat again)* Yeah. At least when I'm fighting, I feel stronger. I count on me, only me.

SUE J: What's it like to say that, Nancy? Your voice sounds kind of flat right now when you say that—"I count on me, only me."

NANCY: It feels fine. Well . . . *(pause, voice softer),* it feels a bit empty, I guess.

SUE J: *(I lowered and slowed down my voice, to help her connect with the experience.)* Can you help Will understand this battle that goes on inside of you—wanting to trust and being terrified to put yourself in Will's hands, and wanting to be invulnerable and show him that he can't deceive you or hurt you? Wanting to trust, but then making sure that he's never going to trick you into letting your guard down? *(Pause)* Can you show him what that internal battle looks like? Can you help him understand *(motioning toward Will)*?

NANCY: *(She leaned toward Will. Her voice was soft and intense.)* This struggle goes on all the time. I start to believe you, and then I just have to stop. It feels dangerous. Then I see something suspicious—you're smiling at another woman, something like that. I feel–I'll show you. You can't hurt me. I won't let you hurt me. I'll never be shattered again. *(Tears)*†

> †*I find the term "shattered" an interesting choice of words. I can't help wondering why Nancy chose this particular word to use. Was it representative of something more significant in her life?*

SUE J: Can you say that again, Nancy? "I'll never be shattered again."

NANCY: Yes. That's it. Never again.

SUE J: So you pick up your machine gun and wipe him out first, hmm?

WILL: *(To Nancy)* But I'm not dangerous! I never knew all that was going on inside of you. *(He threw up his hands in a gesture of exasperation.)*

NANCY: *(Looking up at him, pause, soft voice)* But you're so closed.

SUE J: And it's hard to trust a stranger, right? And when we start to trust them, our suspicions remind us of the danger that we could be in.

NANCY: Yes. That's it, that's it.

WILL: *(In a more assertive tone)* Well, you're so harsh with me. I get pushed into a corner. You tell me who I am, and there's no place to move. I'm on trial, and I'm tired.

SUE J: So then it's hard to open up and show her who you are, yes? She's so fierce, she looks so dangerous to you, and you can't figure out how to do it right. *(Will nodded).* Can you tell her *(motioning toward Nancy)?*

WILL: Maybe I don't open up enough, but, I just can't. No matter how much I want to.

SUE J: You would like to open up, but Nancy is pretty intimidating for you, pretty fierce, yes?

WILL: Yes, I don't want this to fail. I've never really felt close to anyone, and I would go through fire for that possibility.

Sessions 5–7

I took the image of fire and framed the scenario in terms of both of them walking through fire to get to each other. I attempted to use tracking, reflecting, evoking questions, heightening their statements and expanding them with conjectures to work with the fear behind Nancy's attacks and generally defended stance, and the sense of failure and helplessness behind Will's passive withdrawal. I framed the cycle and the fear—for her of betrayal, and for him of rejection—as robbing them of the closeness that neither of them had ever experienced, but that both of them longed for. The expressive tasks I introduced also brought this expanded experience into the dialogue, where it then expanded the interaction. As the cycle deescalated, they began to have hope for the relationship and to spend more time together.

In the middle stage of therapy, my concern is to help partners change their interactional positions with each other. For Will, this involved helping him become more actively engaged and assertive in the relationship, and also then more responsive to Nancy. On Nancy's side, this process involved helping her to organize her responses around her fears and longings, rather than her anger and her contempt.

Session 8

Will talked of trying to help Nancy with her fear, but said that he couldn't reassure Nancy when he was "being shot at." He elaborated on his frustration and his "devastation" when she called him derogatory names. I heightened this image and framed him as trying to stand and hold out his hand in the face of her disapproval, which for him was like a "hail of bullets." Nancy wept at this point and said that sometimes she let down her guard for a moment but then became afraid and attacked him. We pieced together an image of Will tired and overwhelmed, trying to shout over Nancy's doubts and fears, and then feeling defeated and helplessness. He then spoke of "numbing out" and "shutting down," despairing of ever getting close. His fears about himself also arose at this point, and he asked

Nancy, "Am I that unlovable?" He then began to assert that he was not such a dreadful, unacceptable person. The session continued:

SUE J: What's that like for you to say that, Will? To say, "I don't deserve all this. *(Pause)* I just touch the wound you have (pause), I'm not that bad. I can't keep proving myself to you." *(His eyes filled with tears.)* What's happening, Will?

WILL: I cower like a wimpy puppy. It's overwhelming. She despises me. *(long pause)* All I hear is that I don't have the goods.

SUE J: You despair—maybe feel like no one will or can really love you?

WILL: Yes. *(He leaned forward and cupped his head in his hands.)*

SUE J: And you numb out, hmm? And then it's so risky to be open and to reach for her.

WILL: Yeah! *(He looked up and raised his voice.)* I want to open up. *(I motioned for him to tell Nancy.)* I want to open up, but I can't handle your attacks. It's like my mother choosing my brothers and leaving me with my dad all over again. What was wrong with me that she left me?

SUE J: You start to feel like a failure, like you're defective and helpless, yes? That this must be about you being unlovable, hmm? And then you cower more, I guess. But there's some part of you—a little part that says you don't deserve all this rage, all these judgments, and that you don't want to keep proving yourself, hmm?†

> †*Dr. Johnson nicely uncovered one of Will's schemas that, like Nancy's schema in session 4, reverted to issues with his family of origin. Perhaps Will was also projecting some of the anger he felt for his mother onto Nancy. I think that it would have been important at some point to help him differentiate these schemas, perhaps by using some imagery through which he could visualize addressing these issues directly with his mother. This might have been especially helpful for him to do in Nancy's presence.*

WILL: Right. She has no right to say those things to me. I'm not an expert on closeness, but I don't want to be gunned down. It's hard for me to take a stand, but . . .

SUE J: But part of you is into refusing to prove yourself and refusing to swallow Nancy's rages. The same part that says that you are not an unlovable person—that you don't deserve her accusations, just like you didn't deserve to be left with your father, yes? [I expand and heighten his shift to a more assertive stance.]

WILL: Right. *(He looked straight at Nancy.)*

SUE J: So can you tell her that, Will, please?

WILL: *(To Nancy, in a clear voice)* I'm not a sexual predator. I'm not your image of evil male betrayer. I'm a rather insecure guy who isn't sure how to be close and give you what you need. I think I've let you down there, but I don't deserve this. And I don't want to be intimidated and live my whole life trying to prove to you that I'm not your first husband.

SUE J: What do you want from Nancy, Will? Will you tell her?

WILL: I want you to take a deep breath in those times when you get scared and talk to me about that. Not to go and get your gun right away. I'm not going to be intimidated. I'm tired of it; it's enough now. I'm not a criminal. I don't deceive people, and I'm sick of being nailed to the wall.

SUE J: How do you feel as you say this, Will?

WILL: I feel good. *(He smiled at me.)* I want to learn to be close and not spend my time cowering behind a rock feeling bad about myself.

SUE J: This feels really important—you saying, "I'm not going to cower and hide. I want to learn to be close. I want you to put your gun down." It feels good to stand up and say who you are and that you want respect, hmm? Nancy, what's happening for you here? Can you tell Will?

NANCY: *(Her eyes were on Will's face; she sighed and spoke very quietly.)* I know I have accused you unjustly, I know *(becoming teary)*.

SUE J: What's happening, Nancy?

NANCY: *(Whispering)* I don't believe him.

SUE J: You don't believe him?

NANCY: That he wants to learn to be close to me. *(Raising her voice and looking away)* I'm replaceable. If I left, 2 weeks later he would have someone else.

SUE J: Right. Let me slow this down a little, so much is happening here. [I gave them a replay of the process as I saw it]. First, Will is coming out and talking about how he gets intimidated by your accusations and definitions of him—how they bring up all his fears about himself and make it hard for him to come close. He wants you to put your gun down, so he can learn to stand beside you. He knows he has been hard for you to see, to lean on. Second, on one level, you know you hurt him and you even know your accusations are inaccurate, but part of the pain—the wound that gets you wild and fierce—is a dreadful doubt, a fear that you don't really matter to him. Is that it? *(She nodded.)* [I formulate her attachment panic.]

WILL: *(To Nancy, very emphatically)* You are my home, the center of my life. *(Nancy's eyes widened in disbelief as she stared at Will.)*

SUE J: *(Leaning forward toward Nancy)* You don't believe you're that special to him, Nancy? That he is fighting to be with you, trying to hang in, even when you get your gun out?

NANCY: *(Looking from me to Will, turning her head as if she was disoriented)* Well, I guess, maybe. I've never felt I was special to anyone, but maybe he is trying, fighting.

We ended the session here.

Session 9

Will continued to emerge and to assert his need for respect and acceptance. Between sessions 8 and 9, he began to spend less time watching TV and playing sports, and became more accessible to Nancy. An incident also occurred at home in which he was able to stay engaged rather than withdraw when she became jealous, and to reach out to her and reassure her. In session 9, I continued to encourage Nancy to accept as legitimate Will's experience as outlined above (step 6 of EFT), and his refusal to cower and be defeated by her rage. Will then went on to expand on his general withdrawal in the relationship and to place it in a context of his fear of rejection and need for positive confirmation of his worth from Nancy. He placed this in the context of his own fears about himself, associated with his mother's choosing to take his brothers and leave him behind when he was a child. At that point, he stated that he had decided he was "second-rate," and was able to grieve for this loss with Nancy in the session. His expression of grief and her soothing response constituted a new kind of interaction for this couple. Will was also able to talk about the fact that openness and closeness were "unknown territory" for him—territory that, in and of itself, evoked a paralyzing lack of confidence and efficacy—but that he was learning and wanted to learn with Nancy.

The central focus of therapy now became Nancy's deep distress and her related need for, as I phrased it, "barbed wire around her." My intention at this point was for Nancy to move into steps 5 to 7 of EFT, where she could risk being vulnerable and could own and express her attachment needs.†

> † *Once again, Dr. Johnson was right on target here; she identified the important emotional vulnerabilities of both spouses. It strikes me that adding the cognitive component of actually restructuring thought content through the assimilation of new evidence that each spouse gained from the other would only have enhanced the reframing process, without diminishing from the emotional focus that Dr. Johnson so artfully demonstrated here.*

Session 10

Nancy started by saying that she felt closer to Will and that they had done more together, and Will agreed.

SUE J: So, Nancy, I'd like to go back to the incident you just described, about the fear that comes up. You said that Will complimented his tennis partner and you immediately got hot. Is that what you said?

NANCY: Yes, it's so powerful. It really takes nothing to activate that fear. It's like instant desperation, and I get my guns out and I blaze away and we're off into the cycle.†

> †*First of all, I don't know whether I would have accepted such a statement from Nancy at face value. The statement "It really takes nothing to activate that fear" was erroneous. She actually exerted a great deal of energy in activating such a fear, albeit to some degree unconsciously. This could have been another excellent juncture at which to make Nancy aware of the fact that her cognitions—namely, her automatic thoughts—were contributing significantly to the activation of her fear response.*

SUE J: Desperation. From playing tennis to desperation, in a flash.

NANCY: Right. And then I want him to prove it, to prove his innocence, to prove I should trust him. So I push him—I push him to prove he is trustworthy.

SUE J: But he can't, can he? Not right then and maybe never. He doesn't argue real well under fire. And only you can face the fear and decide to risk depending on Will. He can't do it, can he? The only one who can decide to put the gun down and risk trusting him is you, isn't it?

NANCY: *(Soft voice, hands over her chest)* I don't like that . . . the image . . . of putting the gun down.

SUE J: What happens to you when you picture that?

NANCY: I feel exposed, naked, at risk.†

> †*Second, when Nancy stated that she didn't like the image of "putting down her gun" and that it made her feel at risk, perhaps the use of an alternative image—such as holstering her gun, instead of putting it down—might have helped her reduce her sense of vulnerability.*

SUE J: He could really shatter you then, hmm? What would he do? What is your most terrible fear around that?

NANCY: *(Long pause; she was very quiet and very still.)* I don't know.

SUE J: You don't know? *(Pause)* Maybe it's hard to touch?

NANCY: *(Very quiet voice; twisting her scarf as she spoke)* When I drive home at night, I sometimes leave early, 'cause I imagine Will will be there at home making love with some woman. I know it's not true, but I drive home early anyway. *(She sobbed.)*

SUE J: *(Pause until Nancy's sobs subsided)* You drive home, full of fear, compelled to check out if this dreadful image of betrayal is true?

NANCY: Yes. *(Weeping)* I just get obsessed with it, so I drive. The first time I thought Will was flirting with someone, I kept it inside for 2 months and it got worse and worse. I just have to let it out.

WILL: *(Leaning forward and reading to touch her hand)* My God, how awful. I can't imagine driving home with that scene in my head.

NANCY: Maybe it comes from my first marriage, only it never happened, that scene. I know it's a fantasy. I never tell Will about it when I check on things like that.

SUE J: This is a courageous risk, then, you talking about it right now. Letting him know how much of your life is about trying to decide if he is safe or not. Letting him know how wounded you must have been to be so concerned with this.

NANCY: *(Very quietly)* Yes.

SUE J: What happens to you, Will, when you hear this?

WILL: I want to comfort her, to help her heal from this. I could never do that, betray her like that.

NANCY: *(To Will)* But sometimes when you've been so—so—not there, so distant and superficial, I've felt like I don't exist and I don't matter. Then I'll do anything . . .

SUE J: To get a response from Will? *(Nancy nodded).*†

> † *I wonder whether Nancy's perception of Will's being "not there, distant" was accurate, or whether it was more of a distortion on Nancy's part. Cognitive-behavioral therapists use the gathering of evidence to substantiate what one spouse claims to see in the other. It's not clear how a therapist using the EFT approach would do this. I would think that this would have been an important issue in this case, since if Nancy was basing her actions on a misperception, this would have had a profound impact on the course of future change.*

SUE J: Anything to stop that sense that you don't matter, hmm? You fight to exist, not be treated as nothing and betrayed again, yes? Any response is better than nothing, yes? You fight to have Will respond to you so you know you matter to him, is that it? [Here I used a classic attachment frame for her behaviors.]

NANCY: *(Sighing)* Right. *(Pause)* But now, I guess *(pause)*, he isn't really the enemy, is he?

SUE J: I don't think so. I think I remember him saying something about going through fire for closeness with you.

NANCY: *(Looking up at Will and weeping)* I can't believe anyone would do that—that anyone would go through fire to be with me.

SUE J: It's hard for you to believe you are that precious and irreplaceable to Will?

WILL: *(Addressing both me and Nancy)* We both have such self-doubts, it's amazing we ever got this far. We've both been so afraid.

SUE J: Well, it's taken a lot of struggling and courage, but I guess you both long for something. How can Will help you feel safe in this relationship, Nancy?

NANCY: He has been recently. He's more affectionate, and he pays more attention to me, and he talks more. He's less distant now.

SUE J: So you don't have to poke at him to see if he's there, to check if he sees you?

NANCY: Right. I'd try to force him to talk to me, to be closer, but then he'd just withdraw more . . . and then I'd be alone.

SUE J: How can he help you with your fears, your doubts that you're precious to him.

NANCY: *(Giggling)* Look at me the way he's looking now.

SUE J: Can you ask him for what you need?

NANCY: *(Turning to Will)* I need you to stay close, make time for me, and let me in.

WILL: I'm trying. I haven't looked after you the way I wanted to. I was all caught up in my own problems.

Final Sessions

After this session, the process of Nancy's asking for her needs to be met and Will's responding continued. The spouses began a new cycle of confiding in and supporting each other in regard to their attachment fears and insecurities. Nancy began to talk about her jealousy as having "evaporated," and the couple began to move into step 8 of EFT. Step 8 involves finding pragmatic solutions to ongoing problems—for example, how much time Will spent at the gym.†

† *This step sounds similar to the type of homework assignments that cognitive-behavioral therapists use with couples. The manner in which it was introduced in this particular context sounds a bit more subtle than it may be in a cognitive-behavioral approach. This type of intervention appears to be very important in solidifying new behaviors and insuring against the regression into maladaptive patterns.*

I consolidated the couple's new positions in the last session of therapy (session 12) by summarizing the therapy process and the contrast between the present and past interactions (step 9 of EFT).

CONCLUDING COMMENTS

In terms of change ingredients in EFT, it is important to note that the expansion and reorganization of key affective responses prime a redefinition of the relationship and new interactive behaviors, rather than some kind of emotional release or catharsis. Labeling emotions and discussing them from a detached distance are also not effective; there is an element of discovery in the EFT process, and this requires an active engagement in one's experience. Research suggests (Foa & Kozak, 1986; Borkovec, Roemer, & Kinyon, 1995) that using imagery elicits physiological responses that abstract words does not. These responses then activate associative memory and meaning networks, and allow the reprocessing of affect and the alleviation of distress.

What is unique about EFT? First, it uses newly formulated emotional responses to prime new interactions and new interactions to evoke new emotional experiences. It consistently looks both "within and between," at how people construct context and how context influences people. Second, because of its focus on discovering and reorganizing inner experience, it is essentially personal in a field that has been accused of becoming impersonal and obsessed with technique (Nichols, 1987). The therapist has to become comfortable with affect, and to have a positive trust that clients can discover new elements in their emotional experience and so construct new adaptive responses. This process can occur in family relationships, not just with couples—for example, between a mother and a daughter (Johnson, in press-b).

Third, EFT focuses on and actively uses affect to change interactional positions and redefine attachment relationships, in a field that has often neglected the role of emotion or simply seen it as part of the problem rather than part of the solution. Fourth, EFT validates dependency needs in a culture that has consistently pathologized such needs (Jordan, Kaplan, Miller, Stiver, & Surrey, 1991). Adult love is seen in attachment terms, and EFT focuses upon partners' needs for comfort, caring, safety, and contact. Most of all, EFT reflects the humanistic tradition in its assumption that when people struggle with their basic human needs for security and contact and their other basic emotions, this is also a time of potential growth and transformation. For me as a therapist, it is a privilege and a delight to be part of this process.

AUTHOR'S REPLY TO EDITOR'S COMMENTS

The editor's first question (p. 455) is why I focus on "what happens" in a relationship in the beginning of therapy, rather than focusing on the individual partner's "exact thoughts" and beliefs. The answer is simply that I want to identify the interactional patterns that define the relationship and to determine how each partner views these patterns. This is step 2 of the EFT process. In step 3, I typically explore specific emotions or beliefs. EFT also attempts to modify beliefs—specifically, the working models of self and other that are part of the attachment system. In the transcripts presented in this chapter, the partners' definitions of self (as unworthy or unlovable or ineffective in eliciting love and caring) and of other (as dangerous and undependable) are apparent. These beliefs are modified in EFT by new emotional experiences, rather than by insight or rational challenges. Minuchin and Fishman (1981) suggest that cognitive constructions per se are rarely powerful enough to evoke change in complex interactional systems, and that increasing the affective component compels clients' attention and intensifies therapeutic messages. Engagement in emotional experiencing has also been found to predict the successful disconfirmation of negative beliefs in therapy (Silberschatz, Fretter, & Curtis, 1986).

The EFT therapist does not usually pursue family-of-origin frames in depth (see the editor's comments on p. 462). The focus is on the present relationship and on ways to create new healing interactions in the present context. Past experience in relationships is used, however, to validate partners' present responses and ways of protecting themselves. In relation to Will, I greatly preferred that he deal with Nancy than with his mother, especially since at this particular time in the session he was beginning to assert himself with Nancy. From my perspective, the crucial elements of past experiences are enacted in the present relationship and are most effectively addressed there.

I like the idea of giving Nancy an alternating image of holstering her gun (p. 465, bottom). It is consonant with EFT, because it would have stayed close to Nancy's experience while modifying her original image just slightly, to evoke more safety for her and lessen her anxiety.

In relation to whether Nancy's view of Will's distance was a "distortion" (p. 466), it was clear to me from observing the couple in the sessions that Will had great difficulty becoming emotionally engaged with Nancy. He also freely acknowledged this difficulty and its effects on his wife. Will presented as a typical "distancer" or "stonewaller," as described by Gottman (1994). The question of distortion is an interesting one. From a constructionist, experiential perspective, understanding a client's idiosyncratic meanings and how he or she comes to formulate them is part of the therapy process, but these meanings—no matter how unusual they may be—are not generally viewed as "distortions."

In regard to the last comment, concerning homework assignments (p. 468), the EFT therapist does not generally use homework in the same way as cognitive-behavioral therapists do; by and large, change is considered to take place in the session. In step 8 of EFT, partners are generally able to reach pragmatic agreements of the kind that are directly facilitated in cognitive-behavioral approaches, and such agreements do seem to solidify new behaviors. In EFT, we view this ability to negotiate as arising from the resolution of highly charged issues about the security of the relationship—issues that usually contaminate pragmatic negotiations in distressed couples.

The question of integrating EFT with other approaches has been addressed elsewhere (Johnson, 1996). EFT can be seen as sharing some common ground with narrative approaches, at least at particular times in the change process—especially in step 2, where the identification of the cycle is similar to the narrative intervention of "externalizing the problem." As for the integration of cognitive-behavioral therapy with EFT interventions, in one outcome study of EFT (James, 1991), the addition of particular cognitive-behavioral components (in this case, communication training) did not enhance the effectiveness of EFT. However, one way to look at the issue of integration is to consider the fact that all successful therapies must be adapted to many different kinds of clients and therefore must be flexible in their application. Highly cognitive clients may tend to give the therapist what they think—their automatic thoughts, rather than their feelings. The EFT therapist tries to start by going to meet people where they are, and so would track such thoughts and try to adapt to such a client's style. However, it is also assumed in EFT that this would not be sufficient to create lasting change.

There are two main difficulties in the way of integrating EFT with cognitive-behavioral therapy. The first would be that EFT views relationships in attachment terms, rather than from the exchange perspective used in cognitive-behavioral approaches to couple therapy, which focus upon fostering rational negotiation and behavioral contracts. The second difficulty is that the EFT therapist assumes that the most efficient and effective path to reorganizing attachment behavior is through affect and new affectively primed interactions, and the interventions of cognitive-behavioral therapy would detract from this focus. As the field of couple therapy develops, we may move toward a time when we can target particular relationship issues and problems and can identify specific change strategies and approaches that fit these issues and problems, rather than trying to integrate different models of therapy.

REFERENCES

Alexander, J. F., Holtzworth-Munroe, A., & Jameson, P. (1994). The process and outcome of marital and family therapy: Research review and evaluation. In A. Bergin & S. Garfield (Eds.), *Handbook of psychotherapy and behavior change* (4th ed., pp. 595–607). New York: Wiley.

Borkovec, T., Roemer, L., & Kinyon, J. (1995). Disclosure and worry: Opposite sides of the emotional processing coin. In J. Pennebaker (Ed.), *Emotion, disclosure, and health* (pp. 47–70). Washington, DC: American Psychiatric Press.

Bowlby, J. (1969). *Attachment and loss: Vol. 1. Attachment.* New York: Basic Books.

Bowlby, J. (1988). *A secure base.* New York: Basic Books.

Dessaulles, A. (1991). *The treatment of clinical depression in the context of marital distress.* Unpublished doctoral dissertation, University of Ottawa.

Dunn, R. L., & Schwebel, A. I. (1995). Meta-analytic review of marital therapy outcome research. *Journal of Family Psychology, 9,* 58–68.

Foa, E., & Kozak, M. (1986). Emotional processing of fear: Exposure to corrective information. *Psychological Bulletin, 99,* 20–35.

Gordon-Walker, J., Johnson, S., Manion, I., & Cloutier, P. (1996). Emotionally focused marital interventions for couples with chronically ill children. *Journal of Consulting and Clinical Psychology, 64,* 1029–1036.

Gordon-Walker, J., & Manion, I. (1997). *Emotionally focused marital therapy for the parents of chronically ill children: A two year follow-up study.* Manuscript in preparation.

Gottman, J. (1994). An agenda for marital therapy. In S. M. Johnson & L. S. Greenberg (Eds.), *The heart of the matter: Perspectives on emotion in marital therapy* (pp. 256–296). New York: Brunner/Mazel.

Gottman, J., & Levenson, R. W. (1986). Assessing the role of emotion in marriage. *Behavioral Assessment, 8,* 31–48.

Greenberg, L. S., & Johnson, S. M. (1988). *Emotionally focused therapy for couples.* New York: Guilford Press.

Greenberg, L. S., Rice, L. N., & Elliott, R. (1993). *Facilitating emotional change: The moment-by-moment process.* New York: Guilford Press.

Hazan, C., & Shaver, P. (1987). Conceptualizing romantic love as an attachment process. *Journal of Personality and Social Psychology, 52,* 511–524.

James, P. (1991). Effects of communication training component added to an emotionally focused marital therapy. *Journal of Marital and Family Therapy, 17,* 263–276.

Johnson, S. M. (1996). *The practice of emotionally focused marital therapy: Creating connection.* New York: Brunner/Mazel.

Johnson, S. M. (in press-a). Emotionally focused couple therapy: Straight to the heart. In J. Donovan (Ed.), *Short-term couple therapy.* New York: Guilford Press.

Johnson, S. M. (in press-b). Listening to the music: Emotion as a natural part of systems theory. *Journal of Systemic Therapies.*

Johnson, S. M., & Greenberg, L. S. (1988). Relating process to outcome in marital therapy. *Journal of Marital and Family Therapy, 14,* 175–183.

Johnson, S. M., & Greenberg, L. S. (Eds.). (1994). *The heart of the matter: Perspectives on emotion in marital therapy.* New York: Brunner/Mazel.

Johnson, S. M., Hunsley, J., Greenberg, L. S., & Schlindler, D. (1997). The effects of emotionally focused marital therapy: A meta-analysis. Manuscript submitted to *Clinical Psychology.*

Johnson, S. M., & Talitman, E. (1997). Predictors of success in emotionally focused marital therapy. *Journal of Marital and Family Therapy, 23,* 135–152.

Johnson, S. M., & Williams-Keeler, L. (in press). Creating healing relationships for traumatized couples: The use of emotionally focused marital therapy. *Journal of Marital and Family Therapy.*

Jordan, J. V., Kaplan, A. G., Miller, J. B., Stiver, I. P., & Surrey, J. L. (1991). *Women's growth in connection: Writings from the Stone Center.* New York: Guilford Press.

Minuchin, S., & Fishman, H. (1981). *Family therapy techniques*. Cambridge, MA: Harvard University Press.

Minuchin, S., & Nichols, M. P. (1993). *Family healing*. New York: Free Press.

Nichols, M. P. (1987). *The self in the system*. New York: Brunner/Mazel.

Rogers, C. (1951). *Client-centered therapy*. Boston: Houghton Mifflin.

Silberschatz, G., Fretter, P., & Curtis, J. (1986). How do interpretations influence the process of psychotherapy? *Journal of Consulting and Clinical Psychology, 54*, 646–652.

Simpson, J. A., Rholes, W. S., & Nelligan, J. S. (1992) Support giving and support seeking within couples in anxiety-provoking situations: The role of attachment styles. *Journal of Personality and Social Psychology, 62*, 434–446.

SUGGESTED READINGS

Bowlby, J. (1969). *Attachment and loss: Vol. 1. Attachment*. New York: Basic Books.

Bowlby, J. (1988). *A secure base*. New York: Basic Books.

Greenberg, L. S., & Johnson, S. M. (1988). *Emotionally focused therapy for couples*. New York, Guilford Press.

James, P. (1991). Effects of communication training component added to an emotionally focused marital therapy. *Journal of Marital and Family Therapy, 17*, 263–276.

Johnson, S. M. (1996). *The practice of emotionally focused marital therapy: Creating connection*. New York: Brunner/Mazel.

Johnson, S. M. (in press). Listening to the music: Emotion as a natural part of systems theory. *Journal of Systemic Therapies*.

Johnson, S. M. , & Greenberg, L. S. (Eds.). (1994). *The heart of the matter: Perspectives on emotion in marital therapy*. New York: Brunner/Mazel.

Jordan, J. V., Kaplan, A. G., Miller, J. B., Stiver, I. P., & Surrey, J. L. (1991). *Women's growth in connection: Writings from the Stone Center*. New York: Guilford Press.

Nichols, M. P. (1987). *The self in the system*. New York: Brunner/Mazel.

Silberschatz, G., Fretter, P., & Curtis, J. (1986). How do interpretations influence the process of psychotherapy? *Journal of Consulting and Clinical Psychology, 54*, 646–652.

Chapter 20

Epilogue

FRANK M. DATTILIO

> It behooves all of us to continue being students. My
> recommendation is that we free ourselves to look anywhere
> to what seems to fit. This makes each of us continually
> growing entities.
> —Virginia Satir (in Satir & Baldwin, 1983, p. ix)

The best part of putting this book together has been the opportunity to work with so many outstanding contributors. The hardest has been trying to describe the commonalities between cognitive-behavioral strategies and the various other models of therapy, while at the same time honoring their uniqueness. There is no doubt that cognitive-behavioral strategies have a great deal to offer, but it is unfair to say that all modalities of couple and family therapy do pretty much the same thing.

Once upon a time, like many neophyte therapists, I was so enthusiastic about my approach that I believed it to be all things to all people. I was convinced that because of its empirical support, cognitive-behavioral therapy was superior to the other approaches that I had read about. In a grandiose way, I regarded it as the "be all to end all."

Fortunately, time and experience has taught me many things. One is that cognitive-behavioral strategies are not always effective and are not for everyone. For example, individuals with serious intellectual impairment, severe psychopathology, or those from certain cultural backgrounds that discourage alternative thinking styles are not ideal candidates for a cognitive-behavioral approach. Upon discovering that this approach couldn't be all things to all people, I began to explore other models of therapy and the possibility of integrating these models with cognitive-behavioral strategies. I began to incorporate some of the philosophies and theories of other models into my own approach. At this point, it became evident to me that integration was possible with some models but not with others.

Of course, I was not the first one to make this discovery. Family therapy itself was at one time divided into various distinct schools almost like warring camps, each of which proclaimed its own truth. To some degree, this provided the impetus for theorists to begin exploring aspects of integrating theories. Today, most therapists would agree that no one modality has a patent on truth or is uniquely effective in working with diverse cultures or populations. Therefore, the need to consider exploring the best combination of differing orientations in a systematic fashion is paramount to the achievement of success with a wide variety of cases.

Cognitive-behavioral therapy has always been a modality that remains open to change, since it has so many "noncognitive elements," such as attention to emotional issues and psychoanalytic principles. Likewise, cognitive-behavioral therapy's central mechanism of action (cognitive change) is shared with other models of treatment. In a general sense, because most approaches to couples and families involve human communication, the majority of therapies may be said to be "cognitive." For similar reasons, most therapies can be considered behavioral as well, because communication is behavior and all behavior is communicative. And because the human condition involves emotions, most psychotherapies address emotion to a significant degree. Consequently, any particular therapy can be viewed through a variety of lenses—as cognitive, behavioral, emotional, and so on. Several therapists have gone a step further and suggested that behavior, cognitions, emotions, physiological components, and interpersonal components are tightly linked, so that if any one element changes during the course of therapy, all change (Horowitz, Weckler, & Doren, 1983; Leventhal, 1984; Rachman, 1981).

It's not surprising, then, that cognitive-behavioral strategies would be integrateable to some degree with a the majority of other models of couple and family therapy. The extent to which this is possible, however, depends on how certain strategies are integrated and whether they can be presented so as not to contradict the underlying philosophy of treatment.

I was quite pleased to learn that most of the therapeutic models described in this text appear to be compatible and integrateable with cognitive-behavioral strategies. Strategic family therapy is perhaps one of the modalities most receptive to the use of cognitive-behavioral strategies because it too utilizes problem-solving strategies and collaborative reframing. Although strategic therapists may not necessarily use such techniques for the same reasons cognitive-behavioral therapists use them, the eventual goal with both approaches is to facilitate change. James Keim (Chapter 6), who has worked closely with two of the foremost figures in strategic family therapy, Cloé Madanes and Jay Haley, has underscored the compatibility in his author's reply. Regardless of the differences that exist between cognitive-behavioral therapy and the strategic approach, the two allow for the appropriate blending of modalities—primarily because both models regard the family as a system and view the therapist as having a direct role in facilitating change.

The same holds true for the contextual and solutions-focused approaches. Even though the solution-focused approach places less emphasis on the emotional component in treatment, both the solution-focused and contextual approaches are oriented toward behavioral change. David Ulrich (Chapter 7) states the similarity between the contextual and cognitive-behavioral approaches succinctly in his author's reply. The style of the respective approaches differ, but they have the same goals. Insoo Kim Berg and Michael Hoyt (Chapter 9), two well-respected pioneers of the solution-focused approach, provide readers with nice guidelines for avoiding potential conflicts between cognitive-behavioral strategies and their modality. Of particular note is how they streamline their goal by cutting to the core with the couple presented in their case. Their comments suggest that cognitive-behavioral strategies could bog down their attempt to achieve a solution at an earlier point in the treatment process. At the same time, some of the principles of solution-focused therapy are similar to those of cognitive-behavioral therapy—for instance, the directiveness of both approaches.

Other approaches lend themselves quite well to the cognitive-behavioral strategies. For example, integrative marital therapy (Chapter 10), transgenerational family therapy (Chapter 11), and imago relationship therapy (Chapter 17) are clearly compatible, since all three adhere somewhat to a social learning model. The transgenerational approach is particularly compatible with the cognitive-behavioral concept of the family schema and how this schema contributes to family dysfunction. In fact, I was surprised to find Laura Giat Roberto's approach in Chapter 11 more cognitive-behavioral in nature than I had anticipated.

As Cheryl Rampage describes her model of feminist therapy (Chapter 15), I am astounded at how strongly influenced it is by cognitive-behavioral theory. She targets perceptions and beliefs in much the same fashion as cognitive-behavioral therapists do. I was extremely impressed with Dr. Rampage's chapter, particularly since it provided me with a clearer perception of what feminist family therapy is all about.

Paula Hanson-Kahn and Luciano L'Abate's model of cross-cultural family therapy (Chapter 12) is also quite integrative. It is open to focusing on cognitive change and the modification of behavior; this is especially promising to anyone wishing to blend cognitive-behavioral strategies with their approach. Of course, the particular cultural aspects of the couple or family must be amenable to cognitive restructuring. One of the particular limitations of the cognitive approach is that some cultures place a limit on the challenging of automatic thoughts and schemas, especially when such thoughts and schemas pertain to a religious belief or a basic, long-standing tenet of the culture's philosophy. I was quite impressed with how Hanson-Kahn as the therapist and Dr. L'Abate as the consultant managed to do effective work in such a difficult case, involving a culture that so strongly values stability and tradition.

It became apparent during my exchanges with the chapter authors that the collaborative potential of cognitive-behavioral therapy is frequently misunderstood. Depending on the style of a cognitive-behavioral therapist, it need not always be as directive and "concrete" as it is commonly thought to be. One example of this confusion can be seen in the chapter on psychoanalytic couple therapy (Chapter 18)—particularly in Fred Sander's surprise at how analytic my comments appeared. That is, at times my suggestions appeared to him to be nondirective and explorative. This was the chapter that I was initially most worried about and, quite frankly, I anticipated the strongest rebuttal from Dr. Sander. The issue of directiveness is also highlighted in the chapters on the narrative solutions and internal family systems approach. With his internal family systems approach (Chapter 14), Richard Schwartz tends to encourage the members of a couple or family to take more of a leadership role. In a sense, then, individuals take more responsibility much earlier in the treatment process. I like that, since it calls into question the couple's or family's motivation to change early in the treatment. Some styles of cognitive-behavioral therapy are more compatible than others with Schwartz's approach, in that they heavily stress the need for client responsibility. The issue of responsibility appears to be the same in the narrative solutions approach described by Joseph Eron and Thomas Lund (Chapter 16). The goal is to motivate the clients to rethink their views of themselves and others on their own; this is designed to enhance the empowering process. The long-range goal of cognitive-behavioral therapy is also to empower clients through having them restructure their views in a collaborative manner. This, once again, can vary according to the personality and style of the therapist. However, the process by which the goal is obtained in the course of treatment varies widely and may make the differences between whether or not the approach is effective. This is something that has made me seriously rethink the structural application of cognitive-behavioral therapy with certain cases, particularly those in which the enhancement of empowering might be more effective.

I certainly anticipated in the course of editing this text that some modalities would be much less amenable than others to the integration of cognitive-behavioral strategies. Three such approaches in particular are social constructive/narrative couple therapy (Chapter 13), experiential family therapy (Chapter 8), and the pure behavioral approach (Chapter 4). I was somewhat surprised by Terry MacCormack and Karl Tomm's reply regarding the intrusion of my comments, since it was my impression that the social constructivist movement bases a good deal of its philosophy on cognitive concepts. In fact, Dr. Tomm highlights the cognitive aspects of his approach whenever describing his modality of treatment. Their particular style is very different from the cognitive-behavioral approach; they espouse a more nondirective, almost passive approach. Yet, I was impressed with how effective it was with the case described in their chapter. In fact, even the entire method of conceptualizing the case gives clients the leeway to accept or reject the therapist's involvement in the treatment process and evolve more on their own. Although any client has the option of doing this in therapy, it is my opinion that for most approaches it would mark the termination of treatment. Cognitive-behavioral therapy is based largely on the notion that the couple or family has to buy into the fundamental tenet of the approach or its effectiveness diminishes. It appears that at times almost the opposite is the case with the social constructive/narrative approach and the experiential approach. This is not to say that these modalities necessarily employ paradox; however, they reject structure almost outright. Clearly, the concrete and directiveness that characterize cognitive-behavioral therapy in even its most passive forms are considered the most potent aspect of the modality. David Keith (Chapter 8) describes the therapist's subtle role nicely in his chapter, which is so artistically written.

As for the pure behavioral approach (Chapter 4), although behavioral interventions are undoubtedly integral to cognitive-behavioral therapy, it appears that cognition is almost a hinderance to the pure behaviorist. Indeed, cognitive strategies slow down the process of behavioral treatment, according to Marion Forgatch and Gerald Patterson. This has been a topic of hot debate in some of the recent literature, particularly among behaviorists who turn cognitive. Although I maintain the utmost respect for Drs. Forgatch and Patterson, I feel that their approach is too rigid by excluding a cognitive component. In so doing, it may exclude the types of families that would benefit from the challenging of cognitions, especially in cases where distorted perceptions are having a profound impact on the relationship.

I agree with Drs. Forgatch and Patterson that the empirical evidence supporting the effectiveness of a cognitive component is weak. Yet, there are cases in which the problem tends to be more a matter of distorted thought and perception than a matter of pure behavior; in such cases, I believe that the problem cannot be reached by focusing solely on behavior. Despite the absence of empirical support, cognitive interventions may still be successful, and I hope that in time more empirical outcome studies will bear this out.

Like the narrative solutions approach and the internal family systems approach, structural family therapy (Chapter 5) underscores the notion that the couple or family members must actually take the responsibility for change. Thus, in structural family therapy, the focus is almost entirely on the clients. By using "enactments," structural family therapists turn over the reins to family members themselves. At the same time, the therapist can

also be very directive, even aggressive at times, particularly when enactments break down. For example, in one instance during the case of Philip
and Lauren, Dr. Minuchin used a line of questioning that he learned from
Murray Bowen when he encourages the couple to use concrete details to
make them think. In a sense, Drs. Minuchin and Nichols suggest that during
some periods of emotional volatility, they will utilize cognitive strategies,
albeit within a completely different framework than traditional cognitive-
behavioral therapist's would. They do not go into the same detail that
cognitive-behavioral therapists would, but the intentions of addressing
cognition are still tacitly implied.

The same holds true for the emotionally focused approach (Chapter
19). In my opinion, Susan Johnson places too much emphasis on the
cognitive-behavioral approach as interfering with important affect and
derailing the process of focusing on the attachment aspects of relationships.
Although I believe that Dr. Johnson raises a cogent point, I still personally
contend that there are ways to blend these techniques compatibly. Once
again, there needs to be a moderation in the use of cognitive-behavioral
principles if they are to be blended with an emotionally focused approach.
This is a case where the degree of intensity of cognitive-behavioral strategies
may be varied at the therapist's discretion; they may prove to be most
effective if used in a unique and creative fashion.

Interestingly, during the process of soliciting endorsers for the book,
one of the colleagues who was asked to provide an endorsement declined,
stating in his reply, "Your attempt to force the various authors into your
framework reminded me of Cinderella's stepsisters' efforts to force their
feet into the glass slipper." Maybe he has a point! I truly hope I have not
portrayed myself as proposing congitive-behavioral therapy to do the same
things that every other modality does. This was not my intention. It's just
that sometimes we don't know whether or not a shoe will fit unless we try
it. In a sense, perhaps, this book served as an initial course of trial and
error in exploring the appropriateness of cognitive-behavioral strategies
with various modalities.

In summary, what we may conclude from this attempt to integrate the
use of cognitive-behavioral strategies with other therapeutic modalitites is
that such strategies are appropriate sometimes and innappropriate at other
times. What is most striking, however, is that each approach has distinct
characteristics of its own. It may not be possible to integrate various
models completely with cognitive-behavioral therapy without losing a vital
element in what they do, but at the very least cognitive-behavioral strategies
may be worth considering as a adjunct to treatment. In conclusion, then,
clinicians wishing to utilize cognitive-behavioral strategies should be thoroughly familiar with their own modalities of treatment and should use the
techniques proposed in this text in a manner that is respectful to the basic
tenets of their own theoretical orientations and style of therapy.

REFERENCES

Horowitz, L. M., Weckler, D. A., & Doren, R. (1983). Interpersonal problems and symptoms: A cognitive approach. In P. C. Kendall (Ed.), *Advances in cognitive-behavioral research and therapy* (Vol. 2, pp. 81–125). New York: Academic Press.

Leventhal, F. (1984). A perceptual motor theory of emotion. In K. R. Scherer & P. Ekman (Eds.), *Approaches to emotion* (pp. 271–291). Hillsdale, NJ: Erlbaum.

Rachman, S. (1981). The primacy of affect: Some theoretical implications. *Behaviour Research and Therapy, 19,* 279–290.

Satir, V. M., & Baldwin, M. (1983). *Satir step by step: A guide to creating change in families.* Palo Alto, CA: Science & Behavior Books.

Index